Multilingual Aspects of Speech Sound Disorders in Children

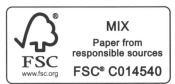

MIX
Paper from responsible sources
FSC
www.fsc.org
FSC® C014540

COMMUNICATION DISORDERS ACROSS LANGUAGES
Series Editors: Dr Nicole Müller and Dr Martin Ball, *University of Louisiana at Lafayette, USA*

While the majority of work in communication disorders has focused on English, there has been a growing trend in recent years for the publication of information on languages other than English. However, much of this is scattered through a large number of journals in the field of speech pathology/communication disorders, and therefore, not always readily available to the practitioner, researcher and student. It is the aim of this series to bring together into book form surveys of existing studies on specific languages, together with new materials for the language(s) in question. We have launched a series of companion volumes dedicated to issues related to the cross-linguistic study of communication disorders. The series does not include English (as so much work is readily available), but covers a wide number of other languages (usually separately, though sometimes two or more similar languages may be grouped together where warranted by the amount of published work currently available). We have been able to publish volumes on Finnish, Spanish, Chinese and Turkish, and books on multilingual aspects of stuttering, aphasia, and speech disorders, with several others in preparation.

Full details of all the books in this series and of all our other publications can be found on http://www.multilingual-matters.com, or by writing to Multilingual Matters, St Nicholas House, 31-34 High Street, Bristol BS1 2AW, UK.

Multilingual Aspects of Speech Sound Disorders in Children

Edited by
Sharynne McLeod and Brian A. Goldstein

MULTILINGUAL MATTERS
Bristol • Buffalo • Toronto

Library of Congress Cataloging in Publication Data
A catalog record for this book is available from the Library of Congress.
Multilingual Aspects of Speech Sound Disorders in Children/Edited by Sharynne McLeod and Brian A. Goldstein.
Communication Disorders Across Languages: 6
Includes index.
1. Speech disorders in children. 2. Bilingualism in children. 3. Multilingual persons.
I. McLeod, Sharynne. II. Goldstein, Brian.
RJ496.S7M845 2011
618.92855–dc23 2011035422

British Library Cataloguing in Publication Data
A catalogue entry for this book is available from the British Library.

ISBŃ-13: 978-1-84769-513-0 (hbk)
ISBN-13: 978-1-84769-512-3 (pbk)

Multilingual Matters
UK: St Nicholas House, 31-34 High Street, Bristol BS1 2AW, UK.
USA: UTP, 2250 Military Road, Tonawanda, NY 14150, USA.
Canada: UTP, 5201 Dufferin Street, North York, Ontario M3H 5T8, Canada.

The policy of Multilingual Matters/Channel View Publications is to use papers that are natural, renewable and recyclable products, made from wood grown in sustainable forests. In the manufacturing process of our books, and to further support our policy, preference is given to printers that have FSC and PEFC Chain of Custody certification. The FSC and/or PEFC logos will appear on those books where full certification has been granted to the printer concerned.

Typeset by Datapage International Ltd.
Printed and bound in Great Britain by Short Run Press Ltd.

Contents

Part 2: Multilingual Speech Acquisition

Part 3: Speech-Language Pathology Practice

Contributors

Martin J. Ball [ˈmɑtɪn ˈʤeɪ ˈbɔl] RP ∼ [ˈmɑɹtn̩ ˈʤeɪ ˈbɑl] GenAm
Department of Communicative Disorders, University of Louisiana at Lafayette, USA
Martin J. Ball is Hawthorne-BoRSF Endowed Professor at the University of Louisiana at Lafayette, USA. His main research interests include socio-linguistics, clinical phonetics and phonology, and the linguistics of Welsh, and he has published widely in these areas. He is an honorary Fellow of the Royal College of Speech and Language Therapists.
Email: mjball@louisiana.edu

Ruth Huntley Bahr [ruθ hʌntlɪ baɚ]
Department of Communication Sciences and Disorders, University of South Florida, Tampa, FL, USA
Ruth Huntley Bahr is a Professor in the Department of Communication Sciences and Disorders at the University of South Florida (USF). Her research interests focus on metalinguistic knowledge in bilingual and bidialectal children as they learn to read and spell.
Email: rbahr@usf.edu

Avivit Ben-David [aviˈvit ben daˈvid]
Department of Communication Disorders, Hadassah Academic College, Jerusalem, Israel
Department of Communication Disorders, Tel-Aviv University, Israel
Avivit Ben-David is a speech-language pathologist with a PhD in linguistics from Tel-Aviv University, Israel. She is a Senior Lecturer at the Department of Communication Disorders, Hadassah College, Jerusalem, and a teaching instructor at the Department of Communication Disorders, Tel-Aviv University. Her research focuses on phonological acquisition and disorders in Hebrew and Palestinian Arabic phonological acquisition.
Email: avivitb@hadassah.ac.il

B. May Bernhardt [ˈbi ˈmeɪ ˈbɚnˌhɑɹt]
School of Audiology and Speech Sciences, University of British Columbia, Vancouver, Canada
B. May Bernhardt is a Full Professor and speech-language pathologist at the University of British Columbia. She researches and teaches in the areas of child language acquisition, with a primary focus on phonological acquisition, assessment and intervention. One current project is investigating protracted phonological development across several diverse languages.
Email: may.bernhardt@audiospeech.ubc.ca

Françoise Brosseau-Lapré [fʁɑ̃sˈwɑz ˈbʁɔso ˈlæpʁe]
School of Communication Sciences and Disorders, McGill University, Canada
Françoise Brosseau-Lapré is a registered speech-language pathologist and has worked with children with communicative impairments since 2002. She is currently completing a doctoral degree at McGill University under the supervision of Dr Rvachew. Her research focuses on developing more effective assessment and intervention procedures for francophone children with speech sound disorders.
Email: francoise.brosseau-lapre@mail.mcgill.ca

Pamela Sau Ping Cheung [ˈpæmələ sɐu pʰiŋ ˈtsœŋ]
Child Assessment Service, Hong Kong Special Administrative Region, China
Pamela Cheung is a registered speech and language therapist working in the Child Assessment Service in Hong Kong. She has ample experience in working with pediatric clients with developmental disabilities. She is particularly interested in historical sound change in society and speech sound development in children. Email: pspcheung@hotmail.com

Pi-Yu Chiang [pi y tɕjaŋ]
Department of Foreign Languages, National Taiwan Normal University, Taiwan
Pi-Yu Chiang is an Assistant Professor in the Department of Foreign Languages at National Taiwan Normal University in Taiwan. Her research is concerned with speech perception, speech production and phonological awareness in Mandarin-speaking children learning English as a second or foreign language. Email: piyu.chiang@gmail.com

Kathryn Crowe [ˈkæθɹən ˈkɹou]
National Acoustic Laboratories, Sydney, Australia
Charles Sturt University, Bathurst, Australia
Kathryn Crowe is a research speech-language pathologist working on the Longitudinal Outcomes of Children with Hearing Impairment (LOCHI) study at the National Acoustic Laboratories, Sydney, Australia, and is focused on better understanding multimodal and multilingual children with hearing loss. She has experience working with children and adults with hearing loss at all levels of education. Email: kathryn.crowe@nal.gov.au

Meghan Clayards [mɛɡən kleɪɑɹdz]
School of Communication Sciences and Disorders, McGill University, Canada
Meghan Clayards is an Assistant Professor in the School of Communications Sciences and Disorders and the Department of Linguistics at McGill University. Her research concerns phonetic variability in production and its role in shaping acoustic phonetic cue weights in perception.
Email: meghan.clayards@mcgill.ca

Martine Coene [maʁˈtinə ˈkunə]

Language and Communication, Applied Linguistics, Vrije Universiteit Amsterdam, Netherlands

Martine Coene is Professor of Applied Linguistics at the Vrije Universiteit, Amsterdam. She is mainly concerned with developmental language disorders, especially those resulting from hearing impairment. Her recent research focus is on prosodic reception in cochlear-implanted deaf children and, more particularly, how it influences the development of grammar. Together with Sue Peppé, she has adapted the PEPS-C to Dutch (Flemish). Email: mmr.coene@let.vu.nl

Madalena Cruz-Ferreira [mɐdɐˈlɛnɐ ˌkruʃˈfɐejrɐ]

Independent scholar, Singapore

Madalena Cruz-Ferreira holds a PhD in Linguistics and Phonetics from the University of Manchester, UK, and works on multilingualism, child language, phonology and intonation, and the language of science. Her recent books include *Three is a Crowd¿* (Multilingual Matters, 2006), *Multilingual Norms* (Peter Lang, 2010) and *Multilinguals are ...¿* (Battlebridge, 2010). Email: madalena@beingmultilingual.com

Barbara L. Davis [baɹbaɹə deivɪs]

Department of Communication Sciences and Disorders, The University of Texas at Austin, Austin, Texas, USA

Barbara Davis is the Houston Harte Centennial Professor of Communication at The University of Texas at Austin. Her research focuses on cross-language studies of typical speech acquisition, viewed as emergence of a complex system. She studies typically developing children, children with hearing impairment and children with severe speech disorders. Email: babs@mail.utexas.edu

Jan Edwards [ˈdʒæn ˈɛdwɚdz]

Department of Communicative Disorders, University of Wisconsin-Madison, Madison, WI, USA

Jan Edwards is a Professor of Communicative Disorders at the University of Wisconsin, Madison. Her research focuses on lexical and phonological development of children learning different first languages, including children with both typical and atypical language development. Email: jedwards2@wisc.edu

Annette V. Fox-Boyer [ɑˈnɛtə ˈfɔks bɔɐˈje]

Department of Speech and Language Pathology, University of Applied Sciences Fresenius, Hamburg, Germany

Annette Fox-Boyer trained and worked as a speech and language pathologist (SLP) in Germany before furthering her education with an MSc in neuropsycholinguistics and a PhD entitled 'The acquisition of phonology and the classification of speech disorders in German-speaking children', at the Department of Speech at the University of Newcastle upon Tyne in north-east England. In 2003, she became Professor of Speech Therapy at the first university for SLP in Germany. Email: fox-boyer@hs-fresenius.de

Christina Gildersleeve-Neumann [kɹɪsˈtinə ˈɡɪldɚsliv ˈnumən]
Portland State University, Portland, OR, USA
Christina Gildersleeve-Neumann, PhD, CCC-SLP, is Associate Professor in the Department of Speech and Hearing Sciences at Portland State University in Portland, Oregon. Dr Gildersleeve-Neumann has published papers on bilingual development in Spanish-English and Russian-English children and on treatment efficacy in children with speech sound disorders. She worked as a bilingual speech-language pathologist for three years in the public schools. Email: cegn@pdx.edu

Brian A. Goldstein [ˈbɹɑɪən ˈɡoldstin]
Temple University, Philadelphia, PA, USA
Brian Goldstein, PhD, CCC-SLP, is Professor in the Department of Communication Sciences and Disorders at Temple University. Dr Goldstein is well published in the area of communication development and disorders in Latino children, focusing on phonological development and disorders in monolingual Spanish and Spanish-English bilingual children. He is a Fellow of the American Speech-Language-Hearing Association.
Email: briang@temple.edu

Helen Grech [hɛlɛn ɡrɛk]
Department of Communication Therapy, Faculty of Health Sciences, University of Malta, Malta
Helen Grech, PhD, is a speech-language pathologist and educational audiologist. She heads the Department of Communication Therapy and is Deputy Dean of the Faculty of Health Sciences at the University of Malta. As a research fellow at the University of Limerick, Ireland, she completed the standardization of a Maltese-English speech and language assessment. Email: helen.grech@um.edu.mt

Isabelle Hesling [izabɛlə ɛslɪŋ]
UMR-CNRS 5231, Laboratoire d'Imagerie Moléculaire et Fonctionnelle, Université Bordeaux2, France
Isabelle Hesling is a Senior Lecturer at Bordeaux University in France and was awarded a doctorate in linguistics and speech science in 2000. She has been interested in prosody for the last 15 years. Her main research concerns

the integration of speech prosody in bilingualism and in speech pathologies, such as autism and aphasia, using both behavioral studies and fMRI. She has adapted the PEPS-C to the French language with Sue Peppé.
Email: isabelle.hesling@wanadoo.fr

Yvette Hus [i'vɛt hʌs]
TAV College, Language Intervention Technicians Training Program, Montreal, Canada
Yvette Hus, PhD, is a speech-language pathologist specializing in literacy disabilities in culturally and linguistically diverse children and adolescents, and a coordinator-instructor at TAV College in the language intervention paraprofessional training program. She is a long-standing member of and a frequent presenter at the International Association of Logopedics and Phoniatrics and the Multilingual Affairs Committee conferences.
Email: yhus@videotron.ca

David Ingram [devɪdɪŋɡɹəm]
Department of Speech and Hearing Science, Arizona State University, USA
David Ingram is a Professor in the Department of Speech and Hearing Science at Arizona State University. His research interests are in language acquisition in typically developing children and children with language disorders, with a cross-linguistic focus. The language areas of interest are phonological, morphological and syntactic acquisition.
Email: David.Ingram@asu.edu

Ghada Khattab [ˈɣaːda χɑˈtˤːɑːb]
Newcastle University, Newcastle Upon Tyne, UK
Ghada Khattab is a Lecturer at Newcastle University (UK). Her research interests include monolingual and bilingual phonological acquisition, sociolinguistics and Arabic linguistics. She has published papers on clinical sociolinguistics, the role of phonetic accommodation in bilinguals and Arabic speech acquisition. Email: ghada.khattab@ncl.ac.uk

Minjung Kim [ˈmɪndʒʌŋ ˈkɪm]
Department of Human Communication Studies, California State University, Fullerton, USA
Minjung Kim completed her PhD at the University of Washington and is a certified member of the American Speech-Language and Hearing Association. She is an Assistant Professor in the Department of Human Communication studies, California State University-Fullerton. Her research interests include cross-linguistic and multilingual studies of speech sound development and disorders in children. Email: minjungk@fullerton.edu

Sophie Kern [sofi kəɹn]
Laboratoire Dynamique du Langage, Institut des Sciences de l'Homme, Lyon, France
Sophie Kern is Researcher at the CNRS Laboratory Dynamique du Langage in Lyon, France. Her research projects cover very early language development in a cross-linguistic perspective with a special focus on babbling and first words. With colleagues, she adapted and normed the MacArthur-Bates Communicative Development Inventories for French. She is also co-editor of a volume on *Emergence of Linguistic Abilities* (Cambridge).
Email: Sophie.Kern@univ-lyon2.fr

Pastora Martínez-Castilla [pasˈtɔra marˈtinɛθ kasˈtiʝa]
Universidad Nacional de Educaciœn a Distancia, Spain
Pastora Martínez-Castilla is concerned mainly with developmental communication disorders, specifically language and cognition in Williams syndrome (WS). At the Universidad Autónoma de Madrid, she is involved in research as well as therapies for individuals with WS all over Spain (Unidad de Apoyo Psicológico al Síndrome de Williams). Currently, she is a Lecturer of Psychology at the Madrid Open University. In collaboration with Dr Sue Peppé, she has adapted the PEPS-C battery for use in Spanish.
Email: pastora.martinez@psi.uned.es

Felix Matias [filɪks matias]
Department of Communication Sciences and Disorders, University of South Florida, Tampa, FL, USA
Felix Matias is a Clinical Instructor in the Department of Communication Sciences and Disorders at University of South Florida. He is originally from Puerto Rico and has extensive experience in the assessment and treatment of bilingual (Spanish-English) children. Email: fmatias@usf.edu

Karen Mattock [kæɹen mætʰɒk]
Department of Psychology, Lancaster University, UK
Karen Mattock is a Research Council UK Fellow at the Department of Psychology, Lancaster University, UK. She investigates the development of speech perception, babbling and word learning in infancy, and how these are influenced by exposure and experience with language(s) in the first years of life. Email: k.mattock@lancaster.ac.uk

Thóra Másdóttir (Þóra Másdóttir) [ˈθouːˌra ˈmauːsˌtouhtɪɹ̥]
The National Hearing and Speech Institute of Iceland
The University of Iceland, Medical Department (division of Speech and Language Pathology)
Thóra Másdóttir has an MA degree as a speech and language pathologist from Indiana University, Bloomington, USA. She received a PhD degree

from Newcastle University in the UK in 2008. In her research, she focuses mostly on typical and disordered speech development in Icelandic-speaking children. Email: thoramas@hti.is

Sharynne McLeod [ˈʃæˌɹən məˈklaʊd]
Charles Sturt University, Bathurst, Australia
Sharynne McLeod, PhD, is Professor of Speech and Language Acquisition at Charles Sturt University in Australia. She is editor of the *International Journal of Speech-Language Pathology*, vice president of the International Clinical Linguistics and Phonetics Association, and a Fellow of both the American Speech-Language-Hearing Association and Speech Pathology Australia. Her recent books include *The International Guide to Speech Acquisition* (Cengage), *Speech Sounds* (Plural) and *Interventions for Speech Sound Disorders in Children* (Paul H. Brookes). Email: smcleod@csu.edu.au

Inger Moen [ˈiŋeʀ ˈmuːən]
Department of Linguistics and Scandinavian Studies, University of Oslo, Oslo, Norway
Inger Moen is Professor of Linguistics at the University of Oslo. Her field of study is clinical linguistics and phonetics. One of her ongoing research projects is an investigation of production and perception of prosody in various clinical populations. She collaborated with Sue Peppé on the translation of PEPS-C into Norwegian. Email: inger.moen@iln.uio.no

Benjamin Munson [ˈbɛndʒəmən ˈmʌnsn̩]
Department of Speech, Language, and Hearing Sciences, University of Minnesota, Minneapolis, MN, USA
Benjamin Munson is an Associate Professor of Speech-Language-Hearing Sciences at the University of Minnesota, Minneapolis. His research focuses on production-perception dynamics, relationships among word learning, speech production and speech perception, and the production and perception of socially meaningful variation in speech by children with typical development, children with atypical language development and normal adults. Email: munso005@umn.edu

Sean Pert [ʃɔːn pɜːt]
NHS Heywood, Middleton and Rochdale Primary Care Trust, UK
Sean Pert is a speech and language therapist with a special interest in bilingualism and speech and language impairment. He completed his PhD at Newcastle University researching intrasentential code switching in Pakistani heritage children and the process of the insertion of alien verbs. He has published several research papers, book chapters and assessments on bilingualism. Email: seanpert@speechtherapy.co.uk

Sue Peppé [su ˈpɛpe]
Speech and Hearing Sciences, Queen Margaret University, Edinburgh, Scotland, UK
Sue Peppé has specialized for 20 years in the assessment of prosody and intonation in communication disorders. Following her MA at University College, London, she spent several years working there on intonation in the Survey of English Usage with Randolph Quirk and others. She then devised the procedure *Profiling Elements of Prosody in Speech-Communication* (PEPS-C) with Dr. Bill Wells and Dr. Joanne Cleland, and was awarded a doctorate in Speech Sciences in 1998 for a thesis entitled 'Investigating linguistic prosodic ability in adult speakers of English'. This test, available in French, Spanish, Flemish, Norwegian and five versions for English regional accents, has been used in several publicly funded studies of prosody in adults and children. For the last 10 years, she has been a Research Fellow at Queen Margaret University, Edinburgh, specialising in prosody in autism.
Email: sue.peppe@gmail.com

Raúl F. Prezas [ˈraul ˈpɾesas]
Texas Christian University, Fort Worth, Texas, USA
Grand Prairie Independent School District, Grand Prairie, Texas, USA
Raúl F. Prezas is an Assistant Professor in the Department of Communication Sciences and Disorders at Texas Christian University in Fort Worth, Texas. He specializes in the area of Spanish phonology, including the assessment and treatment of monolingual Spanish and bilingual Spanish-English children. In addition to his research and work in the university clinical setting, Dr. Prezas serves as a bilingual speech-language consultant for the Grand Prairie Independent School District in Grand Prairie, Texas.
Email: r.prezas@tcu.edu

Raúl Rojas [ˈraul ˈroxas]
University of Texas at Dallas, Callier Center for Communication Disorders, Dallas, Texas, USA
Raúl Rojas is a Postdoctoral Research Scientist/Fellow at the University of Texas at Dallas, Callier Center for Communication Disorders, in Dallas, Texas, USA. His research focuses on child language from a longitudinal and processing perspective, specifically bilingual language development in typically developing children and in children with language impairments. Dr. Rojas, a certified speech-language pathologist, has provided bilingual (Spanish-English) speech-language pathology services in multiple settings, including schools and early intervention. Email: raul.rojas@utdallas.edu

Susan Rvachew [ˈsuzən ɹəˈvæʃu]
School of Communication Sciences and Disorders, McGill University, Canada
Susan Rvachew is an Associate Professor in the School of Communications Sciences and Disorders at McGill University. Her research is concerned with

the relationship between speech perception and speech production in typical and atypical language acquisition and the development of interventions for children with speech sound disorders.
Email: susan.rvachew@staff.mcgill.ca

Shelley E. Scarpino [ˈʃɛli skɑɹˈpino]
The Richard Stockton College of New Jersey, Pomona, NJ, USA
Shelley Scarpino, PhD, CCC-SLP, is Assistant Professor in the Department of Speech Pathology and Audiology at The Richard Stockton College of New Jersey. Her research focuses on speech sound development and disorders in monolingual and bilingual children, the relationships among speech, language and early literacy skills, and clinical service delivery issues pertaining to culturally and linguistically diverse populations.
Email: shelley.scarpino@stockton.edu

Isabelle Simard [izabɛl simaʁ]
ORTHO FUN I: Les petits Cocos, Montréal, Québec, Canada
Isabelle Simard is the creator, owner, manager and clinician of *ORTHO FUN I: Les petits Cocos*, a private speech-language pathology (SLP) practice for multilingual children in *Montréal*. Polyglot since childhood, as well as determined to aid the multilinguals from her birthplace, she studied abroad, has completed three degrees (linguistics and SLP) at the Université de Montréal and regularly partakes in numerous international conferences. While fluent in five languages, she currently conducts therapy in 17.
Email: simardisabelle@hotmail.com

Joseph P. Stemberger [ˈʤousəf ˈpʰi ˈstemˌbɚgɚ]
Department of Linguistics, University of British Columbia, Vancouver, Canada
Joseph P. Stemberger is a Full Professor at the University of British Columbia. He researches and teaches in the areas of phonology, phonetics and morphology, with particular foci on children's language development and adult psycholinguistic studies. Two current projects are focusing on phonological acquisition in Zapotec and, with Dr. Bernhardt, protracted phonological development across diverse languages.
Email: Joseph.Stemberger@ubc.ca

Carol Stoel-Gammon [ˈkɛɹəl ˈstolgæmən]
Department of Speech and Hearing Sciences, University of Washington, Seattle, USA
Carol Stoel-Gammon, PhD, is Professor Emerita in the Department of Speech and Hearing Sciences at the University of Washington. Her research interests include prelinguistic vocal development, cross-linguistic

phonological acquisition, and early speech and language in children with typical and atypical patterns of development. Email: csg@u.washington.edu

Carol Stow [ˈkaɹəɫ stəʊ]
NHS Heywood, Middleton and Rochdale Primary Care Trust, UK
Carol Stow leads a team of speech and language therapists working with bilingual children in their mother tongue. Her PhD focused on identifying speech disorders in Pakistani heritage children. She teaches and writes on issues relating to delivering an equitable service to bilingual children. Email: carolstow@speechtherapy.co.uk

Carol Kit Sum To [kæɹəl kit sɐm tou]
Division of Speech and Hearing Sciences, The University of Hong Kong, Hong Kong Special Administrative Region, China
Carol To is an Assistant Professor in the Division of Speech and Hearing Sciences at The University of Hong Kong and a speech and language pathologist. Her research focuses on assessment and intervention of speech and language disorders in children with disabilities, including speech sound disorders, autism spectrum disorders and language disorders. Email: tokitsum@hotmail.com

Seyhun Topbaş [ˈséjhun ˈtopbaʃ]
Department of Speech and Language Therapy, Institute of Health Sciences; Education, Training and Research Centre for Speech and Language Pathology, Anadolu University, Eskisehir, Turkey
Seyhun Topbaş, PhD, is a Professor of Speech and Language Pathology, and is one of the pioneers of the profession in Turkey. She led the foundation of the formal research center and initiated the Masters and Doctorate Degree programs at Anadolu University. She has authored numerous papers and chapters in international and national journals. She is a member of the International Issues Board of the American Speech-Language-Hearing Association (ASHA), a member of the International Clinical Phonetics and Linguistics Association (ICPLA) and on the editorial board of *Clinical Linguistics and Phonetics*. Email: stopbas@anadolu.edu.tr

Karla N. Washington [ˈkɑɹlə ˈwɔʃɪŋtən]
University of Cincinnati, USA
Karla Washington completed her PhD at the University of Western Ontario, London, Canada. She is a registered speech-language pathologist and has recently completed a federally-funded postdoctoral fellowship in pediatric outcome measurement at the Bloorview Research Institute, Toronto, Canada. She has specialized training in child language development and disorders and uses the lens of the ICF/ICF-CY to guide her clinical and research practices. Email: washink2@ucmail.uc.edu

Cori Williams [ˈkɔɹi ˈwɪljəmz]
School of Psychology and Speech Pathology, Curtin University, Perth, Australia
Curtin Health Innovation Research Institute, Curtin University, Perth, Australia
Cori Williams studied Australian Aboriginal linguistics at the Australian National University, and wrote a grammar of an Indigenous language spoken in the north-west of New South Wales. After training as a speech pathologist at Curtin University, she completed a PhD looking at news told by Aboriginal and non-Aboriginal children in urban classrooms. She is currently an Associate Professor and acting Head of the School of Psychology and Speech Pathology at Curtin University in Perth, Australia.
Email: c.j.williams@curtin.edu.au

Acknowledgments

First, we would like to thank the authors for their participation in this project. Without the work they are doing in their research and speech-language pathology settings, this book would not have been possible. They have shown us that we know significantly more about speech sound disorders in multilingual children than we initially believed. We are indebted to them for their efforts and for working within our editing guidelines to ensure a consistent book despite the number of authors.

We would like to acknowledge those children and their families who participated in the research summarized in this volume. It is our sincere hope that the information presented here allows for more appropriate speech-language pathology services to be delivered to multilingual children around the world.

We thank Nicole Müller and Martin J. Ball, the editors for this series of books at Multilingual Matters. We also thank the editorial staff at Multilingual Matters. You have made our lives significantly easier.

From Sharynne: To David, Brendon and Jessica – thanks for your enthusiasm about (and accompanying me on) my travels to meet and work with multilingual children, researchers and speech-language pathologists around the world. Your insights are invaluable.

From Brian: To Linda, Lauren and Jenna – thanks for your love, support and understanding, especially of my need to work on the book, even during Thanksgiving. You keep me grounded.

Foreword

Speech, as a funnel for language, is a primary and powerful means of connecting with others. Speech sounds are the basic substance of spoken communication. The mastery of these sounds and their rules of assemblage is a cumulative process of successive approximations. This process begins in infancy and continues through early childhood. Speech acquisition by children is marked by 'developmental errors' – normal child speech that misses the adult target. Developmental errors are the result of linguistic and physiological factors. The linguistic factors, including the sounds, their frequency of appearance and the permissible ways for combining them into words, vary across languages and dialects. As such, expectations for a child's speech are based on speech community standards as well as the performance of age peers who share similar language-learning experiences. For some languages and dialects, there is robust normative data on speech sound development; for many more languages, there are no such standards.

For most children learning one, two or more languages, speech sound development progresses smoothly, reflecting a symbiotic relationship with language: more sophisticated ideas are expressed in increasingly clear speech. The sound systems of the ambient languages are 'mastered' and speech is easily understood, providing a powerful tool for socialization and learning. However, for an important subset of children the acquisition of speech is anything but seamless. Children who lag behind their peers in the acquisition of speech are at significant social and educational disadvantage. Early identification of their struggles, adequate description of what is 'wrong' with the child's speech sound system and a plan to remediate the identified challenges is needed. Speech-language pathologists have this responsibility. There are now excellent evidence-based resources to guide professional actions with monolingual English-speaking children with speech sound disorders. Evidence and resources that guide professional actions with bilingual or multilingual children with suspected speech sound disorders have been largely absent. Yet, bilingualism and multilingualism are increasingly recognized as the rule rather than the exception.

Bilingualism and multilingualism describe the presence of more than one language in a society or within an individual. A majority of the global population and societies are bilingual or multilingual. Some children learn one language at home and different languages in the school and broader community. Other children may experience two or more languages in their homes. Some of these languages are considered 'prestige' or hold more power and privilege in the broader society; all are equal in terms of linguistic adequacy and essential to optimally meet functional needs of everyday life for multilingual children. As with children who learn only a single language, a small but important subset of bilingual and multilingual learners will also show evidence of a speech sound disorder. In order to adequately interpret the speech performance of these learners, professionals must understand the child's social or cultural circumstances, the critical features of the target speech systems to be learned as well as the typical developmental pathway. *Multilingual Aspects of Speech Sound Disorders in Children* provides critical information to guide this process.

Multilingual Aspects of Speech Sound Disorders in Children is an expertly edited collection of work from scholars in more than a dozen countries. These international scholars provide a truly global perspective on the acquisition and assessment of speech in many languages, and in many different social contexts. Foundation, research and theoretical chapters provide a meaningful context for understanding speech acquisition and disorders in children acquiring different and multiple languages. Complementing these core chapters are practical applications, illustrating select aspects of clinical practice with multilingual learners in Australia, Canada, Germany, Hong Kong, Israel, Iceland, Jamaica, Korea, Malta, Norway, Turkey, the UK and the USA! McLeod and Goldstein have organized this volume so that it can be read as a rich, meaningful whole, then referred back to in pieces as each chapter provides its own tutorial of sorts with respect to the relevant cultural and linguistic environments for interpreting the information presented.

The sheer breadth of information in this volume is impressive, but beyond this is the richness and practicality of the material. *Multilingual Aspects of Speech Sound Disorders in Children* carefully presents the best information currently available for serving multilingual learners with speech sound disorders, what to do with this information and, importantly, how to go beyond current knowledge constraints. As just one example, speech sampling tools available in different languages are described in Chapter 13. Building on this 'what's there' information, Chapter 14 addresses gaps in available tools and how to create clinical tools to fill this gap – a necessary skill for professionals who work in multilingual contexts. For both assessment and intervention of speech sound disorders in children learning multiple languages, this resource provides a much-needed springboard for clinical actions.

Multilingual Aspects of Speech Sound Disorders in Children addresses the complex issues of detecting and treating speech skills that fall below community and developmental expectations in learners of multiple languages. Given the prevalence of multilingualism, the significance of speech sound disorders and the general absence of resources for clinical professionals who serve children who speak languages other than or in addition to English, the information contained in this volume fills a basic need. *Multilingual Aspects of Speech Sound Disorders in Children* should prove the essential reader for students, professionals and clinical researchers interested in using current evidence to best serve children with suspected speech sound disorders who are acquiring two or more languages.

Kathryn Kohnert, PhD
Professor
Speech-Language-Hearing Sciences
University of Minnesota, USA

Preface

Multilingual Aspects of Speech Sound Disorders in Children aims to translate research into clinical practice for people working with multilingual children with speech sound disorders. Children with *speech sound disorders* are defined as those who have articulatory and/or phonological delay or disorder, as well as those with childhood apraxia of speech. Children with speech sound disorders are one of the largest groups of children on speech-language pathologists' caseloads (Broomfield & Dodd, 2004; Mullen & Schooling, 2010). A number of books have been written about *monolingual* children with speech sound disorders from a variety of language backgrounds; however, this book focuses on *multilingual* children with speech sound disorders from across the globe.

A broad definition of *multilingualism* has been used within *Multilingual Aspects of Speech Sound Disorders in Children*, so that the range of those who fit under this construct are included. This is in line with authors such as Valdés and Figueroa (1994: 115), who propose a continuum of proficiencies: bilingualism 'rather than being an absolute condition is a relative one. Bilingual individuals can be both slightly bilingual or very bilingual'. Terminology that is encompassed within our broad definition of multilingualism includes: bilingual, multilingual, simultaneous bilingual, sequential bilingual, bilingual first language acquisition (BFLA), culturally and linguistically diverse (CALD), English language learner (ELL), non-English speaking background (NESB), non-French speaking background (NFSB), etc., language other than English (LOTE), language other than Icelandic (LOTI), etc.

Multilingual Aspects of Speech Sound Disorders in Children explores both multilingual and multicultural aspects of children with speech sound disorders. The book is divided into three sections:

(1) Foundations
(2) Multilingual speech acquisition
(3) Speech-language pathology practice

The introductory chapter discusses the importance of considering multilingual children with speech sound disorders. Subsequent chapters consider how the disorder manifests in different languages, cultural contexts and speakers, then chapters address speech acquisition, diagnosis, assessment and intervention for children with speech sound disorders.

A unique feature of this book is the translation of research into clinical practice. There are 12 research chapters that primarily focus on a topic and describe available research across a wide range of languages. These are supplemented by 17 chapters that translate research into practice, providing vignettes for specific geographical, cultural or linguistic contexts. By including these two different styles of chapters, information has been drawn from across the globe to provide exemplars of the multitude of issues when working with multilingual children with speech sound disorders. The epilogue chapter draws together the rich content of the book.

The 44 authors come from 16 different countries: Australia, Canada, Hong Kong Special Administrative Region (China), France, Germany, Iceland, Israel, Malta, The Netherlands, Norway, Spain, Singapore, Taiwan, Turkey, UK and USA. The languages in focus include: Australian Sign Language, Cantonese, English, German, Hebrew, Icelandic, Jamaican Creole, Korean, Maltese, Norwegian, Spanish and Turkish. Overall, there are 112 languages and dialects mentioned in the book: Albanian, American Sign Language, Amharic, Arabic (various dialects), Armenian, Athabaskan languages, Australian Indigenous languages, Australian Sign Language (Auslan), Austronesian languages, Basque, Bini, British Sign Language, Bulgarian, Burmese, Cantonese, Catalan, Chinese, Creole, Czech, Danish, Dutch, English (various dialects), Estonian, Ewe, Farsi, Finnish, Flemish, French, Fulani, Galician, German, Gilbertese, Greek, Gujarati, Haida, Hawai'ian, Hebrew, Hindi, Hokkien, Hungarian, Icelandic, Inuit, Irish, Italian, Jalapa Mazatec, Jamaican Creole (Patois), Japanese, Khmer, Khoisan language family, Korean, Kurdish, Lahanda, Lao, Latin, Latvian, Limburg, Lithuanian, Lugandan, Malay, Maltese, Mandarin, Mayan languages, Melpa, Mirpuri, Mongolian, Navajo, Norwegian, Oto-Manguean, Pakistani heritage languages, Pawaian, Persian, Polish, Portuguese (Brazilian and European), Punjabi, Putonghua, Quiché, Rabinian, Romanian, Rotokas, Russian, Sami, Samoan, Scottish Gaelic, Serbo-Croatian, Shanghainese, Sindhi, Singlish, Slovene, Southern Min, Spanish (various dialects), Swahili, Swedish, Tagalog, Tamil, Teke, Thai, Tlingit, Tok Pisin, Turkish, Urdu, Vietnamese, Welsh, Western Pahari, Wolof, Xhosa, !Xū, Yucatec, Wolof and Zulu.

The main audience of this book is practicing speech-language pathologists (speech and language therapists, logopaedists, etc.) and graduate students who work with children from around the world. This will include speech-language pathologists who work in schools, preschools, private clinics and health facilities, as well as speech-language pathologists who travel to different nations. Other people who will be interested in this book include phoneticians, linguists, anthropologists, sociolinguists and educators.

Multilingual Aspects of Speech Sound Disorders in Children documents past and present knowledge and practices around the globe, as well as providing recommendations for the future. The authors of the translation to practice chapters have clearly described the *status quo* in their countries and most have described the need for additional attention to be paid to multilingual children. Using this book as a baseline, it will be fascinating to see how world practices change in the future decades as multilingualism and multiculturalism continues to be the way of the world.

References

Broomfield, J. and Dodd, B. (2004) Children with speech and language disability: Caseload characteristics. *International Journal of Language and Communication Disorders* 39 (3), 303–324.

Mullen, R. and Schooling, T. (2010) The National Outcomes Measurement System for pediatric speech-language pathology. *Language, Speech, and Hearing Services in Schools* 41, 44–60.

Valdés, G. and Figueroa, R.A. (1994) *Bilingualism and Testing: A Special Case of Bias*. Norwood, NJ: Ablex.

Sharynne McLeod and Brian A. Goldstein
Bathurst, Australia and Philadelphia, PA, USA

Part 1
Foundations

1 Prologue: Cross-linguistic and Multilingual Aspects of Speech Sound Disorders in Children

David Ingram

Languages mentioned: *Bulgarian, Cantonese, Dutch, English, Estonian, French, German, Greek, Icelandic, Italian, Khoisan language family, Korean, Quiché, Swahili, Swedish, Turkish, Xhosa*

The linguist David Crystal once raised the question of whether or not a monolingual English-speaking speech-language pathologist (SLP) would ever need to know something about Swahili. The answer, of course, is a definite yes, no or maybe. Reasons why she should, include the fact that it is interesting to linguists and SLPs, she might move to a Swahili-speaking country one day, she might develop an interest in Swahili folk music and culture or she might have a Swahili-speaking client on her caseload. Reasons why she should not, include she might not like linguistics, never move to a Swahili-speaking country, care for international music or ever see a Swahili-speaking client. That leaves us with maybe.

The field of speech-language pathology has spent over 30 years trying to figure out whether children who have multiple speech errors and poor intelligibility have speech problems or phonological problems. The late Eric Lenneberg (1962) reported a case study of an 8-year-old boy who had acquired English receptively, but could not speak due to severe anarthria (see also Stromswold, 1994). That probably can be described as a speech disorder. Recently, Caroline Bowen (2009) has written a state-of-the-art book on children with multiple speech errors, entitled *Children's Speech Sound Disorders*. Many of the children discussed in that book sound to me as if they have phonological problems. While Bowen is likely using 'speech' in the general sense of 'speaking', the extent to which phonological problems are exclusively speech based is still an open question, at least for some. The answer to whether or not children have speech or phonological problems then is a definite maybe.

Before we sink into an abyss of indefinity (my word), it should be noted that there are at least two reasons why an SLP should care about languages other than English. One reason is that they are an SLP for clients who speak another language. There are chapters in the present collection that fit into this category. For example, there are discussions of children's speech in numerous languages, including Korean, Icelandic, German and French, among others. The second reason, related to the first, is that they work with clients who are multilingual. Several chapters address this issue as well. SLPs with either of these interests will find this volume of great interest.

What then about the SLP who does not fit either of the above characterizations? Is there any reason for them to take time to learn about multilingual aspects of speech sound disorders? It is to this group that the rest of this chapter is addressed. And here's a hint. The study of multilingual aspects of speech disorders provides the greatest evidence available that speech disorders, in many instances, are phonological disorders.

Let's Talk Greek Dental Fricatives

Let's talk Greek. I am reminded of a cartoon depicting a university student meeting with his professor of classical languages. The confounded professor responds to the student 'it's supposed to sound Greek to you'. So, continuing along in the spirit of David Crystal's comment about Swahili, why should an SLP working with English-speaking children care about Greek? Let's look at one of the more interesting characteristics of Greek phonology. Greek, like English, has the dental fricatives [θ] and [ð]. That of itself is interesting because these are relatively rare in the languages of the world (c.f. Ball, Chapter 5). These two sounds are also among the last sounds acquired in English; for example, they are among Shriberg's late eight sounds acquired (Bleile, 2006; Shriberg, 1993). To understand the nature of these sounds and how they function in English requires an understanding of how they pattern in languages in which they occur.

One possibility that we might consider is that dental fricatives are rare in languages, and that they are rare because they are hard to make. This option is a serious proposal, and has been addressed in linguistics under the general topic of markedness. Sounds that are common in languages, and acquired early, are seen as unmarked or more basic, while those that are rare and later acquired are seen as marked. For purposes of comparison, we can consider the English labiodental fricative [f] as unmarked when compared to dental fricatives. It is relatively common in languages, and is acquired early (cf. Ingram *et al.*, 1980). Also, [f] is a common substitute for [θ]. Similarly, [d] is a common consonant across languages, is acquired early and is often a substitute for [ð]. The sound [d] then is unmarked relative to [ð], which would be a marked counterpart.

To a large extent, the above is true, and would lead to certain predictions about Greek. One prediction would be that dental fricatives should show evidence of being marked in Greek relative to unmarked sounds like [f] and [d]. Secondly, we would expect Greek children to acquire these sounds (i.e. dental fricatives) later, and also to use unmarked sounds as substitutes for them. It turns out, however, that these predictions are false. As reported in Ferguson (1978), the following relations hold. (a) The phoneme /ð/ is used in a much wider range of contexts than /d/. It occurs in word-initial position and intervocalically, as well as clusters. It occurs nearly three times more often than /d/, which is mostly restricted to loan words. The fricative therefore can be interpreted as unmarked in relation to the stop, the opposite of normal expectations. (b) The opposite relation exists for /t/ versus /θ/. The stop is much more common than the voiceless fricative, resulting in an asymmetry between the voiced and voiceless pairs. (c) Based on the limited data available (see the review in Mennen & Okalidou, 2007; Stephany, 1997), dental fricatives are acquired early in Greek, and do not appear to present any undue problems in their acquisition. In fact, a study on Greek children with speech disorders (Petinou, n.d.) found that the children did well with the voiced dental fricative, while having problems with other Greek fricatives (alveolar, palatal and velar, voiced and voiceless pairs).

This ease of production for /ð/ is not restricted to Greek children. A colleague of mine followed his son's English phonological acquisition, and noted that his son's first and only fricative for some time was [ð]. All other fricatives were either avoided or replaced with an [h]. This was verified to me while listening to a recording of his son, who I shall refer to as Ian. Ian was very aware of his difficulties with fricatives, and developed a unique means to avoid words he could not say well. Instead of saying them, he would say the word *lemon*. Here are some excerpts from the recording:

Father: Can you say 'J'.
Ian: Called 'lemon'
Father: Can you say 'zither'?
Ian: Can't say the word.
Father: Say 'sheriff' dida bear.
Ian: 'Lemon!' (loud)
Father: Say 'saxophone'.
Ian: I call them 'lemon [hon]'.

Circumstances such as those just described are an important lesson that phonetic difficulty and articulatory tendencies cannot be taken as absolutes. Children are not just learning how to pronounce. They are learning how to form and store mental representations of words; they are learning a phonological system, not a set of phonological probabilities; and they are learning to approximate the words of the language they are acquiring.

Let's Talk Turkey (with Quiché)

Topbaş (1992, 2007) has extensively studied phonological acquisition in Turkish in both typically developing children and children with phonological disorders. Her data provide opportunities to see what sounds are found to be difficult by both groups of children. A comparison of her studies in

Ingram (2008) noted that both groups showed similar phonetic inventories. One striking feature was that both groups acquired affricates relatively early, especially [ʧ]. The affricate [ʧ] also showed a tendency to be acquired before any fricatives. A discrepancy was found, however, regarding [l]. The consonant [l] is not acquired early in English, and is often glided to a [w] or [j]. In the Turkish data, children showed an early glide [j], which presumably would be available for target /l/ phonemes. Surprisingly, the children with phonological disorders showed an early [l], but not the typically developing children. Barring another explanation, we have a case where the children with disorders were apparently doing better on a sound than typical children, relatively speaking.

It turns out that another rather different study found early acquisition of [ʧ] and [l]. Pye *et al*. (1987) studied the early consonants of five children acquiring Quiché, a Mayan language spoken in Guatemala. No linguist has ever proposed that Quiché and Turkish are related languages, though unrelated languages certainly can share typological similarities. Pye *et al*. found two consonants to be the most frequently used in the early vocabularies of the five children. These were the consonants [l] and [ʧ], the same two sounds noted above for Turkish. Initially, they were stunned by this result, because they had believed, as everyone else at the time believed, that the order of acquisition of speech sounds was determined by phonetic complexity. Wrong. No doubt, phonetic complexity plays a role, but something else was going on.

To explore what else was influencing the early use of [l] and [ʧ], Pye *et al*. looked at the distribution of these two consonants in the words that the Quiché children were acquiring. They found a strong correlation between the order of acquisition of the Quiché consonants by children and their use in the vocabulary that they were acquiring. The interpretation was something like this. If a speech sound plays a prominent role in the vocabulary that the child is learning, then that prominence may, at least in the case of Quiché [l] and [ʧ], lead to earlier acquisition than what might be predicted based solely on phonetic complexity. They labeled this influence *functional load*, a term that has been used in linguistics for many years (Meyerstein, 1970). Functional load refers to the role that a phoneme plays in the phonological system of a language in terms of how often it contrasts with other phonemes. It needs to be distinguished with phonetic frequency, which is how often a sound occurs in spoken language. This difference can be demonstrated with the English fricative /ð/ as it occurs in word-initial position. The English /ð/ only occurs in a small number (less than 20) of grammatical words in word-initial position; e.g. *the, this, that*, etc. It, therefore, has a low functional load. These grammatical words are frequent, so /ð/ has high phonetic frequency. This distinction can be used to account for the differences between how English and Greek children acquire /ð/. In English, the consonant has low functional load, and is acquired late. In

Greek, however, it has high functional load, which can be argued to be the reason for its early acquisition. Importantly, it is also acquired early by Greek children with language impairments (Petinou, n.d.). If this pattern holds up across studies of other languages (e.g. Icelandic), then it is strong evidence that children with errors in their speech have a phonological disorder, since their order of acquisition, albeit delayed, is showing the influence of functional load, not solely phonetic complexity.

Let's Click

As reviewed in Ingram (2008), research across languages shows variations on when children acquire consonants that reflects an interaction between phonetic complexity and functional load. Another example of this interaction is found in the limited research on the acquisition of clicks. Clicks comprise a range of sounds that involve an alteration of airflow (a velaric airstream mechanism), which results in a clicking sound. They occur in a relatively small number of languages in Africa, particularly the Khoisan family, where they constitute a large number of the consonant inventory (cf. Ladefoged, 1992: 138, showing examples of five different clicks in Xhosa). The fact that they do not occur in a wide range of languages suggests that they may be sounds of greater articulatory complexity, though the extent to which that is true is open to debate. It is less controversial, however, that Xhosa has a complex inventory of consonants. Mowrer and Burger (1991) report that Xhosa has 38 consonants and three clicks, which can vary in place and manner, resulting in 12 click allophones. They further point out that the language has the following sounds also not found in English: ejective plosives, a bilabial implosive, a rolled 'r' and both velar and lateral fricatives. Based on this range of complex sounds, one might expect that the Xhosa consonant inventory would be difficult for children to acquire. Mowrer and Burger constructed an articulation test for Xhosa, and gave it to 70 children, divided into seven groups of 10 children each, ranging from 2;5 to 6 years of age. Further, they matched the Xhosa children to 70 English-speaking children. They did not make a prediction in their study, but it would have been a reasonable hypothesis that the Xhosa-speaking children would show a longer course of acquisition than the English-speaking ones, given that their Xhosa inventory was nearly twice as large and contained several more complex consonants. The results, however, did not bear this out. Mowrer and Burger compared 20 consonants in the two languages that were similar. They found that the Xhosa children actually produced fewer errors on the shared consonants than their English counterparts did. Further, the Xhosa children did not show excessive difficulty with the more complex sounds unique to Xhosa. The clicks, for example, were acquired, by and large, by age three.

V, The Sound (Not the Novel)

Studies on the acquisition of [v] vary, but they generally show that it is not an early-acquired sound in English. Shriberg (1993) places it in the middle eight sounds. Studies by Templin (1957) and Ingram *et al.* (1980) show word-initial [v] to be one of the last fricatives acquired. Templin found 6-year-olds still showing only 70% accuracy, and Ingram *et al.* found errors extending into their 5-year-old participants. Thus, from these data, [v] appears to be a phonetically complex sound. Locke (1983) makes exactly this claim, based on his study of the sounds found cross-linguistically in babbling and children's first words. Salus and Salus (1974) also make this case for fricatives in general, although they add the additional factor that it is due to late myelination of the auditory nerve and thus late acquisition of the ability to perceive them.

In Ingram (1988), I examined the acquisition of [v] for three case studies of children acquiring Swedish, Estonian and Bulgarian. For Swedish, larger samples can also be found in Nettelbladt (1983) for 10 children with phonological disorders and 1 typically developing child, and in Magnusson (1983) for 32 children between 3 and 6 years of age. The fricative [v] was found in the inventories of both groups. A similar finding was reported for Italian in Bortolini *et al.* (1993). They compared the early word-initial consonantal inventories of nine typically developing children with nine children with phonological disorders. For the typically developing 2-year-olds, the first fricatives produced were [f], [v], [s] and [z], with [z] being the least frequently used. For the atypical children, ranging in age from 4;9 to 7;1, the fricatives [f], [v] and [s] were used, mirroring order of acquisition for the typically developing children.

So, was Locke (1983) wrong? The answer is a clear yes, no or maybe. Yes, he was correct in that he made a strong case from babbling data that [v] and other late or infrequently babbled sounds are likely to be so because of phonetic complexity. In fact, there was never a claim in the proposal for the role of functional load that phonetic complexity should not also be taken into consideration. The claim was only that there are instances, perhaps not many, where functional load may lead to a sound being acquired earlier in one language than another. It appears incorrect, however, to claim that all the early consonants acquired in children's early words can be predicted solely on the basis of phonetic complexity.

Now, let's look at maybe. More recent research by Stokes and Surendran (2005) shows that the relation between phonetic complexity, functional load and phonetic frequency is complex, and can vary by language, based on their analyses of Dutch, Cantonese and English. They examined these three factors in terms of when sounds are acquired (age of emergence), and for their accuracy of production. Regarding age of emergence, they found that phonetic frequency was the best predictor for Chinese, but that functional load was the best predictor for English. Different interactions emerged for accuracy of production. Phonetic complexity (or ease of production, in their terminology) was the best predictor for English, while it was not for Dutch. They also suggested that phonetic complexity appeared to be predictive of the late acquisition of a subset of complex consonants in Arabic (Amayreh, 2003). Clearly then, the results reported to date are the tip of the iceberg in our understanding of how these factors interact in individual languages, and likely individual children.

Time for Clinical Implications

As stated at the onset, the reasons for multilingual studies include insights into how to approach intervention in monolingual contexts. Foremost, the argument was made that multilingual studies provide a strong case that many children with multiple speech errors have a phonological problem, not just one of an inability to articulate speech sounds. If the problem was solely articulatory, then children should show the same speech errors regardless of their linguistic environment. It has been shown that children studied to date in different linguistic settings do not always show the same speech deficits. Further, the order of acquisition for children with speech deficits looks more similar to that of their typically developing peers than to children with speech deficits acquiring other languages. Intervention with these children requires approaches that see the problem as one of phonological remediation, not just articulatory remediation.

One implication is the way in which the clinician views the role of the environment. In speech intervention, the environment is minimal, consisting of the SLP who leads the child through traditional techniques that have been around since the days of Van Riper (1939). In phonological intervention, the role of the environment is much more critical. This can be exemplified by the approach developed by Hodson (1984) and referred to as cycles. Cycles involve a number of procedures that can be best understood when treatment is seen as influencing the child's phonological development, not just their speech. Treatment begins at the word level, since speech exists to assist children in acquiring words, not vice versa. Children are exposed to a range of words through auditory bombardment, a practice that can be perceived as explicit environmental manipulation to draw the child's attention to the phonological importance of a target phoneme (i.e. its functional load). Production practice also focuses on words, though a smaller set. Further, cycles involve the selection of a range of sounds, not just a single sound that is drilled until a high rate of correct production. Children do not acquire speech by acquiring individual sounds. They acquire sounds systematically by their related phonological features, not randomly. Hodson also does not set explicit criteria for successful productions during the first cycle, since children typically take months to establish underlying presentations, not days.

The importance of recognizing the child as having a phonological deficit influences the way in which assessment is approached. Assessment should not exclusively focus on individual speech sounds. In recent years, more and more arguments are being made that phonological assessment needs to be multidimensional. In Ingram and Ingram (2001), we proposed an approach that examined four levels of the child's phonological system, moving from measures of whole words to measures of individual consonants. More recently, Ingram and Dubasik (2010) revised the Basic Analysis with nine measures used across four levels:

(1) Whole word analysis (three measures): phonological mean length of utterance (pMLU) of target words; pMLU of child words; whole word proximity of child's words to their targets.
(2) Word shape analysis (two measures): number of preferred syllable shapes (e.g. CV, CVC, CVCV); proportion of monosyllabic words.
(3) Analysis of phonetic inventories: (two measures): Articulation Score (PI AS) separately for onset and coda consonant inventories; (PI AS measures the size of each inventory).
(4) Relational analysis (two measures): Articulation Score (R AS) separately for onset and coda consonant inventories; R AS measures the number of matches (correct consonants) for each inventory.

We further demonstrated how children can vary from one another on any of the nine measures, and that any more restricted analysis will miss these variations.

In summary, the multilingual study of phonological acquisition and disorders provides insights not as easily noted if only focusing on the acquisition of a single language. The study of a single language such as English can give the impression that the order of acquisition of speech sounds follows a consistent pattern, predicted by the articulatory complexity of the individual sounds. Cross-linguistic studies, however, show that the order of acquisition is not just the result of articulatory complexity, but also the result of the functional load of each language's phonemes, and also their phonetic frequency. These other factors show an influence on the phonological development of children with speech disorders as well. Phonemes with high functional load in a language will be acquired earlier by both typically developing children and by children with phonological deficits. So, does a monolingual SLP need to be aware of aspects of multilinguistic phonological acquisition. It is concluded here, without indefinity, that the answer is 'yes'!

References

Bleile, K. (2006) *The Late Eight*. San Diego, CA: Plural Publishing.

Bowen, C. (2009) *Children's Speech Sound Disorders*. London: Wiley-Blackwell.

Ferguson, C. (1978) Phonological processes. In J.H. Greenberg (ed.) *Universals of Human Language* (Vol. 2; pp. 403–444). Stanford, CA: Stanford University Press.

Hodson, B. (1984) Facilitating phonological development in children with severe speech disorders. In H. Winitz (ed.) *Treating Articulation Disorders. For Clinicians by Clinicians* (pp. 75–89). Baltimore, MD: University Park Press.

Ingram, D. (1988) [v]: The acquisition. *Language and Speech* 31, 77–85.

Ingram, D. (2008) Cross-linguistic phonological acquisition. In M. Ball, M. Perkins, N. Müller and S. Howard (eds) *The Handbook of Clinical Linguistics* (pp. 626–640). Oxford: Blackwell.

Ingram, D. and Dubasik, V. (2010, November) Multidimensional assessment of phonological similarity between and within children. Seminar presented to the annual meeting of the American Speech-Language-Hearing Association, Philadelphia.

Ingram, D. and Ingram, K. (2001) A whole word approach to phonological intervention. *Language, Speech, and Hearing Services in Schools* 32, 271–283.

Ingram, D., Christensen, L., Veach, S. and Webster, B. (1980) The acquisition of word-initial fricatives and affricates in English by children between 1 and 6 years. In G. Yeni-Komshian, J. Kavanaugh and C. Ferguson (eds) *Child Phonology, Vol. 1 Production* (pp. 169–192). New York: Academic Press.

Lenneberg, E. (1962) Understanding language without ability to speak: A case report. *Journal of Abnormal and Social Psychology* 65, 419–425.

Locke, J. (1983) *Phonological Acquisition and Change*. New York: Academic Press.

Mennen, I. and Okalidou, A. (2007) Greek speech acquisition. In S. McLeod (ed.) *The International Guide to Speech Acquisition* (pp. 398–411). Clifton Park, NY: Thomson Delmar Learning.

Meyerstein, R. (1970) *Functional Load: Descriptive Limitations, Alternatives of Assessment and Extensions of Application*. The Hague: Mouton.

Mowrer, D. and Burger, S. (1991) A comparative analysis of phonological acquisition of consonants in the speech of 2½-6-year-old Xhosa- and English-speaking children. *Clinical Linguistics and Phonetics* 5, 139–164.

Petinou, L. (n.d.) Phonological patterns in two groups of Cypriot Greek-speaking children. Unpublished study.

Pye, C., Ingram, D. and List, H. (1987) A comparison of initial consonant acquisition in English and Quiche. In K.E. Nelson and A. van Kleeck (eds) *Children's Language* (Vol. 6; pp. 175–190). Hillsdale, NJ: Lawrence Erlbaum.

Salus, P. and Salus, M. (1974) Developmental neurophysiology and phonological acquisition. *Language* 50, 151–160.

Shirberg, L.D. (1993) Four new speech and prosody-voice measures for genetics research and other studies in developmental phonological disorders. *Journal of Speech and Hearing Research* 36, 105–140.

Stephany, U. (1997) The acquisition of Greek. In D.I. Slobin (ed.) *The Crosslinguistic Study of Language Acquisition* (Vol. 4; pp. 183–333). Hillsdale, NJ: Erlbaum.

Stokes, S. and Surendran, D. (2005) Articulatory complexity, ambient frequency and functional load as predictors of consonant development in children. *Journal of Speech, Language, and Hearing Research* 48, 577–591.

Stromswold, K. (1994, January). Language comprehension without language production: Implications for theories of language acquisition. Paper presented at the 18th Annual Boston University Conference on Language Development.

Templin, M. (1957) *Certain Language Skills in Children*. University of Minnesota Institute of Child Welfare Monograph Series 26. Minneapolis, MI: University of Minnesota Press.

Topbaş, S. (1992) A pilot study of phonological acquisition by Turkish children and its implications for phonological disorders. Paper presented to the Sixth International Conference on Turkish Linguistics, Eskisehir, Turkey.

Topbaş, S. (2007) Turkish speech acquisition In S. McLeod (ed.) *The International Guide to Speech Acquisition* (pp. 566–579). Clifton Park, NY: Thomson Delmar Learning.

Van Riper, C. (1939) *Speech Correction: Principles and Methods*. New York: Prentice-Hall.

2 Sociolinguistic and Cultural Considerations when Working with Multilingual Children

Madalena Cruz-Ferreira

Languages mentioned: *Arabic, Danish, Dutch, English, French, German, Hokkien, Japanese, Mirpuri, Norwegian, Portuguese, Punjabi, Singapore Standard English, Singlish (Singapore Colloquial English), Spanish, Swedish, Tok Pisin, Turkish, Urdu*

Multilingual Typicality versus Speech-language Disorder

Overarching considerations when working with multilingual children concern the special status that continues to be accorded to multilingualism. Virtually all current knowledge about linguistic and cultural practices draws on monolingual and mono-cultural behaviour, whose *mono* character is glossed over and so tacitly emerges as default. In contrast, research on multilingualism invariably includes explicit reference to *multi* settings, thereby signalling an exceptionality worthy of a dedicated label. Multilingual children are *culturally and linguistically diverse* (CLD), as if monolingual children were, by definition, culturally and linguistically homogeneous; or users of *heritage varieties*, as if monolinguals lacked linguistic heritage.

Labels such as these belie the fact that multilingualism is itself a norm, historically and statistically. They conveniently explain (away) idiosyncrasies necessarily found in a population for whom proper norms, and so properly normed assessment instruments, have yet to be formulated: extant assessment tools are normed from and for monolingual uses of language. Correlating multilingualism, which is the feature shared by such children, with mismatches to norms, and interpreting correlation as causality often results in diagnosing the child with multilingualism itself, for which the remedy is monolingualism (Stow & Dodd, 2003). There is no correlation between multilingualism and disorder (Genesee *et al.*, 2004), but there is evidence that therapy delivered in a home language will impact the child's other languages (Kohnert, 2007; Stow, 2006). Tragically, the misguided association of multilingualism with disorder finds support from perhaps the least expected sources: Bavin's (2009) recent collection dedicates one chapter to child multilingualism in a section entitled 'Varieties of Development', which otherwise deals with specific language impairment (SLI), autism and genetic disorders. The alternative view, that multilingualism correlates with giftedness, does equal disservice to multilingual children: a gift would not be labelled a gift if it were typical.

Multilingualism has mostly been treated as a special case of monolingualism, on the assumption that multilingualism is what Cruz-Ferreira (2006: 14ff) termed 'dual monolingualism' or, more generally, multi-monolingualism, a simple addition of languages. At the same time, there is implicit acknowledgement that multilinguals and monolinguals are not the same population. If they were, the common practice of comparing multilinguals to monolinguals, but never the other way around, would have long been abandoned. The issue seems to be a surprising lack of awareness that monolinguals and multilinguals alike use exactly as many languages as required by their everyday needs. This chapter reviews sociolinguistic and cultural issues in multilingual settings, starting with a brief discussion of their relevance for extant assessment tools, and concluding with their implications for clinical work with multilingual children.

Linguistic and Cultural Variation versus Standardised Assessment Tools

Like their monolingual peers, multilingual children acquire language varieties, not languages. The label *language* subsumes the complex set of actual varieties under it. For the same reasons, each assessment instrument is normed from and for one language variety, including where that variety may have acquired (prestige) status as the *standard* form, and come to be identified with the name of the language to which it belongs. Labels like *English*, *American English* or *British English*, whether in speech-language pathology (SLP) clinics or foreign language classrooms, designate languages and countries, abstract entities whose linguistic and political boundaries show little congruity with linguistic behaviour on the ground.

Instruments normed for the particular language (variety) used by a child may be unavailable, an issue that affects monolinguals and multilinguals alike, naturally hampering identification of clinical issues (Stow, 2006). Multilingual children's productions of varieties unaccounted for in assessment norms, and therefore deviating from them, may be attributed to multilingualism itself rather than to language variation, precisely because the child comes labelled, as multilingual and thus special, whereas language variation in the child's environment does not. The norms that can usefully serve as benchmark lie instead in the input available to the child, on which child forms naturally depend. For example, the child form [mɑk] for the English target /mɑːsk/ (mask) shows typical consonant-cluster reduction. Singaporean English-speaking children may produce the form [mɑt] for the same word, apparently showing an additional substitution of [t] for /k/. Awareness of the word's target form in Singapore Standard English, /mɑːs/, explains the child rendition as a typical example of stopping instead. Multilingualism, which is the rule in Singapore, is irrelevant here.

Expectations about presumed default cultural norms complete the assessment equation. Culture, like language, does not necessarily associate with a piece of land (a *nation* or a *region*), although it is informally discussed as if it did: we talk about, e.g. African or Australian *culture*. But there are expectations about which non-linguistic behaviours pattern with which language(s), in that languages capture cultural settings not only through grammar and vocabulary (noun classifiers, forms of address), but also through social perceptions associated with their use. In Singapore, for example, English is the language of science, whereas Hokkien is a *dialect* for use in the army and for rough partying.

Cultural practices become an inherent part of one's identity through socialisation. Telling linguistic and cultural variation apart is therefore not straightforward, although this chapter treats them under separate headings. The patrimony that a child acquires through social interaction and that, in turn, affects individual experiences, which is one definition of culture, includes the language varieties of the community, which is the subject matter of sociolinguistics. Both issues are relevant in clinical settings. Whether linguistic and cultural behaviours are intentional or not, they project images of the user as belonging (or not belonging, or wishing to belong) to a particular social group, which in turn prompts personal judgements about the user and associated linguistic responses from the interlocutor, including a clinical interlocutor. When working with children, their relevance for judgements on which assessment naturally builds is twofold: children behave as they experience behaviour, in ways which, if mentioned at all, may not match textbook and assessment models; and children may have been socialised in adult beliefs about their uses of their languages and about multilingualism itself (MacSwan, 2000), and behave accordingly.

Sociolinguistic considerations in the assessment of multilingual children

Sociolinguistic issues broadly concern the covariance of social and linguistic behaviour. Variables relate to social hierarchy and status (sociolect); geographical location (dialect); perceived (social, age-bound) status of both speaker and listener (register); or idiosyncratic features of individual users (idiolect).

These variants encompass lexis, grammar and accent, and cut across one another in a cline-like rather than discrete fashion. Only recently has their relevance to multilingual settings caught researchers' attention. In order to achieve appropriate pragmatic purposes, multilingual children may use different languages instead of different variants of the same language; and those children whose caregivers predominantly use one language each with them, will show the effects of this language policy in their own productions: in her speech, a female child will naturally use features of male adult uses of the language for which she has predominantly male input, and vice versa (Cruz-Ferreira, 2006; Potowski, 2008).

Within sociolinguistic studies, multilingualism falls under matters of language contact, which can be said to have two core effects. Among languages, contact results in variation (across space) and change (across time), whose twin role in keeping languages alive, and therefore usable, is often underestimated, if not reviled (Burridge, 2010). New varieties that thus emerge, so-called contact varieties, may further rise to full status as (national) languages, once acquired natively, or co-exist in diglossic situations with officially sanctioned variants of the same language. Examples are Tok Pisin in Papua New Guinea, and the two variants of English used in Singapore, Singapore Standard English and Singapore Colloquial English (also called *Singlish*), respectively. Among users, language contact results in multilingualism itself, often surfacing in the form of *mixes*, a label used here as a cover term for *code-switching, code-mixing* and *borrowing*, to describe utterances containing features of more than one language.

Mixes are a *multilingual norm* of language use (Cruz-Ferreira, 2010; Pert, 2007). They have had a mixed fate in the literature on multilingual acquisition, being taken as evidence of linguistic shortcoming and linguistic proficiency, of language separation and language confusion, and of typical versus atypical developmental progress. Bullock and Toribio (2009) provide a recent survey of this topic. When the same data give rise to paradoxical interpretations such as these, the problem lies, of course, in data analysis. The issue is that extant assessment norms, which are all monolingual, fail to identify the typicality of multilingual mixes.

Typical mixing is rule governed, thus amenable to linguistic description. Lanvers (2001) found stable functions in child mixes, matching adult-like mixing, in longitudinal German-English conversational data from two simultaneous bilinguals aged 1;6 to 2;11. The children's mixes signalled emphasis and appeal, conversation topic change and so-called vocabulary gaps. It should be added here that in cases where a particular word is inaccessible in one language, for reasons that may include developmental immaturity, using fillers from the same language or from another language amounts to the same repair strategy: multilinguals resort to (so-called) mixes, and monolinguals to (unnamed) sets of all-purpose words like *thingamajig*, as argued in Cruz-Ferreira (2006). This study draws on a database from three trilingual siblings, spanning their first 10 years of life. The children are simultaneous bilinguals in

Portuguese and Swedish, and acquired English through schooling in Hong Kong and Singapore from ages 3 to 7, respectively. The study further showed that not only the choice of language(s) incorporated in mixes, but also the choice itself to switch language, regardless of the languages involved, served pragmatic communicative purposes. Pert (2007) sampled patterns of mixing among 167 typically developing Pakistani heritage children living in the UK, aged between 2;6 and 7;2, whose home languages were Mirpuri, Punjabi or Urdu, to conclude that atypical mixing, or lack of mixing, may assist in the identification of language development disorder, particularly SLI, among this population.

Teenagers, an age group well known for adopting specific, mostly self-empowering and peer-oriented forms of speech (Stenström *et al.*, 2002), were found to use mixes as markers of identity and protest (Jørgensen, 1998, 2005). Jørgensen's research targets second-generation immigrants to Denmark, who use Turkish and Danish to follow, reject or modify the mixing habits of their home and peer communities for different purposes. Importantly, Jørgensen concludes that adolescent linguistic behaviour, whether monolingual or multilingual, shares patterns across the board.

Phonetic mixes from adult multilinguals have deserved active attention under labels like *foreign accent* (including the common misnomer 'speaking with an accent': all varieties of all languages must be spoken with an accent), but remain underrepresented in the literature on multilingual acquisition. The bulk of extant research addresses segmental sounds (vowels and consonants). In the USA, Pearson and Navarro (1998) studied the productions of 11 simultaneous Spanish-English bilinguals (mean age: 3;0) in words representing typical segmental features of each language in the children's environment. Although conceding difficulties in distinguishing foreign accent from phonological immaturity, the study concludes that brief and isolated features of the former can be observed in developing bilinguals. Khattab (2009) reports data from three simultaneous Arabic-English bilinguals, second-generation immigrants to the UK, aged 5, 7 and 10, respectively, who regulated their production of segmental Arabic-accented English, in otherwise mixed or English-only utterances, to compensate their perception of their own language (non)dominance, to create distinct identities when using English at home or with monolingual English-speaking peers and, overall, to establish themselves as multilinguals. As Pearson and Navarro (1998) made clear, phonetic mixes must be carefully distinguished from developmental phonological processes (also called *common mismatches* or *error processes*). The latter designate standard differences between child speech sound productions and adult targets, commonly involving substitution, addition, omission and simplification. They account for regularities across children and languages, thus providing robust benchmarks against which to assess developing pronunciations, but they concern segmental productions only.

Cruz-Ferreira (1999, 2006) studied multilingual suprasegmental features of language (prosody), including intonation, rhythm, stress and tempo, which are necessarily present in any speech, at any age. Drawing on the Portuguese-Swedish-English database mentioned above, the first study reports that prosodic mixes, i.e. using the prosody of one language with the segmentals of another, reflect multilingual acquisitional strategies, in that they serve the purpose of testing, across languages, meaningful patterns encountered in one language. The second study details the crucial role of developmental prosody, both as conveyor of linguistic meaning and indicator of language identity from before the one-word stage.

Cultural considerations in the assessment of multilingual children

Among multilinguals, non-linguistic behaviour is likely to show features of culture contact, parallel to language contact, which surface as cultural mixes. Body language, including posture, facial expressions and hand and head gesturing, has a grammar of its own, which depends on social and cultural idiomacy, as reported in Cruz-Ferreira (2006) for Portuguese-Swedish simultaneous bilinguals. Voice gestures, as they may be termed, signal meaning too. Different languages are spoken with characteristic articulatory settings, typifying habitual and language-specific configurations of the vocal tract, and with characteristic tones of voice. These are culture bound, indicating politeness and sex-appropriate uses (Yuasa, 2008), or expressing emotion (Tanaka *et al.*, 2010). Non-linguistic sounds, gestures or postures may be rude or playful, instrumental or expressive, depending on the observer's cultural norms, or even pass unremarked where the child may have intended them as significant.

Gesturing is inherent to communicative competence, and an indicator of typical linguistic and/or cognitive development. According to Schopler and Mesibov (1985), autistic children prefer instrumental to expressive gestures. Nicoladis *et al.* (1999) reported correlation between the development of certain types of gestures and mean length of utterance (MLU) in French and English, among five simultaneous bilinguals aged 2;0–3;6. Rowe and Goldin-Meadow (2009) found disparity in the use of gestures among 50 English monolingual children, aged 1;2, from different socio-economic status (SES), which matched disparity in their vocabulary size at school entry, at age 4;5.

Researching story telling among Dutch monolingual and immigrant children, van Hell *et al.* (2003) found that predictors of narrative competence, whether quantitative (length) or qualitative (coherence), correlated with the children's cultural familiarity with a topic rather than with their knowledge of Dutch. In the USA, Minami (2008) asked 40 simultaneous bilinguals, aged 6–12, to narrate a picture storybook in both Japanese and English.

Adult Japanese and American evaluators, respectively, rated high stories that were lengthy, contained a large and varied vocabulary and were told in the past tense. But what defined a 'good story' for each set of evaluators was not so much its linguistic packaging as whether the narrator managed to convey cultural features that identified a story as a good Japanese story or a good English story. For example, Japanese judges appreciated the report of temporal sequences of action devoid of evaluative and/or emotional comments, whose presence, in contrast, was highly valued by American judges.

The same phonetic utterance may evoke quite different meanings for users of different languages, whether co-occurring with culture-specific body language or not. One example reported for the children in Cruz-Ferreira's (2006) study, at around age 1;0, is the sound [m]. Uttered on a high-rising tone, together with pointing behaviour, it signals a wh-question in a Portuguese exchange. In a Swedish context, accompanied by a brief nod, it signals assent. In the absence of visual or verbal clues, due to disorder or other reasons, utterances of this kind that rely entirely on idiomatic prosody are difficult to interpret. Luthy (1983) removed all contextual clues from 14 American English intonation signals and played them to adult learners of English, who either missed or misinterpreted much of their non-lexical meanings. Silence itself is significant: in some Western(-like) communities, it is interpreted as absence of (adequate) speech, or of response to speech; among Asians and Nordic Europeans, silence is the presence of an event that is culturally relevant. Among Nordic Europeans, for example, it expresses respect for the speaker's message and conversational turn, until the speaker signals turn yielding (Cruz-Ferreira, 2006; Nakane, 2007; Tulviste *et al.*, 2003; Li Wei *et al.*, 2005).

Peppé and colleagues developed prosodic assessment tools for child users of different languages (Peppé, 2009a; Peppé *et al.*, 2010). Suspected atypical prosody can be gauged against a listener's prosodic expectations, with the proviso that mismatches need not necessarily reveal disorder, in that they can reflect sophisticated uses of prosody instead (Peppé, 2009b). Cruz-Ferreira's (1999) study showed that mismatches can also signal multilingual acquisitional strategies: if multilingualism were factored out of the assessment equation for these children, their productions would be found deviant.

Clinical Implications for Work with Multilingual Children

Findings such as these prove not only the fundamental inadequacy of descriptive accounts of single languages to approach multilingualism, but also that the particular languages involved in multilingualism are not an issue: the issue concerns the uses that children make (or not) of their overall linguistic resources. Among adults working with multilingual children, these studies are a call to raise awareness of sociolinguistic and cultural variability, and to exercise analytical flexibility. In one crucial sense, linguistic and social development amounts to acquiring communicative competence for the benefit of specific adult interlocutors. Acquisition is, in fact, deemed complete when children's use of (their) language(s) matches everyone else's in their surroundings.

Multilingualism means differential use of different languages, disproving the assumption that testing one of the languages of multilinguals provides insight into their overall linguistic ability. In the absence of normed tests for particular languages or language varieties, resorting to translation and/or adaptation of available instruments is often unavoidable, despite concerns about the validity of such practices (Paul, 2007). Two recent studies provide striking examples of the extreme caution that must be observed when modifying tools designed for other uses. Peppé *et al.* (2010) discuss the translation of an English prosodic assessment test, where core uses of English intonation are absent or marginal in Spanish or vice versa, and where uses of lexical tone in Norwegian are non-existent in English. Brebner (2010), adapting an English expressive language test for a different variety of the language, reports a stumbling block in the use of a picture representing something apparently as culturally universal as a cat catching mice: the relative body sizes of cats and common rodents in different parts of the world must be taken into account.

Where the SLP and the child client have no common language, dynamic assessment methods can provide insight into language ability, as opposed to ability in particular languages (Gutiérrez-Clellen & Peña, 2001). Multilingual clinical staff may be called on to act as interpreters (Meyer & Apfelbaum, 2010), and caregivers as sources of information, interpreters and/or deputy therapists in the home setting, although the effectiveness of both parental reports and clinical advice has been questioned on cultural grounds. Stow (2006) and Peña (2007) observed difficulties among Pakistani caregivers in the UK and Mexican caregivers in the USA, respectively, to identify speech issues in their own children, whereas Johnston and Wong (2002) found differential child-rearing beliefs and related verbal interaction practices among Chinese and Western mothers of pre-schoolers, which contrasted with Western-bound advice about children with language delay. Friend and Keplinger (2008) reported distortion of assessment results entailed by forms of engagement with testing methodologies that were assumed as default, but which are culture-bound: children may fail to respond to a common test procedure like touching a named object because their parents forbid them to touch objects that do not belong to them.

For all these reasons, SLPs may find themselves enacting Labov's (1972: 113) Observer's Paradox: *mutatis mutandis*, 'to obtain the data most important for linguistic theory, we have to observe how people speak when they are not being observed'. Children are not routinely socialised in speech-language clinics. Where home, peer and school standards differ, the child may not know which one applies, if at all, in a novel environment, including where the child's cultural upbringing may (dis)allow addressing adults in one or all of their languages, and/or taking initiative to do so. Knowledge of languages other than the language of intervention, or of multilingualism itself, is, in turn, not part of SLPs' routine training. Even clinicians who are multilingual and may envisage practice in multilingual contexts continue to be trained in monolingual frameworks for monolingual purposes. This status quo results in imbalanced referral of multilinguals to speech-language clinics, in two opposite ways: under-referral, from false negatives that take disorder as typical multilingualism (Cruz-Ferreira & Ng, 2010; Stow, 2006) and over-referral, from false positives that take typical multilingualism as disorder. Young language learners, particularly in immigration settings, form a disproportionate percentage of over-referrals (MacSwan & Rolstad, 2006), where *bilingual deficit* in fact often means low ability in a foreign but mainstream language of instruction.

To end this chapter on the same note as it started, the issue is to remove the *multilingual stigma* from children who happen to need more than one language to function appropriately in their environments. What constitutes disorder in multilingual children can only emerge against norms that reflect typical multilingual behaviour, for whose establishment new questions need to be asked: the answers must make multilingual sense. If generalisations about monolingualism have held sway over language uses across the board, there is no reason to assume that generalisations about multilingualism will not. Speech-language assessment concerns *speech and language*, regardless of which languages and how many.

References

Bavin, E.L. (ed.) (2009) *The Cambridge Handbook of Child Language*. Cambridge/New York: Cambridge University Press.

Brebner, C. (2010) The development of the Singapore English Action Picture Test: An expressive language screening assessment for Chinese Singaporean preschool children. In M. Cruz-Ferreira (ed.) *Multilingual Norms* (pp. 323–341). Frankfurt: Peter Lang.

Bullock, B.E. and Toribio, A.J. (eds) (2009) *The Cambridge Handbook of Linguistic Code-switching*. Cambridge: Cambridge University Press.

Burridge, K. (2010) Linguistic cleanliness is next to godliness: Taboo and purism. *English Today* 26 (2), 3–13.

Cruz-Ferreira, M. (1999) Prosodic mixes: Strategies in multilingual language acquisition. *International Journal of Bilingualism* 3 (1), 1–21.

Cruz-Ferreira, M. (2006) *Three is a Crowd? Acquiring Portuguese in a Trilingual Environment*. Clevedon: Multilingual Matters.

Cruz-Ferreira, M. (ed.) (2010) *Multilingual Norms*. Frankfurt: Peter Lang.

Cruz-Ferreira, M. and Ng, B.C. (2010) Assessing multilingual children in multilingual clinics. Insights from Singapore. In M. Cruz-Ferreira (ed.) *Multilingual Norms* (pp. 343–396). Frankfurt: Peter Lang.

Friend, M. and Keplinger, M. (2008) Reliability and validity of the Computerized Comprehension Task (CCT): Data from American English and Mexican Spanish infants. *Journal of Child Language* 35 (1), 77–98.

Genesee, F., Paradis, J. and Crago, M. (2004) *Dual Language Development and Disorders. A Handbook on Bilingualism and Second Language Learning*. Baltimore, MD: Paul H. Brookes.

Gutiérrez-Clellen, V.F. and Peña, E.D. (2001) Dynamic assessment of diverse children. A tutorial. *Language, Speech, and Hearing Services in Schools* 32, 212–224.

Johnston, J.R. and Wong, M-Y.A. (2002) Cultural differences in beliefs and practices concerning talk to children. *Journal of Speech, Language, and Hearing Research* 45 (5), 916–926.

Jørgensen, J.N. (1998) Children's acquisition of code-switching for power wielding. In P. Auer (ed.) *Code-switching in Conversation: Language, Interaction and Identity* (pp. 237–260). New York: Routledge (Taylor & Francis).

Jørgensen, J.N. (2005) Plurilingual conversations among bilingual adolescents. *Journal of Pragmatics* 37 (3), 391–402.

Khattab, G. (2009) Phonetic accommodation in children's code-switching. In B.E. Bullock and A.J. Toribio (eds) *The Cambridge Handbook of Linguistic Code-switching* (pp. 142–159). Cambridge: Cambridge University Press.

Kohnert, K.J. (2007) *Language Disorders in Bilingual Children and Adults*. San Diego, CA: Plural.

Labov, W. (1972) Some principles of linguistic methodology. *Language in Society* 1 (1), 97–120.

Lanvers, U. (2001) Language alternation in infant bilinguals: A developmental approach to codeswitching. *International Journal of Bilingualism* 5 (4), 437–464.

Li Wei, Miller, N., Dodd, B. and Zhu, H. (2005) Childhood bilingualism: Distinguishing difference from disorder. In M.J. Ball (ed.) *Clinical Sociolinguistics* (pp. 193–206). Malden, MA: Blackwell.

Luthy, M.J. (1983) Nonnative speakers' perception of English 'nonlexical' intonation signals. *Language Learning* 33 (1), 19–36.

MacSwan, J. (2000) The Threshold Hypothesis, semilingualism, and other contributions to a deficit view of linguistic minorities. *Hispanic Journal of Behavioral Sciences* 22 (1), 3–45.

MacSwan, J. and Rolstad, K. (2006) How language proficiency tests mislead us about ability: Implications for English language learner placement in special education. *Teachers College Record* 108 (11), 2304–2328.

Meyer, B. and Apfelbaum, B. (eds) (2010) *Multilingualism at Work. From Policies to Practices in Public, Medical and Business Settings*. Amsterdam: John Benjamins.

Minami, M. (2008) Telling good stories in different languages: Bilingual children's styles of story construction and their linguistic and educational implications. *Narrative Inquiry* 18 (1), 83–110.

Nakane, I. (2007) *Silence in Intercultural Communication. Perceptions and Performance*. Amsterdam: John Benjamins.

Nicoladis, E., Mayberry, R.I. and Genesee, F. (1999) Gesture and early bilingual development. *Developmental Psychology* 35 (2), 514–526.

Paul, R. (2007) *Language Disorders from Infancy through Adolescence: Assessment and Intervention* (3rd edn). St. Louis, MO: Mosby.

Pearson, B.Z. and Navarro, A.M. (1998) Do early simultaneous bilinguals have a "foreign accent" in one or both of their languages? In A. Aksu-Koç, E. Erguvanli-Taylan, A.S.

Ozsoy and A. Kuntay (eds) *Perspectives on Language Acquisition: Selected Papers from the VIIth International Congress for the Study of Child Language* (pp. 156–168). Istanbul: Bogazici University Printhouse.

Peña, E.D. (2007) Lost in translation: Methodological considerations in cross-cultural research. *Child Development* 78 (4), 1255–1264.

Peppé, S. (2009a) PEPS-C (Profiling Elements of Prosodic Systems – Children). http://www.qmu.ac.uk/ssrc/prosodyinasd/PEPS-C.htm.

Peppé, S. (2009b) Why is prosody in speech-language pathology so difficult? *International Journal of Speech-Language Pathology* 11 (4), 258–271.

Peppé, S., Martínez-Castilla, P., Coene, M., Hesling, I., Moen, I. and Gibbon, F. (2010) Assessing prosodic skills in five European languages: Cross-linguistic differences in typical and atypical populations. *International Journal of Speech-Language Pathology* 12 (1), 1–7.

Pert, S. (2007) Bilingual language development in Pakistani heritage children in Rochdale, UK: Intrasentential codeswitching and the implications for identifying specific language impairment. Unpublished doctoral dissertation, University of Newcastle.

Potowski, K. (2008) "I was raised talking like my mom": The influence of mothers in the development of MexiRicans' phonological and lexical features. In M. Niño-Murcia and J. Rothman (eds) *Bilingualism and Identity: Spanish at the Crossroads with Other Languages* (pp. 201–220). Philadelphia, PA/Amsterdam: John Benjamins.

Rowe, M.L. and Goldin-Meadow, S. (2009) Differences in early gesture explain SES disparities in child vocabulary size at school entry. *Science* 323 (5916), 951–953.

Schopler, E. and Mesibov, G. (eds) (1985) *Communication Problems in Autism*. New York: Plenum.

Stenström, A-B., Andersen, G. and Hasund, I.K. (2002) *Trends in Teenage Talk. Corpus Compilation, Analysis and Findings*. Amsterdam: John Benjamins.

Stow, C. (2006) The identification of speech disorders in Pakistani heritage children. Unpublished doctoral dissertation, University of Newcastle.

Stow, C. and Dodd, B. (2003) Providing an equitable service to bilingual children in the UK: A review. *International Journal of Language and Communication Disorders* 38 (4), 351–377.

Tanaka, A., Koizumi, A., Imai, H., Hiramatsu, S., Hiramoto, E. and de Gelder, B. (2010) I feel your voice: Cultural differences in the multisensory perception of emotion. *Psychological Science* 21 (9), 1259–1262.

Tulviste, T., Mizera, L., De Geer, B. and Tryggvason, M.-T. (2003) A silent Finn, a silent Finno-Ugric, or a silent Nordic? A comparative study of Estonian, Finnish, and Swedish mother-adolescent interactions. *Applied Psycholinguistics* 24 (2), 249–265.

van Hell, J.G., Bosman, A.M.T., Wiggers, I. and Stoit, J. (2003) Children's cultural background knowledge and story telling performance. *International Journal of Bilingualism* 7 (3), 283–303.

Yuasa, I.P. (2008) *Culture and Gender of Voice Pitch. A Sociophonetic Comparison of the Japanese and Americans*. London: Equinox.

3 Translation to Practice: Sociolinguistic and Cultural Considerations when Working with the Pakistani Heritage Community in England, UK

Carol Stow, Sean Pert and Ghada Khattab

Languages mentioned: English, Mirpuri, Punjabi, Urdu

Context

The Pakistani heritage community is the second largest and most widely dispersed minority ethnic community in England and Wales (Office for National Statistics, 2001). The majority of the community originate from the west Punjab region of Pakistan and the Mirpur District of Azad Kashmir, areas with a long history of internal and external migration driven by economic, political and social factors. During the 1950s and 1960s, the textile towns in northern England sent recruitment officers to the area in response to labour shortages in the UK (Khan, 1991) and the original community clustered around discreet geographic areas, establishing shops and supermarkets to meet their specific needs. The population now consists of third generation children born to parents who were themselves born and raised in England, and members newly arrived from Pakistan, usually as marriage partners. The community retains strong links with their extended families and villages in Pakistan and extended holidays to Pakistan are routine. Satellite television allows access to Pakistani television programmes and there are local and national radio stations broadcasting in the main community languages.

Languages spoken

Three main mother tongue languages are spoken within the community: Mirpuri, Punjabi and Urdu, along with varying degrees of English proficiency. Language use usually reflects both the geographic area of origin and social status of the individual's family. There is a perceived hierarchy with Urdu, the official language of Pakistan, seen as the highest status language, followed by Punjabi and finally Mirpuri, a language associated with the more rural, poorer areas in Pakistan. Mirpuri has no written form, leading professionals, members of the public and politicians to incorrectly label Mirpuri speakers as 'illiterate' (see, e.g. Gulzar & Manthorp, 2009: 7). As literacy is not an option available to Mirpuri speakers, a more accurate description would be 'pre-literate'. Grosjean (1982) remarked on the propensity of dominant groups to attack the language of minorities by referring to them as dialects, thereby linking them to the negative connotations associated with dialects by non-linguists. Urdu and Punjabi speakers frequently describe Mirpuri as 'just a dialect' and, possibly as a result, many Mirpuri speakers self-report as Urdu or Punjabi speakers, despite not being able to understand those languages (Pert, 2007; Stow, 2006). Within the Pakistani heritage community reported on here, there is an expectation of bilingualism and intrasentential code switching is typical of adult bilingual-to-bilingual speech.

The Clinical Context

Cultural considerations in the clinical situation

Parents and caregivers prefer face-to-face or verbal methods of communication. It is best practice to ask a bilingual assistant/interpreter to telephone the parents prior to the first appointment. This contact will clarify which language the family actually speaks and also reassures non-English speakers that a mother tongue speaker will always support them at the appointment. In addition, those families unfamiliar with speech-language pathology services will have an opportunity to ask about what to expect. One frequent theme is anxiety around being unable to speak fluent English. When the appointment takes place in an obviously medical or educational environment, parents and children may attempt to use only English, as they perceive the environment as an exclusively English setting. Reassurance that the speech-language pathology team is there to support the child to use their mother tongue skills will usually circumvent such misunderstandings.

As the community (typically) has low levels of literacy in their Pakistani heritage languages, any advice or therapy programmes are best discussed verbally and, if necessary, recorded onto an audio format rather than simply distributing printed information leaflets or therapy advice in English.

Code switching

Code switching between a Pakistani heritage language and English is the model provided by parents to their children. It is unsurprising that children typically use code switching. However, as young children generally use ethnic identity to guess adult speakers' language, they are less likely to use their full language repertoire when confronted with a white monolingual speaker. It is therefore crucial to commence the session with the bilingual assistant talking to the parents and child in their mother tongue, thereby establishing the speakers present and the environment as a mother tongue setting. The use of a mother tongue greeting or praise will help the child to see the clinician as a mother tongue speaker, despite the visual disparity in appearance.

There is evidence that children use their longest and most grammatically sophisticated utterances when employing code switching (Pert & Letts, 2006). Intrasentential code switching, or truly bilingual utterances, means that the child is able to use his/her full range of vocabulary and linguistic skill. Inexperienced clinicians may interpret bilingual utterances as signs of language disorder, especially when large proportions are in English but the frame is in Mirpuri; e.g. 'boy flowers smell kar-na pija' (boy flowers smell do-ing + male is + male).

In order to fully analyse a child's utterances and discuss with the bilingual assistant if a particular utterance is disordered or merely code switched, the original data must be preserved. For this reason, during the session, the bilingual assistant must transcribe the child's utterances verbatim (without online translation) and these data must form the basis of the clinical record. Following the session, time for translation, analysis and discussion are crucial. This may be supplemented by audio or video recordings.

Speech assessment

Code switching is not isolated to one Pakistani heritage language and English. Code switching may take place between any of these languages. Lexical items from different languages are often seen as synonyms. This is recognised in the assessment of speech with the *Bilingual Speech Sound Screen* (BiSSS) tool (Stow & Pert, 2006), where a single recording form lists the transcriptions for each tested item in all three Pakistani heritage languages.

Different patterns of adult–child interaction

Assessment and therapy is a formal form of adult–child interaction developed within a western context. Within the Pakistani heritage community, different modes of interaction are found. In many families, children are not expected to initiate communication with adults, and when addressed by an adult, children are expected only to give a concise and prompt response, not always verbal. As a result, children may fail to respond because of these pragmatic differences, or offer a non-verbal response such as eye pointing. Non-responder numbers were so high they form part of the normative data for BiSSS.

Delivering therapy

Parents may fail to engage in therapy activities, as they perceive the child's difficulties to have a medical basis and would prefer an overtly medical solution (e.g. a medicine or injection). Highlighting the link between speech and language skills and educational success may motivate parents to engage in the therapy process. Therapy activities that expect the parent to interact with the child may be less successful than those where the child's older siblings take the lead. There is evidence that parents in the community have a highly directive communication style with children (Stow, 2006) and older children typically spend more time interacting with their siblings and engaging them in play-related activities than adults do.

In summary, when working with the Pakistani heritage communities in the UK, it is important to bear a number of sociolinguistic aspects in mind and to approach clinical therapy accordingly. For instance, the proclaimed spoken languages of the community may not be their actual native language(s), so some investigative work is required to establish the target language(s) for therapy. Bilingual assistants/interpreters can then be employed to facilitate the use of the home language(s) in the clinic. Furthermore, if the nature of discourse in the community is bilingual/multilingual, it is essential to factor code switching into assessment and subsequent therapy. Finally, when planning home activities to support therapy, an understanding of patterns of interaction among family members in a particular culture can alleviate potential breakdown of home support.

References

Grosjean, F. (1982) *Life with Two Languages: An Introduction to Bilingualism*. Cambridge, MA: Harvard University Press.

Gulzar, S. and Manthorp, S. (2009) Black and white and colour: Films made by or about black and minority ethnic communities. http://www.yorkshirefilmarchive.com/files/yfa/BlackWhiteColourMono1_1.pdf. Accessed 18.1.11.

Khan, F. (1991) The Urdu speech community. In S. Alladina and V. Edwards (eds) *Multilingualism in the British Isles, Africa, the Middle East and Asia* (Vol. 2; pp. 128–140). London: Longman.

Office for National Statistics (2001) *Census 2001*. http://www.statistics.gov.uk. Accessed 18.1.11.

Pert, S. (2007) Bilingual language development in Pakistani heritage children in Rochdale UK: Intrasentential codeswitching and the implications for identifying specific language impairment. Unpublished doctoral thesis, University of Newcastle upon Tyne.

Pert, S. and Letts, C. (2006) Codeswitching in Mirpuri speaking Pakistani heritage preschool children: Bilingual language acquisition. *International Journal of Bilingualism* 10, 349–374.

Stow, C. (2006) The identification of speech disorders in Pakistani heritage children. Unpublished doctoral thesis, University of Newcastle upon Tyne.

Stow, C. and Pert, S. (2006) *Bilingual Speech Sound Screen: Pakistani Heritage Languages*. Winslow: Speechmark.

4 Translation to Practice: Sociolinguistic and Cultural Considerations when Working with Indigenous Children in Australia

Cori J. Williams

Languages mentioned: Aboriginal English, Australian English, Indigenous languages

Context

The Aboriginal people of Australia share a history of conflict with a colonising power, which has had far-reaching consequences. These consequences continue to be felt today (Trudgen, 2000). Health issues are endemic, and include extreme incidence of otitis media that extends beyond childhood (Couzos *et al.*, 2001; Williams *et al.*, 2009). Educational levels for Aboriginal children fall well below those of their non-Aboriginal peers (Commonwealth of Australia, 2007) and Aboriginal people are over-represented in the justice system (Australian Human Rights Commission, 2009).

Languages Spoken by Aboriginal Australians

Although it is reported that over 400 languages (Australian Bureau of Statistics, 2010) are spoken in Australia, the sociolinguistic context of the country as a whole is one in which English is the language of the dominant community, the language of education, power and influence. For Aboriginal children, the sociolinguistic context includes both language shift and a history of language loss. Of the estimated 750 indigenous dialects spoken in Australia at the time of colonisation, only 18 are still spoken by people from all age groups (Australian Institute of Aboriginal and Torres Strait Islander Studies, 2005). The sociolinguistic context in which Aboriginal children grow up differs with geographical location and the language(s) spoken in the home.

Aboriginal English (AE) is the first language for the majority (around 88%) of the Aboriginal population, most of whom live in urban areas. AE is a non-standard dialect of English, which differs from Standard Australian English (SAE) in non-trivial ways (Malcolm *et al.*, 1999). The characteristics of AE vary along a continuum from *light* varieties (more similar to SAE) to *dark* or *heavy* varieties (less similar to SAE) (Butcher, 2008). These characteristics encompass all language areas. Although AE is recognised by at least some state education systems (see resources produced by the Department of Education, Western Australia), support for the acquisition of SAE may not be available in the classroom setting. In rural and remote areas of Australia, the sociolinguistic context for Aboriginal children may include a creole or one or more indigenous languages (Wigglesworth & Simpson, 2008), and SAE as the language of education. Children who grow up speaking indigenous languages may have little exposure to SAE before entering the education system. Bilingual education is not provided (Simpson & Wigglesworth, 2008) and federal benchmarking literacy and numeracy testing is carried out in SAE.

Characteristics of Australian Indigenous Languages and Culture

Australian indigenous languages share a number of characteristics (see Blake, 1987, for more detailed information). These include:

- phonological systems which have nasals and plosives at up to six places of articulation, non-phonemic voicing of stops, no fricatives or affricates, as few as three vowels;
- morphologically complex (case marking) syntax with relatively free word order;
- complex pronoun systems (singular, dual and plural marking, free and bound forms);
- complex verb systems;
- no articles.

Cultural and linguistic characteristics shared by Aboriginal people regardless of geographical location and first language have also been identified. Shared language characteristics include pragmatic and discourse characteristics, which differ from those of SAE. Within Aboriginal interactions, expectations regarding eye contact differ from expectations in non-Aboriginal interactions. Many reports indicated that questions are used in culture-specific ways; for example, direct questioning is not always appropriate (Eades, 1982). However, more recent research has not supported this contention (Moses & Yallop, 2008). Extended oral text is produced within a framework that assumes a high level of shared cultural knowledge, and therefore does not require the use of detail in the linguistic expression (Sharifian, 2001). This may mean that non-Aboriginal listeners (such as teachers) will find it difficult to understand the texts (Sharifian *et al.*, 2004).

Shared cultural characteristics relate to ways of being in the world, and to the rich cultural and spiritual life of the people. The concept of *shame* means that Aboriginal people are not comfortable in situations that draw attention to them as individuals (Eades, 1996). In one-to-one therapy situations, this may be evident in an apparent lack of engagement. The need to fulfil cultural obligations, such as attendance at funerals and important ceremonies, may affect attendance at appointments, which may result in the withdrawal of services if there is a lack of understanding by the service provider.

The provision of culturally and linguistically appropriate intervention for Aboriginal children remains challenging. Recruitment and retention of speech-language pathologists (SLPs) in rural and remote Australia is difficult, particularly in the very remote areas, which are home to some Aboriginal children. The remoteness means that services are available, if at all, on an occasional basis. Little information about speech and language acquisition in Aboriginal children is available to guide assessment and intervention. Partnerships with linguists are needed to support the provision of appropriate services in remote areas where children speak an indigenous language as the first language. Partnerships with indigenous people (health workers, interpreters and caregivers) are needed regardless of location. Such partnerships will not only assist the SLP in developing cultural understanding and facilitate communication, but also allow consideration of indigenous teaching strategies that may be beneficial in working with Aboriginal children (Lowell, 1995).

References

Australian Bureau of Statistics (2010) *Yearbook Australia, 2009–10.* http://www.abs.gov. au/AUSSTATS/abs@.nsf/Lookup/1301.0Feature+Article7012009%E2%80%9310.

Australian Human Rights Commission (2009) *2009 Social Justice Report.* Sydney: Author.

Australian Institute of Aboriginal and Torres Strait Islander Studies (2005) *National Indigenous Language Survey Report.* Canberra: Author.

Blake, B.J. (1987) *Australian Aboriginal Grammar.* London: Croom Helm.

Butcher, A. (2008) Linguistic aspects of Australian Aboriginal English. *Clinical Linguistics and Phonetics* 22 (8), 625–642.

Commonwealth of Australia (2007) *National Report to Parliament on Indigenous Education and Training.* Canberra: Author.

Couzos, S., Metcalf, S. and Murray, R. (2001) *Systematic Review of Existing Evidence and Primary Care Guidelines on the Management of Otitis Media in Aboriginal and Torres Strait Islander Populations.* Canberra: Commonwealth of Australia.

Eades, D. (1982) You gotta know how to talk ... Information seeking in south-east Queensland Aboriginal society. *Australian Journal of Linguistics* 2, 61–82.

Eades, D. (1996) Communicative strategies in Aboriginal English. In J. Maybin and N. Mercer (eds) *Using English from Conversation to Canon* (pp. 28–31). Oxon: Routledge.

Lowell, A. (1995) *Communication and Learning in an Aboriginal School: The Influence of Conductive Hearing Loss*. Batchelor: Batchelor College.

Malcolm, I., Haig, Y., Konigsberg, P., Rochecouste, J., Collard, G., Hill, A. and Cahill, R. (1999) *Two Way English. Towards More User-friendly Education for Speakers of Aboriginal English*. Perth, Australia: Education Department of Western Australia.

Moses, K. and Yallop, C. (2008) Questions about questions. In J. Simpson and G. Wigglesworth (eds) *Children's Language and Multilingualism. Indigenous Language Use at Home and at School* (pp. 30–55) London: Continuum International.

Sharifian, F. (2001) Schema-based processing in Australian speakers of Aboriginal English. *Language and Intercultural Communication* 1 (2), 120–134.

Sharifian, F., Rochecouste, J. and Malcolm, I.G. (2004) 'But it was all a bit confusing…': Comprehending Aboriginal English texts. *Language, Culture and Curriculum* 17 (3), 203–228.

Simpson, J. and Wigglesworth, G. (2008) Introduction. In J. Simpson and G. Wigglesworth (eds) *Children's Language and Multilingualism. Indigenous Language Use at Home and at School* (pp. 1–12). London: Continuum International.

Trudgen, R. (2000) *Why Warriors Lie Down and Die*. Parap: Aboriginal Resource and Development Services.

Wigglesworth, G. and Simpson, J. (2008) The language learning environment of preschool children in Indigenous communities. In J. Simpson and G. Wigglesworth (eds) *Children's Language and Multilingualism. Indigenous Language at Home and School* (pp. 13–29). London: Continuum International.

Williams, C.J., Coates, H.L., Pascoe, E.M., Axford, Y. and Nannup, I. (2009) Middle ear disease in Aboriginal children in Perth: Analysis of hearing screening data, 1998–2004. *Medical Journal of Australia* 190 (10), 598–600.

5 Vowels and Consonants of the World's Languages

Martin J. Ball

Languages mentioned: *Albanian, Arabic, Burmese, Cantonese, Chinese, Danish, Dutch, English (various accents), Ewe, Farsi, Finnish, French, German, Gujarati, Haida, Hawai'ian, Hebrew, Hindi, Hungarian, Icelandic, Inuit, Irish, Italian, Jalapa Mazatec, Japanese, Khmer, Korean, Latvian, Mandarin, Melpa, Norwegian, Pawaian, Polish, Portuguese, Rotokas, Russian, Scottish Gaelic, Sindhi, Spanish, Swedish, Tamil, Teke, Thai, Tlingit, Turkish, Vietnamese, Welsh, Xhosa, !Xū, Zulu*

Introduction

Speech-language pathologists (SLPs), whether working with monolingual or multilingual clients, are likely to hear a wide range of speech sounds from children with speech sound disorders. Indeed, they may encounter sounds not found in natural language at all. In this chapter, the range of consonants and vowels found in natural language will be explored, and different types of phonological systems described. In the following section, the number of consonants and vowels refers to the number of contrastive phonological units (i.e. phonemes) rather than the total number of perceptible different sounds (or phones). For this reason, slant brackets are generally employed for phonetic symbols and are to be understood as denoting the phonological units of the language and variety concerned. There are different ways of counting the phonemes of a language, thus not all researchers agree on the size and make-up of phonological systems. For example, the 18 vowels of General American pronunciation (GenAm) described in Ball and Müller (2005) could be expanded greatly if every vowel $+/ɹ/$ combination is deemed to be a separate r-colored vowel phoneme, and if the $/j/+/u/$ combination is counted as a diphthong. In later sections, when types of consonants and vowels are discussed, sounds are given in square brackets (following the sources of the information), and no claim is made about the contrastive nature of the sound unless otherwise specified. In the following discussion, segment length, tone and syllabic stress are not covered because they are deemed suprasegmental aspects of speech and are discussed in Peppé (Chapter 6).

Phonological Systems

The phonological systems of languages can be large (e.g. 141 units in !Xū) or small (e.g. 11 in Rotokas) (both described in Maddieson, 1984).

The consonant and vowel inventories can be fairly evenly balanced. For example, RP English (received pronunciation, or the standard variety in England) has 24 consonant phonemes and 20 vowel phonemes, whereas GenAm is reckoned to have 24 consonant and 18 vowel phonemes (Ball & Müller, 2005). On the other hand, systems can be unbalanced, e.g. Haida with 46 consonants and 3 vowels and Pawaian with 10 consonants but 12 vowels (though it is rare to find more vowels than consonants) (these examples from Maddieson, 1984).

Both consonant and vowel systems may be examined in terms of their internal make-up. Thus, most of the languages of India (both Indo-European and Dravidian) have a number of retroflex consonants (Maddieson, 1984); Polish has a large number of fricatives (9; Ladefoged & Maddieson, 1996), whereas Australian Aboriginal languages generally lack fricatives (Maddieson, 1984); languages such as English only have pulmonic egressive consonants, while Zulu has pulmonic egressive, glottalic egressive and ingressive (ejectives and implosives) and velaric ingressive (clicks) (Maddieson, 1984). In terms of vowels, we may find systems with monophthongs only (e.g. Turkish; Maddieson, 1984), and others with large numbers of diphthongs (e.g. northern Welsh with 13 contrastive diphthongs; Ball & Williams, 2001).

Research on phonological systems has led to the positing of phonological universals (Greenberg *et al.*, 1978). For example, if a language has voiced obstruents, it will also have voiceless ones (but not vice versa); if a language has front rounded vowels, it will also have front unrounded ones (but not vice versa); if a language has diphthongs, it will also have monophthongs (but not vice versa). Such universals allow us to determine which sounds and groups of sounds are marked and which are unmarked. Bowen (2010), among others, has discussed the implications of markedness in target selection in treating children with speech disorders.

Consonants

In this and the following section on vowels, the discussion will concentrate on sounds not found within English and will list their use in languages that may be encountered in speech clinics in multilingual clients or clients who speak little or no English. However, as noted in Ball *et al.* (2009), most of these non-English sounds may also be encountered in the disordered speech of clients whose target system is English.

Place of articulation

Several places of articulation used in natural language are absent from the English phonological system. Ball *et al.* (2009), however, illustrate the use of all the places described below in the disordered speech of clients with English as their target language.

Retroflex articulations involve the under surface of the tongue tip or blade articulating against the postalveolar or prepalatal region (Ball & Rahilly, 1999). While most English varieties do not use this place of articulation,[1] it is commonly encounteredin the languages of India and many speakers of English from India use the retroflex place of articulation instead of the alveolar (Wells, 1982). Examples of retroflex consonants in a variety of languages are as follows:

Plosives: Hindi टाल (postpone), [ʈal], डाल (branch) [ɖal];
Nasal: Tamil வண்டி (cart) [ʋaɳɖi];
Lateral: Tamil வாள் (sword) [ʋaɭ];
Flap: Hindi लरका (boy) [lərka];
Fricatives: Chinese 杀 *sha* (to kill) [ʂaɹ], 让 *rang* (to assist) [ʐaɳɣ].[2]
(All examples from Ball *et al.*, 2009.)

English does have one palatal consonant (the glide /j/). However, palatal plosives, fricatives, nasals and laterals occur in several languages commonly encountered by English-speaking SLPs. Examples of these sounds are as follows:

Plosives: Albanian *gyuha shqipe* (Albanian language) [ˈɟuha ˈʃcipɛ] (Zymberi, 2007);
Fricatives: German *ich* (I) [ɪç];[3] Latvian *ģimene* (family) [ɟimene] (Praulinš & Moseley, 2009);

Nasal: Spanish *mañana* (tomorrow) [maɲana];
Lateral: Italian *gli* (the + masculine plural nouns) [ʎi].

The uvular place of articulation is also not found in English. It can be used with plosives, fricatives, nasals and trills. Examples include:

Plosives: Arabic قهوه (coffee) [qahwa], Farsi غر (cave) [ɢar] (IPA, 1999);
Fricatives: Welsh *bach* (small) [bɑχ]; German *rot* (red) [ʁot] (although the trill may also be used);
Nasal: Inuit *saarnii* (his bones) [saːɴiː] (IPA, 1999);

Trill: French *rue* (road, street) [ʀy] (although the fricative may also be used).
Finally, it can be noted that the pharyngeal place of articulation is also absent from English. Pharyngeal fricatives are found in Arabic:
سعل (coughed) [saʕala]; حروب (wars) [ħuruwb] (Ball *et al.*, 2009).

Arabic also uses pharyngealization, where tongue root retraction is added to sounds made at other places of articulation. For example: ثن (figs) [tin] ~ طن (mud) [tˤin] (Ball *et al.*, 2009).

Manner of articulation

English uses six manners of articulation (or seven if one classifies glides and liquids separately rather than grouping them as approximants).

However, some of these manners are restricted as to the places of articulation they occur with. Some of the non-English manner–place combinations are examined here together with manners not utilized in English, and it should be noted that most of these combinations have been found in the English target speech of clients in the speech clinic (Ball *et al.*, 2009).

Plosives

Several plosives not found in English were dealt with in the previous subsection. Not covered were the glottal stop and the epiglottal plosive. Glottal stops occur regularly in several varieties of English, e.g. before vowels in vowel initial words (*ounce* [ʔaʊns]) and for intervocalic /t/ in accents in the southeast of England (*better* [bɛʔə]) (Wells, 1982). However, it is difficult to argue that the glottal stop is a contrastive sound of English (i.e. a phoneme). Nevertheless, the transcription of the glottal stop will be important clinically to distinguish between a deletion process and one of glottal replacement. Further, several languages use the glottal stop as a contrastive unit: Hawai'ian *ha'a* (dance) [haʔa] (Pukui & Elbert, 1992); Arabic ﺳﺎﻝ (asked) [saʔala] (Ball *et al.*, 2009). The epiglottal plosives are rarely reported, although Ladefoged and Maddieson (1996) report them in some languages of the Caucasus region and Africa, and note that they may be allophones of pharyngeal fricatives in Arabic and Hebrew.

Affricates

Affricates may be made at a wide range of places of articulation other than those found in English. A few examples will illustrate some of this range: German *pfeiffen* (to whistle) [p͡faɪfən]; Italian *zona* (zone) [d͡zona]; Hungarian *gyár* (factory) [ɟ͡ʝaːr]; and Tlingit *dlaa* (to settle) [d͡ɮaa] (all Ball & Rahilly, 1999).

Fricatives

Although English has fricatives at five places of articulation, several others are not employed. The retroflex, palatal and pharyngeal places have been dealt with above, but several others occur in commonly encountered languages. Considering the bilabial fricatives, Spanish has [β] as an allophone of /b/ in word medial and final positions (though the frication is not especially strong): *Habana* (place name) [ha'βana], while both [ɸ] and [β] occur in Ewe (a major language of Ghana and neighboring areas), e.g. *e fa* (he polished) [éɸá], *εvε* (Ewe) [εβέ] (Ladefoged & Maddieson, 1996).

Velar fricatives are encountered in some Scottish and Ulster-Scots varieties of English (*loch/lough* (lake) [lɔx]), but otherwise prove difficult for English speakers to produce and perceive. Examples of these sounds in commonly encountered languages include: Spanish: *agua* (water) [aɣwa] (although the frication here may be minimal); Russian: *хоккей* (hockey) [xokej]; and Polish: *suchy* (dry) [suxi] (Ball *et al.*, 2009).

Lateral fricatives made at the alveolar place of articulation are commonly encountered realizations of target /s, z/ in children with so-called lateral lisps. However, they also occur as contrastive units in many languages. Examples include Welsh: *llall* (other) [ɬaɬ] and Zulu: *isihlahla* (tree) [isiɬaɬa], *dla* (to eat) [ɮa] (Dent & Nyembezi, 1988).

Nasals

The labiodental nasal [ɱ] is an allophone of English /m/ in words such as *triumph* and *comfy*, and of /n/ in words such as *invent* and *infuse* (see Ball & Müller, 2005), i.e. when preceding a labiodental fricative. This sound occurs as an allophone in many other languages in just such contexts. It is not known as occurring as an independent phoneme (except in the language Teke, which contrasts /m/ and /ɱ/; Maddieson, 1984).

Approximants

English has only one contrastive lateral consonant – the alveolar – albeit with clear and dark allophones. Laterals at the retroflex and palatal positions have already been described, leaving the velar lateral. This can occur in some southern US accents for a dark-l: Texas English *school* [skuʟ]. Ladefoged (2005) describes velar laterals in Melpa, a language of New Guinea, one of the few that has these sounds as phonemes.

There are several central approximants in natural language other than those found in English. The labiodental approximant (often found in error as a realization of target English /ɹ/) is found, for example, in Hindi (although a bilabial variant may also be used): नवाँ (ninth) [nʊʋɑ̃] or [nɔβɑ̃] (Ladefoged & Maddieson, 1996). The labiopalatal glide is found in French: *huit* (eight) [ɥit], and the velar glide in Korean, among others, e.g. Korean 의사 (doctor) [ɰiza] (adapted from the International Phonetic Association (IPA), 1999). Both these sounds have been recorded as being used in disordered speech for target English sounds (see Ball *et al.*, 2009).

Trills and taps

Whereas some varieties of English use these sounds (e.g. both trilled and tapped-r in Scottish English, and the intervocalic flapping of /t/ in north American and Australian English, see Wells, 1982), phonemically contrastive trills and taps are usually considered lacking from standard varieties other than Scottish. However, these sounds are common in many frequently encountered languages. For example, Spanish contrasts a trilled and tapped apical-r: *perro* (dog) [pɛro], *pero* (but) [pɛro] (Ball *et al.*, 2009); and as noted earlier, French and German may use a uvular trill realization for their rhotic. The bilabial trill is rare, however, in natural language, as are labiodental flaps. The retroflex flap was dealt with above.

Voiceless trills may occur contrastively in some languages. For example, Welsh contrasts a voiced apical trill with its voiceless equivalent: *riwl* (measuring ruler) [rɪul], *rhuwl* (order, grouping) [r̥ɪul].

Phonation

Voiceless sonorants

English has voiceless and voiced obstruents, but lacks voiceless sonorant consonants except as allophonic variants of the voiced ones (Ball & Müller, 2005 e.g. approximants in clusters with voiceless obstruents, /sm-, sn-, pɹ-, kl-, tw-, pj-/). However, voiceless nasals and voiceless approximants may occur contrastively with voiced equivalents in some languages.

For example, voiceless nasals occur in Burmese contrasting with voiced ones: ၃ (nose) [n̥á] with ၃ (pain) [ná]; Burmese also contrasts voiced and voiceless lateral approximants (Ladefoged & Maddieson, 1996). Icelandic voiceless lateral can be seen in *sæll* (a greeting) ['sait̥l̥] (personal communication, Sveinn Haraldsson, 4 May 2010). Some varieties of English (including Scottish and Irish) still contrast a voiced and a voiceless labiovelar approximant, e.g. *witch* ~ *which* /wɪtʃ/ ~ /ʍɪtʃ/ (Wells, 1982).

Aspiration

English fortis plosives are usually pronounced with a relatively long lag in the voice onset time, resulting in audible aspiration. This is especially so when in initial position in a stressed syllable (except when following /s/), and less so in other positions. Following /s/, they are unaspirated (Ball & Müller, 2005). In other languages (e.g. French, Spanish, Italian, Dutch) fortis plosives are always unaspirated (Harris & Vincent, 1988; IPA, 1999). In languages such as German, Turkish, Thai, Welsh and Irish, fortis plosives are generally aspirated (Petrova *et al.*, 2006). Icelandic is one of the languages that exhibits preaspiration, in that a period of voicelessness precedes the closure for the fortis stop: *löpp* (foot) [lœʰp] (personal communication, Sveinn Haraldsson, 4 May 2010).

It is possible to find aspiration not only with fortis, but also with lenis stops (although phonetically, aspiration with voiced plosives involves the use of murmur phonation during the voice onset lag). Hindi has four contrastive plosives (voiceless and voiced aspirated and unaspirated) at four places of articulation (bilabial, dental, retroflex and velar): पाल (nurture) [pal], फाल (hair) [pʰal], बाल (knife blade) [bal] and भाल (brow) [bʱal] (IPA, 1999).

Non-pulmonic airstreams

Ball and Müller (2007) describe the full range of non-pulmonic egressive airstreams and note that virtually all of these are recorded in the literature as occurring in disordered speech of clients whose target language is English. Here, however, there is space to simply exemplify the commonest non-pulmonic consonants in languages that have them as contrastive units. Implosives are found in a wide range of languages, including the languages of sub-Saharan Africa, some south American languages, many languages in

South East Asia and Sindhi, spoken in Pakistan and northern India (Ball & Rahilly, 1999). Ejectives are found in many indigenous languages in both North and South America, and languages in the Caucasus and in Africa (Ball & Rahilly, 1999). Clicks are mainly restricted to southern Africa and are found in the Khoi-San languages and some Bantu languages (Ball & Rahilly, 1999).

All three types of non-pulmonic consonants can be illustrated in Xhosa, which has several clicks as well as a bilabial implosive and several ejectives. Examples include *uxolo* (excuse me) [uk‖ɔlɔ]; *nceda* (please) [ŋ|ɛda]; and *ukubona* (to see) [uk'uɓɔna] (Doke, 1954).

Vowels

As noted earlier in the chapter, English has a comparatively large vowel system in terms of both monophthongs and diphthongs. However, there are several vowel types not found, which will be illustrated in this section.

Front rounded vowels

Front rounded vowels have been described in the literature as occurring in the disordered speech of English target clients (Ball et al., 2010). French has front rounded vowels, e.g. *tu* (you, singular) [ty], *peu* (a little) [pø] and *peur* (fear) [pœʁ]. German also: *Rübe* (turnip) [ʀybə], *Müller* (miller) [mʏlɐ], *Röhre* (pipe) [ʀøʀə] and *können* (be able to) [kœnən] (all these examples from Ball et al., 2010). Other commonly encountered languages that have at least some front rounded vowels include Dutch, Swedish, Danish, Norwegian, Finnish, Hungarian, Turkish, Korean and Chinese (IPA, 1949, 1999).

Back unrounded vowels

Ball et al. (2010) also report on back unrounded vowels occurring in the disordered speech data of clients whose target language is English, but they may also be found in commonly encountered languages. Vietnamese, Turkish, Thai, Korean, Japanese and Chinese have all been described as having at least one back unrounded vowel (IPA, 1949, 1999), and Vietnamese has three: *từ* (forth) [tɯ], *tơ* (silk) [tɤ] and *âng* (favour) [ʌŋ] (Nguyễn, 1987).

Central vowels

High central vowels are quite common in natural language, with opener ones less so. For example, Russian *высь* (height) [vɨsʲ] and Welsh *tŷ* (house) [tɨː] have the unrounded close central vowel (Ball et al., 2010), and the rounded one is found, for example, in Norwegian: *butt* 'blunt' [bʉt] (Haugen, 1987). Swedish has *full* (full) [fɵl] (Haugen, 1987), and other central vowels have been used in regional varieties of English: New Zealand English *comma* [kɒmə] (Bauer *et al.*, 2007) and south Walian English *shirt* [ʃɐt] (Ball *et al.*, 2010). The low central vowel [ɐ] has been described in Khmer (Jacob, 1968), Cantonese and Portuguese (IPA, 1999), and it was seen above in the German example *Müller* (miller) [mʏlɐ].

Diphthongs

Diphthongs can occur with a closing movement of the tongue in the vowel area, an opening one or centering; they may be rising (most emphasis on the final part) or falling (most emphasis on the initial part) (Ball & Rahilly, 1999). Also, triphthongs may occur if the tongue glides through an intermediate position within the timing slot for a single syllable. As noted in Ball *et al.* (2010), non-English diphthongs can be found where neither the start nor the end position (and lip shape) coincide with an English vowel, and where one or both of these positions (and lip shape) do coincide with English sounds but English does not use that diphthong. Examples of both of these can be found below (and in the disordered speech of clients with English as their target, as illustrated in Ball *et al.*, 2010).

Diphthongs in Scottish Gaelic include [ei], [əi], [ai], [ui], [iə], [uə], [ɛu], [ɔu], [au] and [ia] (Gillies, 2009); in Mandarin [ɤu], [iɤu], [iɛ], [yɛ], [ia], [ua] and [uai] (Li & Thompson, 1987); and in Vietnamese [iɜ], [uɜi], [iu], [eu], [ɛu], [iɜu] and [iɜu] (Nguyễn, 1987).

Nasalized vowels

In the context of a following nasal stop, English vowels are somewhat nasalized, but the language lacks phonemically contrastive nasalized vowels (Ball & Müller, 2005). However, a variety of speech clinic clientele use fully nasalized realizations of vowels (Ball *et al.*, 2010), as will speakers of languages where contrastive nasalized vowels are found. These include French *un* (a, one, masculine) [œ̃], *bon* (good, masculine) [bɔ̃]; Portuguese *cão* (dog) [kãũ]; and Hindi में (in) [mẽ] (IPA, 1999).

Phonation and vowels

Vowels are generally voiced, but Ladefoged and Maddieson (1996) note that in some languages they can be pronounced with creak or murmur, or even be voiceless. Some varieties of French use a voiceless pronunciation of word final high vowels: *oui* (yes) [wi̥], while Gujarati contrasts voiced and murmured vowels, and the Central American language Jalapa Mazatec contrasts voiced, murmured and creaky vowels (all Ladefoged & Maddieson, 1996).

Sounds Unattested in Natural Language

The clinician may be faced with a client with a speech sound disorder who uses sounds that are not found in natural language. Such sounds may be consonants using novel places of articulation (e.g. dentolabial, bidental, linguolabial,[4] labioalveolar, velopharyngeal) or novel manners of articulation (e.g. percussives, simultaneous medial and lateral fricatives, nareal fricatives.[5]) These unattested sounds are transcribed via the Extensions to the International Phonetic Alphabet (extIPA: see Ball & Müller, 2005, and appendix), and examples of their use with clinical speech data are given in Rutter *et al.* (2010).

For example, audible nasal escape is described in Howard (1993: 307–308). She gives the following examples from a 6-year-old girl with a repaired cleft palate, who used palatal fricatives accompanied by audible nasal escape: *nose* [ɴəʊɕ̃], *sugar* [ˈɕʊʔə] and *sock* [ɕ̃ɒʔʰ].

Conclusion

A child with speech sound disorder may realize a target sound with the wrong allophone of the phoneme concerned, with a sound that belongs to a different phoneme of the target language variety or with a sound from outside the target system altogether. Clients who are bi- or multilingual may use sounds from any of their language systems, or from none, for a particular target. Finally, clients may use sounds not recorded in any natural language. For all these reasons, clinicians need to be aware of the full range of consonant and vowel systems found in the languages of the world, and at least some of the commonly encountered sounds unattested in natural language.

Notes

(1) Although /ɹ/ for some English varieties (e.g. northern Irish) can be retroflex, causing the following /z/ to be retroflex also in plurals of /ɹ/ final words, e.g. *speakers* /spikɚz/ [spikəɻz].
(2) These two transcriptions contain tone marks: [˥] high level tone; [˥˩] high falling tone.
(3) Generally, examples from German, French, Spanish, Italian, Welsh and English are part of the author's own linguistic knowledge and therefore not further referenced.
(4) Although this place is found in a very few natural languages see Ball & Müller, (2005).
(5) Also termed audible nasal escape.

References

Ball, M.J. and Müller, N. (2005) *Phonetics for Speech Pathology*. Mahwah, NJ: Lawrence Erlbaum.
Ball, M.J. and Müller, N. (2007) Non-pulmonic egressive speech sounds in disordered speech: A brief review. *Clinical Linguistics and Phonetics* 21, 869–874.
Ball, M.J. and Rahilly, J. (1999) *Phonetics. The Science of Speech*. London: Arnold.
Ball, M.J. and Williams, B. (2001) *Welsh Phonetics*. Lewistown, NY: Edwin Mellen Press.

Ball, M.J., Müller, N., Rutter, B. and Klopfenstein, M. (2009) My client's using non-English sounds! A tutorial in advanced phonetic transcription. Part I: Consonants. *Contemporary Issues in Communication Sciences and Disorders* 36, 133–141.

Ball, M.J., Müller, N., Klopfenstein, M. and Rutter, B. (2010) My client's using non-English sounds! A tutorial in advanced phonetic transcription. Part II: Vowels and diacritics. *Contemporary Issues in Communication Sciences and Disorders* 37, 103–110.

Bauer, L., Warren, P., Bardsley, D., Kennedy, M. and Major, G. (2007) New Zealand English. *Journal of the International Phonetic Association* 37, 97–102.

Bowen, C. (2009) *Children's Speech Sound Disorders*. Hoboken, NJ: Wiley.

Dent, G. and Nyembezi, C. (1988) *Scholar's Zulu Dictionary*. Pietermaritzburg: Shuter and Shooter.

Doke, C.M. (1954) *The Southern Bantu Languages*. London: Oxford University Press, for the International African Institute.

Gillies, W. (2009) Scottish Gaelic. In M.J. Ball and N. Müller (eds) *The Celtic Languages*. (2nd edn; pp. 230–304). London: Routledge.

Greenberg, J., Ferguson, C. and Movarvcsik, E. (eds) (1978) *Universals of Human Language. Volume 2, Phonology*. Stanford, CA: Stanford University Press.

Harris, M. and Vincent, N. (1988) (eds) *The Romance Languages*. London: Routledge.

Haugen, E. (1987) Danish, Norwegian and Swedish. In B. Comrie (ed.) *The World's Major Languages* (pp. 157–179). London: Croom Helm.

Howard, S. (1993) Articulatory constraints on a phonological system: A case study of cleft palate speech. *Clinical Linguistics and Phonetics* 7, 299–317.

International Phonetic Association (1949) *The Principles of the International Phonetic Alphabet*. London: The International Phonetic Association.

International Phonetic Association (1999) *Handbook of the International Phonetic Association*. Cambridge: Cambridge University Press.

Jacob, J. (1968) *Introduction to Cambodian*. Oxford: Oxford University Press.

Ladefoged, P. (2005) *Vowels and Consonants*. Oxford: Blackwell.

Ladefoged, P. and Maddieson, I. (1996) *The Sounds of the World's Languages*. Oxford: Blackwell.

Li, C. and Thompson, S. (1987) Chinese. In B. Comrie (ed.) *The World's Major Languages* (pp. 811–833). London: Croom Helm.

Maddieson, I. (1984) *Patterns of Sounds*. Cambridge: Cambridge University Press.

Nguyễn, D.-H. (1987) Vietnamese. In B. Comrie (ed.) *The World's Major Languages* (pp. 777–796). London: Croom Helm.

Petrova, O., Plapp, R., Ringen, C. and Szentgyörgyi, S. (2006) Voice and aspiration: Evidence from Russian, Hungarian, German, Swedish, and Turkish. *The Linguistic Review* 23, 1–35.

Praulinš, D. and Moseley, C. (2009) *Colloquial Latvian* (2nd edn). London: Routledge.

Pukui, M.K. and Elbert, S.H. (1992) *New Pocket Hawaiian Dictionary*. Honolulu, HI: University of Hawaii Press.

Rutter, B., Klopfenstein, M., Ball, M.J. and Müller, N. (2010) My client's using non-English sounds! A tutorial in advanced phonetic transcription. Part III: Prosody and unattested sounds. *Contemporary Issues in Communication Sciences and Disorders* 37, 111–122.

Wells, J.C. (1982) *Accents of English* (3 vols). Cambridge: Cambridge University Press.

Zymberi, I. (2007) *Colloquial Albanian* (2nd edn). London: Routledge.

6 Prosody in the World's Languages

Sue Peppé

Languages mentioned: *Arabic, Athabaskan languages, Australian Indigenous languages, Austronesian languages, Bini, Burmese, Cantonese, Dutch, English, Finnish, French, Fulani, Gilbertese, Hawai'ian, Hebrew, Hindi, Hungarian, Icelandic, Italian, Japanese, Khmer, Korean, Lahanda, Lao, Latvian, Limburg, Lithuanian, Lugandan, Malay, Maltese, Mandarin, Mayan languages, Mongolian, Navajo, Norwegian, Oto-Manguean, Polish, Portuguese, Punjabi, Putonghua, Rabinian, Romanian, Russian, Serbo-Croatian, Shanghainese, Slovene, Spanish, Swahili, Swedish, Thai, Turkish, Vietnamese, Western Pahari, Wolof, Yucatec*

Introduction: Scope of the Topic

In considering speech sound disorders in children who are multilingual to some degree in a number of different countries, some of the disorders may originate in, or be affected by, the prosodic characteristics of a language that is in the child's repertoire (or frequently used in the child's home). Competence in more than one language may of course be complete: in such cases, cross-language interference is unlikely to be apparent. Incomplete competence, where one language is more familiar or dominant than the other, is the topic here, considering the dominant language as the first language (L1) and the transference of prosodic characteristics from the L1 to the second language (L2). This chapter will aim to give some indications of the effects of L1 prosodic transference: the relevance of crosslinguistic prosodic differences to various types of bilingualism, and how the effects of transference can impact on speech sound disorders in bilingual children. Such effects may range from observable differences that barely affect comprehension, to complete misunderstanding; the concern here will be with misunderstanding or lack of intelligibility.

Space will limit the scope: first, research into crosslinguistic prosodic variation is sparse, and research into the effect of L1/L2 interference on the prosody of bi- and multilinguals is scarcer. Second, to consider enough languages adequately, several books would be necessary rather than one chapter; for further information about prosodic variation, the reader can consult e.g. Fox (2000), Hirst and di Cristo (1998), Jun (2006), Ladd (1996) and McLeod (2007). Third, space will also preclude any treatment of vocal quality, and the effects of variation in the way voice is used across languages. Fourth, articulatory settings (e.g. raised or lowered larynx or labial protrusion) can be language specific and can affect the quality of vowels and consonants, but these too are beyond the scope of the chapter. Similarly, it will not be possible to discuss the effect of cultural differences realised through the use of prosody.

Table 6.1 indicates how languages considered in this volume can be described in terms of the prosodic categories considered here. Generalisations about prosody, however, do not necessarily apply across all varieties of a language. (Varieties and dialects, whether regionally, ethnically or sociologically determined, are also often known as 'accents', but that term will be reserved for describing accented syllables to avoid confusion.) Some prosodic realisations, like segmental ones, can apply across languages, but diverge within them according to variety or dialect; for example, the intonation of English statements (in unmarked situations) is falling for some varieties, such as southern British and older populations, but rising for others, such as Australian and younger populations.

Terminology

The term *prosody* will be used to designate the whole field of intonation and suprasegmental phonology. This will cover the ways in which pitch, loudness and length interact to affect the linguistic meaning of words and sentences, and to some extent their paralinguistic meaning, i.e. their affective impact.

It is important to distinguish between the forms of prosody and their communicative function, because the relationship is not one-to-one. There is a great temptation to assume that the exponents of the forms of prosody are similar to those of one's native language; for example, stress may be realised by higher pitch in one language and lower pitch in another. This chapter will give some indications where such assumptions are made. The basic elements of prosody – the pitch of spoken syllables, their duration (or length) and their perceived loudness – combine into clusters that may be considered as the forms of prosody, such as stress, accent and tone; the exponency of these forms, i.e. the combinations of elements that they comprise, vary across languages (see 'Aspects of prominence' for examples). There are also different aspects of pitch to consider, e.g. *tone* (on-syllable pitch change, see 'Tone and tone languages'); *syllable-initial pitch*, or the pitch at which a syllable begins; and *pitch span*, or the extent of frequencies included in syllables or utterances. Such subdivisions of pitch have their own effects on communication and it is helpful to think of them individually. Prosodic elements and forms are, however, typically multifunctional. Following Crystal (1969), we can say that they operate within different systems for different communication functions. In English, for instance, relatively high syllable-initial pitch can indicate the start of a new phrase as well as the onset of a stressed syllable, whereas in Chinese, high

Table 6.1 Crosslinguistic prosodic variation

Language	Vowel reduction in unstressed syllables	Word stress: position (fixed) or free (variable)	Rhythm: syllable or stress timed	Accent: dynamic/ melodic	Lexis: conveyed by tone	Questions: rise/fall
English	Yes*; not north UK, African	Free	Stress	Dynamic	No	Rise
Dutch	Yes	Free	Stress	Dynamic	Some Limburg words	Rise
Icelandic	Yes	First	Stress	Dynamic	No	Rise
Swedish, Norwegian	Yes	Free	Stress	Dynamic	Some words	Rise
French	No	Free	Syllable	Dynamic	No	Rise
Portuguese	No	Free	Syllable	Dynamic	No	Rise
Spanish	No	Free	Syllable	Dynamic	No	Rise
Italian	No	Free	Syllable	Dynamic	No	Rise
Finnish	No	First	Syllable	Dynamic	No	Rise
Hungarian	Some	First	Unclear	Dynamic	No	Fall
Hebrew	Yes	Last	Stress	Dynamic	No	Rise
Turkish	No	Free	Syllable	Dynamic	No	Rise
Maltese	Yes	Free	Stress	Dynamic	No	Rise
Chinese Putonghua	Some	Free	Stress	Dynamic	Mainly	Rise
Chinese Cantonese	Some	Free	Syllable	Dynamic	Mainly	Rise
Korean	No	Free	Unclear	Melodic	No	Rise
Japanese	No	Free	Moraic	Melodic	No	Rise

*Yes = feature present; no = feature absent.

syllable-initial pitch would indicate a particular lexical tone, but not the start of a new phrase or topic. The communicative functions conveyed by these elements and forms, and the way they vary across languages, will be explored further below.

Crosslinguistic Prosodic Differences

Cross-language variation in prosodic forms gives languages their characteristic sound: they function as part of a language's identity. Such differences may be unfamiliar and cause, at least initially, a mild processing delay to the hearer. They may also cause some confusion as to the meaning of utterances, but again this is likely to be transient and to last only while the hearer tunes in (if the speaker's prosody remains consistent). From a clinical point of view, the difference is important when it affects intelligibility and accuracy of communication, or when it is assumed to indicate an individual pathology when it would be more appropriate to consider that it is characteristic of another language. Singled out for attention here are manifestations of stress, accent and speech rhythm. The actual effect of interference from L1 prosodic characteristics on L2 realisations in bilinguals, especially in bilinguals with speech sound disorders, has been little researched; some unsupported tentative suggestions for likely effects are made here.

Aspects of prominence

Stress and accent

The term *stress* will be used here to mean the relative prominence assigned to certain syllables in a word, and the term *accent* to mean prominence at phrase or sentence level; the difference between these in terms of exponency (see, e.g. Beckman, 1986; Ladd, 1996: 155ff; Sluijter & van Heuven, 1996) will not be discussed here. Some languages have fixed stress, in that stress is placed always on a given syllable in a word, although this rule may well be contravened in loanwords. In Icelandic, Czech, Finnish and Hungarian, for example, stress is on the first syllable; in Hebrew and Moroccan Arabic on the last; in Polish, Swahili and many Austronesian languages on the penultimate; and in Greek on the antepenultimate (Goedemans & van der Hulst, 2005). Most languages, including Germanic and Romance languages, Maltese and Turkish, have free or variable stress placement, but L1 languages with fixed stress may be likely to cause prosody transference problems, because the L1 fixed stress pattern could transfer to an L2 with free stress or fixed stress on a different syllable. French has no word stress, but has accent on the final or penultimate syllable of a phrase, which can give rise to unusual stress placement in L2.

Other aspects of crosslinguistic prosodic variation can cause misperception of stress or accent, the phonetic-prosodic exponency of which can vary across languages. In *dynamic accent* languages, such as English, accent or stress on a syllable is manifested by boosted pitch, additional length and extra loudness. In Japanese, accent is realised only by pitch variation, not by variations of intensity or duration; Japanese is therefore designated a *melodic accent language*. In Welsh, stress occurs on syllables that are lower, shorter and less intense than others (Williams, 1985), and this realisation is often carried over into the Welsh varieties of English. To exemplify this, take the English utterance *I saw her parrot on the lawn.* The syllables *saw*, *pa-* and *lawn* are stressed or accented, here represented by capitals: *i SAW her PArrot on the LAWN.* Thus, in Welsh English, the unstressed syllables (*I, her, -rrot, on* and *the*) will be higher in pitch than the accented syllables; if spoken by a child with speech sound disorders and Welsh influence, a hearer with a language in which stress is realised differently (such as Japanese or English) might perceive such syllables as accented when they are not intended to be. Pitch alignment within syllables is another factor that can vary between languages: this can obscure the relative pitch of two adjacent syllables, which may also lead to confusion about where stress or accent occurs.

Vowel reduction

In some languages, vowel quality can be reduced or centralised in the unaccented syllables of a word. Although this variation is, properly speaking, segmental, it is included here because the presence or absence of reduction interacts with prosodic perception. For example, in *I saw her parrot on the lawn*, the above example, *-rrot* is pronounced /ɹət/. If it is pronounced [-ɹɒt], especially where speech sound disorders or L1 realisations of segments suggest words, the full vowel quality will imply that the syllable has potential for carrying stress, and a listener may therefore attempt to parse the word as *parROT*. In this case, no obvious lexical entity other than *parrot* is indicated by the word [pæɹɒt], and in many cases, context will similarly override both segmental and suprasegmental indications, but lack of reduction where it is expected is likely to cause at least a delay in the hearer's interpretation.

Vowel reduction occurs in many languages: Russian, French, German and varieties of English, including southern British, American and Australian. Different languages have different types of reduction, but it is less apparent in Finnish, Hindi, classical Spanish, urban north British and varieties of African-influenced English.

Speech rhythm

There are various ways of considering the speech rhythms of languages, of which the notions of *stress timing* and *syllable timing* are perhaps most useful, although the distinctions are not borne out by acoustic measurement. A few languages, such as Japanese (also Lugandan, Gilbertese and Hawai'ian), are *mora timed*, a mora being defined in terms of rhythm (Abe, 1998). Mora timing resembles syllable timing in that morae are spoken at a roughly constant rate. In stress-timed languages, accented syllables are perceived to occur at roughly regular intervals, interspersed with unaccented ones. In the stress-timed example, *I saw her parrot on the lawn*, unaccented *-rrot on the* is perceived as being uttered in more or less the same amount of time as unaccented *her*. Syllable-timed languages include Hindi, Finnish and Romance languages in general (e.g. French, Spanish, Italian and Romanian), and do not generally include vowel reduction. Stress-timed languages include English, Russian, Arabic and all Germanic languages; tone languages in general also show weak-strong alternation. African-influenced English, however, has some tendency towards syllable timing, and some syllable-timed languages, such as Spanish, show stress timing in some situations and not in others (Alcobar & Murillo, 1998). Speech rhythm in Korean is also a matter of controversy (Jun, 2005). In short, categorisation is not strict, and although speech rhythm is frequently a characteristic feature of a language, it is hard to generalise about the effect of transference of speech rhythm in multilinguals.

Intonation

In general, utterances that are unmarked for particular affective or pragmatic effect usually exhibit *downdrift* or *declination*, that is, each stressed syllable is lower in pitch than the last. This is so frequently a feature in the world's languages that it has been called a prosodic universal.

For the most part, however, intonation varies across languages, and much of the literature on the prosody of the world's languages is devoted to their characteristic intonation, also known as tunes, contours or melodies. For example, Swedish and Norwegian may be perceived as comparatively singsong, perhaps due to the presence of some high unstressed syllables; pitch span is typically larger in British English than in Dutch ('t Hart, 1998). Little space will be devoted here to the features of characteristic intonation for two reasons: first, it requires much description, and second, when such intonation is carried over from L1 to L2, it is not often a major source of misunderstanding or lack of intelligibility, although variation may occasion strong opinions in different cultures as to acceptability. An example of the latter is the furore caused by the *uptalk* (ending a statement with a rise) when it spread around English-speaking countries (see e.g. Ladd, 1996). Moreover, it is fairly rare for tunes to be transferred from L1 to L2 without some L1 segmental characteristics being transferred with it. The combination of the two will usually trigger an assumption by the hearer that the speaker is from another language community; the hearer's consequent adjustments may well include some caution with regard to the functions of the speaker's intonation.

Tone and tone languages

One of the major prosodic differences between languages is the use or non-use of *tone* for lexical distinction. Tone is a term generally used to denote changes of pitch within a syllable: tone can be simple (either rising or falling direction), complex (changing direction within the syllable) or level (unchanging pitch). On-syllable pitch change occurs in all languages, with various uses; in tone languages, the direction of the pitch change (*tone direction*) decides the meaning of a syllable. Tone direction can be fall or rise (simple tones), fall-rise, rise-fall, rise-fall-rise, etc. (complex tones). The meanings designated by tone direction generally apply to lexical distinctions, but in some cases can signal grammatical differences. In the West African (Niger Congo) language Bini, a low tone indicates present tense and high or high-low tones mark past tense (Crystal, 1987).

Estimates of the percentage of tonal languages in the world vary between 40% (Maddieson, 2008) and 60–70% (Yip, 2002). In Europe, there are some simple tone systems, consisting of tonal distinctions for some words: in Norwegian, Swedish and some dialects of Limburg. Heading east, this is also the case for Latvian, Lithuanian, Serbo-Croatian and some dialects of Slovene, whereas Russian, Arabic, Turkish and Semitic languages, including Hebrew, are not tonal. Tone languages are prevalent in sub-Saharan Africa, apart from Swahili, Wolof and Fulani. In the Indian subcontinent, Punjabi, Lahanda, Rabinian and Western Pahari are tonal. Tone languages are numerous in East Asia, including Vietnamese, Thai, Lao and all the Chinese languages, although Shanghainese is only marginally tonal. Some languages in this region, such as Burmese, Korean and Japanese, have simpler tone systems, and some (e.g. Mongolian, Khmer and Malay) are not tonal at all. Australian Indigenous languages and most Austronesian languages are non-tonal. Some of the native languages of North and South America are tonal: they include many of the Athabaskan languages of Alaska and the American Southwest (including Navajo), and the Oto-Manguean languages of Mexico. Mayan languages (in Mexico and Central America) are mostly non-tonal, but there is a simple tone system in Yucatec (the most commonly spoken language in Mexico).

It is notable that children with a tone language as L1 appear to acquire lexical tone distinctions very early in their prosodic development, at least in Cantonese (To *et al.*, 2010) and in Mandarin, well in advance of their mastery of segmental phonemes (Li & Thomson, 1977). This appears also to be the case for Norwegian children (Peppé *et al.*, 2010).

Functions of tone and intonation

Non-tonal languages are often categorised as *intonation* languages, suggesting that intonation (here implying utterance-global pitch features as opposed to pitch change on single syllables) is not used in tone languages. This is somewhat misleading, as both tone and intonation have their uses in both types of languages, but with different functions.

In intonation languages, tone, in the sense of on-syllable pitch change, is most apparent on accented syllables; it does not distinguish lexical meaning, but has other (supra- or post-lexical) functions. It can indicate the imminence of the boundary of a chunk of speech (demarcation function), which may or may not be coterminous with a grammatical structure. In the British school of intonation, the term *nuclear tone*, applied to the nucleus of an utterance, indicates its importance for the sense of completeness; it generally occurs at or near the end of a chunk of speech (which may be a word, a phrase or a complete topic). The occurrence of such a tone can also signal the focal point of an utterance and the end of a conversational turn. Tone is not used in this way in tone languages, although speakers from intonation language backgrounds may fancy they perceive nuclearity. In bilingual tone/non-tone speakers, this may result in misunderstandings involving turn change and the focus of utterances. For purposes of contrastive stress, nuclear tone can be placed prefinally, with subsequent syllables deaccented. In such cases, nuclear tone does not signal phrase-end: this may result in confusion about the focus of utterances. Prefinal accenting occurs readily in Germanic but less so in Romance languages. Accent-placement, its functions and realisation, is the subject of much research (see, e.g. Ladd, 1996; Swerts, 2007).

In intonation languages, tone can, alone, indicate whether an utterance is a question or a statement (illocution function): questions that are independent of grammatical question structure are generally realised with rising pitch, which may be located on a single syllable. This, like declination, is near-universal; an exception is Hungarian (see Ladd, 1996), which has falling intonation for questions: this might be problematic in, e.g. German-Hungarian bilinguals. The converse is not, however, true: statements are not universally uttered with a fall, as indicated in the earlier mention of uptalk. People new to uptalk were allegedly mystified as to whether it expressed a question or not, but this mystification may have owed more to cultural aversion to new usage than to linguistic misunderstanding. In tone languages, and in varieties of English with uptalk, the question/statement distinction is expressed using utterance-level intonation, overall pitch being higher in questions. However, the intonational use of tone can take precedence over lexical use. For example, Ma *et al.* (2006) show that the tone of a final syllable in Cantonese may be changed from its canonical form to a rise in a question.

Tone direction can also indicate the attitude of the speaker (affect function). In English, for example, a rise-fall tone can express enthusiasm or irony and a fall-rise tone can express reservation. The attitudes expressed by such tones can vary from language to language; for example, the fall-rise is not used to express reservation in Spanish (Martínez-Castilla & Peppé, 2008). Vietnamese (Dung *et al.*, 1998) has a system of morphosyntactic markers to express emotions and moods, so intonation has a lesser role; what is often conveyed by intonation in another language is already marked in Vietnamese.

Both tonal and non-tonal languages employ global aspects of intonation, such as the overall pitch of an utterance (high or low) and the pitch range (wide or narrow), not to mention voice quality (resonance, huskiness, etc.) to convey affect. There are too many variations to explore here, but it is true of most languages that the wider the pitch span, the greater the emotional involvement of the speaker.

The implications of these functions of tone and intonation for speakers bilingual between tone and non-tone languages is that there is less potential for misunderstanding than might be expected when the L1 is a tone language, since the practice of conveying post-lexical functions by intonation is common to both types of language. There may, however, be much more difficulty when the L1 is a non-tonal language, since assigning overlapping pitch cues to different linguistic functions in a tonal L2, both in perception and production, requires sophisticated appreciation of pitch distinctions.

Conclusion

In summary, stress patterns, accentuation, speech rhythms and intonation are likely to be transferred from L1 to L2, resulting in some flavour of L1 prosody in the L2; this may also cause some misunderstandings about word meaning, emphasis, turn exchange, demarcation and speaker attitude. In this brief discussion, the focus has been on production, and how L1 prosodic forms and functions can be transferred to the L2. In addition, it needs to be borne in mind that perception of L2 prosody is influenced by native forms, and that this can lead to an emphasising simply of what is perceived to be foreign. For assessment of reception and production of prosody skills, the PEPS-C test (Peppé & McCann, 2003) is available in five regional varieties of English and four other languages: French, Spanish, Flemish and Norwegian (Peppé *et al.*, 2010); the Norwegian version includes tasks to assess lexical tone distinctions.

Finally, it should be remembered that two contradictory influences are at work in the effect on communication of prosody transference in multilinguals. To some extent, listeners are aware of the possibility of prosody transference and discount its effects, allowing factors such as context and facial expression to outweigh their impact, which thus contributes little to misunderstanding or lack of intelligibility. On the other hand, the same people can be ignorant of other prosodic effects and of how much they are influenced by them, e.g. the ways in which it is (wrongly) assumed that prosody operates similarly in all languages, as detailed above. Both factors constitute a reason for increasing awareness of how communication is influenced by prosody.

Acknowledgements

My grateful thanks to both editors and Professor Bob Ladd for indispensable comments on an earlier draft.

References

Abe, I. (1998) Intonation in Japanese. In D. Hirst and A. Di Cristo (eds) *Intonation Systems: A Survey of Twenty Languages* (pp. 360–376). Cambridge: Cambridge University Press.

Alcobar, S. and Murillo, A. (1998) Intonation in Spanish. In D. Hirst and A. Di Cristo (eds) *Intonation Systems: A Survey of Twenty Languages* (pp. 152–167). Cambridge: Cambridge University Press.

Crystal, D. (1969) *Prosodic Systems and Intonation in English.* Cambridge: Cambridge University Press.

Crystal, D. (1987) *The Cambridge Encyclopedia of Language.* Cambridge: Cambridge University Press.

Dung, B.T., Huong, T.T. and Boulakia, G. (1998) Intonation in Vietnamese. In D. Hirst and A. Di Cristo (eds) *Intonation Systems: A Survey of Twenty Languages* (pp. 395–417). Cambridge: Cambridge University Press.

Fox, A. (2000) *Prosodic Features and Prosodic Structure: The Phonology of Suprasegmentals.* Oxford: Oxford University Press.

Goedemans, R. and van der Hulst, H. (2005) Fixed stress locations. In M. Haspelmath, M.S. Dryer, D. Gil and B. Comrie (eds) *The World Atlas of Language Structures* (pp. 62–65). Munich: Max Planck Digital Library. http://wals.info/feature/39. Accessed 20.10.10.

Haspelmath, M., Dryer, M.S., Gil, D. and Comrie, B. (2005) *The World Atlas of Language Structures.* Oxford: Oxford University Press.

't Hart (1998) Intonation in Dutch. In D. Hirst and A. Di Cristo (eds) *Intonation Systems: A Survey of Twenty Languages* (pp. 96–112). Cambridge: Cambridge University Press.

Hirst, D. and Di Cristo, A. (eds) (1998) *Intonation Systems: A Survey of Twenty Languages.* Cambridge: Cambridge University Press.

Jun, S-A. (ed.) (2006) *Prosodic Typology: The Phonology of Intonation and Phrasing.* Oxford: Oxford University Press.

Ladd, D.R. (1996) *Intonational Phonology.* Cambridge: Cambridge University Press.

Li, C.N. and Thompson, S.N. (1977) The acquisition of tone in Mandarin-speaking children. *Journal of Child Language* 4, 185–199.

Ma, J.K., Ciocca, V. and Whitehill, T.L. (2006) Effect of intonation on Cantonese lexical tones. *Journal of the Acoustical Society of America* 320, 3978–3987.

Maddieson, I. (2008) Tone. In M. Haspelmath, M.S. Dryer, D. Gil and B. Comrie (eds) *The World Atlas of Language Structures Online.* Munich: Max Planck Digital Library. http://wals.info/feature/39. Accessed 20.10.10.

Martínez-Castilla, P. and Peppé, S. (2008) Intonation features of the expression of emotions in Spanish: Preliminary study for a prosody assessment procedure. *Clinical Linguistics and Phonetics* 22 (4/5), 363–370.

McLeod, S. (ed.) (2007) *The International Guide to Speech Acquisition.* Clifton Park, NY: Thomson Delmar Learning.

Peppé, S., Martínez-Castilla, P., Coene, M., Hesling, I., Moen, I. and Gibbon, F. (2010) Assessing prosodic disorder in five European languages. *International Journal of Speech-Language Pathology* 12 (1), 1–7.

Peppé, S. and McCann, J. (2003) Assessing intonation and prosody in children with atypical language development: The PEPS-C test and the revised version. *Clinical Linguistics and Phonetics* 17 (4/5), 345–354.

Sluijter, A. and van Heuven, V. (1996) Spectral balance as an acoustic correlate of linguistic stress. *Journal of the Acoustical Society of America* 100 (4), 2471–2485.

Swerts, M. (2007) Contrast and accent in Flemish and Romanian. *Journal of Phonetics* 35 (3), 380–397.

To, C.K.S., Cheung, P.S.P. and McLeod, S. (2011) *Speech sound acquisition of Hong Kong Cantonese.* Manuscript in submission.

Williams, B. (1985) Pitch and duration in Welsh accent perception: The implications for intonation. *Journal of Phonetics* 13, 381–406.

Yip, M. (2002) *Tone.* Cambridge: Cambridge University Press.

7 Translation to Practice: Prosody in Five European Languages

Sue Peppé, Martine Coene, Isabelle Hesling, Pastora Martínez-Castilla and Inger Moen

Languages mentioned: Basque, Catalan, Finnish, Flemish, French, Galician, German, Norwegian, Sami, Spanish, Swedish

Prosody in Five European Languages

This chapter introduces some issues to consider when assessing disorders of prosodic ability (as opposed to segmental speech sound disorders) in speakers of some European languages, and the ways in which prosody can affect speech sound disorders and their diagnosis in multilingual children. Prosodic ability is the capacity to use and interpret variations in pitch, syllable duration and loudness in speech: these factors affect the impact or meaning of spoken utterances. Speech and language therapists/speech-language pathologists (SLPs) rarely attempt remediation of prosodic disorder, but an assessment procedure is available (PEPS-C: Peppé & McCann, 2003); originally in English, this has now been translated into Flemish, Norwegian, French and Spanish. With the common methodology of a translated test, it will be possible to compare milestones in prosodic development, and determine if prosodic deficits in children with communication impairments are cross-linguistically similar. There are, as yet, little data on the instrument, although some preliminary data are given in Peppé *et al.* (2010).

Multilingualism

European countries where English, Flemish, Norwegian, French and Spanish are spoken have comparatively monolingual cultures, although areas near linguistic borders are multilingual: French-Flemish (around Brussels); French-Spanish (southwest France); French-German (northeast France and east Belgium); Spanish-Basque/Catalan/Galician (north Spain); Norwegian-Sami/Finnish (north Norway) Norwegian-Swedish (Norway in general). English speakers can of course be multilingual with many other languages in countries that are primarily English speaking.

Prosody skills

In these European languages, prosody is instrumental in four main areas of communicative function (Roach, 2000). It can indicate: the focal point of an utterance; where utterances and conversational turns begin and end; utterance type (e.g. question or statement); and emotions (affect). Differences of prosodic function (e.g. if there are more/fewer functions in any of the languages), and differences in the prosodic forms used to convey them may have implications for the intelligibility of multilingual children with speech sound disorders.

Cross-linguistic Prosodic Differences

In addition to the functions itemised above, particular pitch patterns (tones) are used to distinguish the lexical meaning of some words in Norwegian, Swedish and in dialects of Limburg in the southeast of the Netherlands and the northeast of Belgium. In this respect, Norwegian, Swedish and the Limburg dialects can be considered as tone languages, although not nearly to the same extent as languages such as Chinese. Tone languages can be considered to sound *singsong*. This quality may be a factor to take into account in children who are multilingual between tone and non-tone languages and have disorders with characteristic *singsong* prosody, as can occur in some manifestations of autism (e.g. Fay & Schuler, 1980). Broadly speaking, Romance languages, such as French and Spanish, differ prosodically from Germanic ones, which include English, Flemish and Norwegian. One of the differences is in speech rhythm (see below); another is in accent placement (see below). Therefore, there is likely to be an effect of prosodic differences in French-Flemish and French-German bilingual children with speech sound disorders. Word accent also differs between Norwegian and Finno-Ugric languages (which include Finnish and Sami), so prosodic interference may contribute to unclear accent placement in children who are bilingual in these languages. Pairings such as French with Spanish, Spanish with Romance minority languages and Norwegian with Swedish are unlikely to be affected in this way.

Speech rhythm

Germanic languages (such as English, Flemish and Norwegian) are stress timed; whereas, Spanish and French are syllable timed (see Peppé, Chapter 6, for clarification of these terms). The effect of this distinction is to produce different manifestations of accent placement, in both whole utterances and in single words (represented here by capitalised syllables). In the French of

French-German bilinguals, speech may sound overly emphatic, having too many stresses. The reverse effect (e.g. in French-German bilinguals when speaking German) would be for speech to sound lacking in stress, with syllables too equal in pitch, length and loudness, making words hard to understand. The effect can be particularly pronounced in the case of French-Germanic bilinguals: French can take accent on syllables such as affixes, which are regarded as *unstressable* in stress-timed languages. Transferred to Germanic languages, this results in unusual word accent patterns (e.g. *allotMENT, simPLY*), hindering intelligibility. An additional factor is that the vowels in English unstressed syllables tend to be reduced, and when given their full value (as in the *-MENT* of *allotMENT*), this can add to the difficulty of interpretation.

Accent placement

Utterance-level accent placement is important for indicating focal points, the ends of phrases and the ends of conversational turns. In Germanic languages, accent can be placed prefinally to focus attention on a particular item (a word or syllable), and subsequent syllables will be deaccented. Final deaccenting is not favoured in Romance languages: the preference is to place accent on the final word, and to change the word order so that the focal item comes at the end. For example, where a Germanic-language speaker might say to a waiter, *I ordered STEAK and chips*, emphasising *steak* and deaccenting *and chips*, to draw attention to the item that is wrong in his order, a Romance-language speaker would prefer to say, *I ordered chips and STEAK*. Transfer of preferences from one language to another can cause misunderstanding as to how phrases are delimited or where the main focus of an utterance occurs. For more information on Romance and Germanic placement of accent, see Zubizarreta (1998) and Swerts (2007).

Affect

As in most of the world, strong affect, negative or positive, is conveyed by wide pitch span in these languages. A rising-falling contour, or wide falling contour from a high initial pitch, conveys positive affect, while a narrow low-pitched contour indicates negative or reserved affect. For Spanish-English differences on the prosodic expression of affect, see Martínez-Castilla and Peppé (2008).

Conclusion

In summary, there are Germanic-Romance prosodic differences that may cause some delay or misunderstanding in hearers, mainly in the placement of accent at word and utterance level. In children with speech sound disorders who are multilingual in these languages, there may, however, be no between-language interference of prosodic systems: problems will depend to a great extent on their proficiency in each of the two languages.

References

Fay, W. and Schuler, A.l. (1980) *Emerging Language in Autistic Children.* London: Edward Arnold.

Martínez-Castilla, P. and Peppé, S. (2008) Intonation features of the expression of emotions in Spanish: Preliminary study for a prosody assessment procedure. *Clinical Linguistics and Phonetics* 22 (4/5), 363–370.

Peppé, S., Martínez-Castilla, P., Coene, M., Hesling, I., Moen, I. and Gibbon, F. (2010) Assessing prosodic disorder in five European languages. *International Journal of Speech-Language Pathology* 12 (1), 1–7.

Peppé, S. and McCann, J. (2003) Assessing intonation and prosody in children with atypical language development: The PEPS-C test and the revised version. *Clinical Linguistics and Phonetics* 17 (4/5), 345–354.

Roach, P. (2000) *English Phonetics and Phonology.* Cambridge: Cambridge University Press.

Swerts, M. (2007) Contrast and accent in Flemish and Romanian. *Journal of Phonetics* 35 (3), 380–397.

Zubizarreta, M.L. (1998) *Prosody, Focus, and Word Order.* Cambridge, MA: MIT Press.

8 Perceptual Considerations in Multilingual Adult and Child Speech Acquisition

Susan Rvachew, Karen Mattock, Meghan Clayards, Pi-Yu Chiang and Françoise Brosseau-Lapré

Languages mentioned: *Arabic, Catalan, English, French, German, Japanese, Spanish*

Perceptual Considerations in Multilingual Adult and Child Speech Acquisition

Approximately 70% of immigrants to Canada do not speak either official language, thus school boards with large immigrant populations experience increasingly multilingual classrooms with, for example, over 40% of students in Toronto speaking a language other than English at home and over 34% of students in Montreal having a mother tongue other than French (Canadian Council on Learning, 2009). This heterogeneity in students' linguistic experience creates diverse challenges to achievement for students in these schools. Consider the example shown in Table 8.1, obtained from a girl (M.S.) aged 5;5, who moved from Egypt in the year prior to enrollment in an English kindergarten program in Montreal (a city in Quebec, Canada, where the majority language is French but a substantial English minority receives schooling in English). The teacher requested a speech assessment to determine if the child's speech patterns reflected her limited exposure to English or more significant difficulties negotiating the transition to a new language. Regardless of the root of the problem, the challenge of planning a course of action to help the child achieve native-like levels of language proficiency in the school language remained. One piece of the puzzle undoubtedly concerns the child's perception of the relevant phonemes. An understanding of how phonemic perception is acquired in first (L1) and second language (L2) acquisition is necessary background to the task at hand.

Second language learning in adulthood

While L2 learning of phonetic categories in children is less well studied, there is an extensive literature on adult perception of L2 phonetic categories.

Table 8.1 Phonetic realization of selected phonemes observed in English words spoken by M.S., an Arabic-speaking girl, aged 5;5, who had been learning English for less than 1 year

Target phoneme	Phonetic realizations
/t/	[t] [d] [tˢ] [tʃ]
/d/	[d] [d̪] [ð]
/tʃ/	[tʃ] [tʰ]
/ʤ/	[ʤ] [tʃ] [ʃ] [ʒ]
/s/	[s]
/z/	[z] [z̥] [s̪]
/θ/	[θ] [f]
/ð/	[d] [d̪]
/ʃ/	[ʃ]

Note. Circle below indicates devoicing. Bridge below indicates dental place of articulation.

Early research (Polivanov, 1931) first noticed that the listener's L1 acts like a filter for discriminating sounds in an L2. A number of theories of L2 learning were developed to describe the interference between L1 and L2: the Perceptual Adaptation Model (Best, 1994), the Speech Learning Model (Flege, 1995) and the Natural Language Magnet model (Kuhl *et al.*, 2008). While differing in their predictions and mechanisms, all hypothesize that it is easier to discriminate sounds in an L2 if they are similar to sounds that *differ* in the listener's L1; however, it is harder to discriminate sounds in an L2 if they are similar (acoustically, phonetically or articulatorily) to the *same* sound in one's L1. For example, English /l/ and /ɹ/ are both similar to a single phone in Japanese transcribed as an approximant /ɹ/ or a flap /ɾ/ depending on the context, making this distinction nearly impossible for native Japanese listeners to distinguish. Applying these principles to M.S., it makes sense that she might confuse /ð/, a phoneme that does not occur in Arabic, with /d/, which is produced at a dental place of articulation in Arabic. On the other hand, if we were to test her, she might prove quite capable of discriminating [θ] from [ð] by assimilating these phones to her own internal representations for the Arabic /s/ vs. /z/ categories.

We caution, however, that it is not enough to simply compare the phonemic inventories of two languages to understand which sounds will be problematic for an L2 learner. It is important to understand which dimensions or acoustic cues a language employs to signal a contrast, and how they use them. Flege and Port (1981) compared Saudi Arabic speakers' and American English speakers' productions of stop consonant voicing. Arabic and English stops appear similar in voicing as they both have aspirated voiceless stops and short-lag voiced stops (Khattab, 2000); however, Flege and Port (1981) found that Arabic and English speakers used different acoustic cues to signal the voicing contrast. In word-initial position before a stressed vowel, Arabic voice onset times (VOTs) were slightly shorter than English VOTs; furthermore, Arabic speakers produced longer closures for voiceless than voiced stops, while English speakers did not. Conversely, for word-final stops before an unstressed syllable, Arabic speakers did not produce a difference in closure duration or preceding vowel length, whereas for English speakers these cues are robustly produced and critical for perception. The same Arabic speakers were asked to produce English stops. Those who resided in the USA for less than a year signaled the voicing contrast in English using the same cues as for Arabic, while those who had been in the country longer shifted toward more English-like pronunciation. English listeners sometimes confused these stops; for example, hearing [d] for /t/, particularly in word-final position where Arabic speakers did not produce cues critical for English. Thus, even where both languages have a stop voicing contrast that is similar at the phonemic level, differences in the phonetic details of the language can interfere with L2 speakers' intelligibility. Referring again to M.S., attention to the details of phonetic implementation of the voicing contrast in Arabic helps to understand the voicing and manner confusions in this child's speech. The voicing confusions most likely reflect the mismatch between the phonetic cues that are used to implement these phonemic categories in Arabic compared to those used by English-speaking transcribers to perceive these categories in English. Conversely, the manner class confusions may reflect the child's efforts to categorize aspiration durations in English that are considerably longer than in her native Arabic.

As the above example highlights, every phonological contrast is potentially signaled by multiple acoustic-phonetic cues, but not all are equally perceptually relevant. Some cues influence perception more than others and the relevance of cues depends on exactly what they are cueing. For example, when discriminating /s/ from /ʃ/ in English, both formant transitions between frication and vowel and the spectral characteristics of the frication are important, but the spectral characteristics of the frication have a much greater influence. On the other hand, when distinguishing /b/ from /d/ in English, formant transitions play a greater perceptual role than the spectral characteristics of the burst (Nittrouer, 2002). Not only are cue weights specific to context, they also differ by language, as we saw in the Arabic-English example. In that example, we also saw that L2 learners improved over time in their ability to appropriately use L2 cues to signal the contrast. In fact, the task of L2 learning more generally could be thought of as learning to attend to and use cues or dimensions that are not relevant in the L1. To return to the example of Japanese speakers learning English /l/ and /ɹ/, Iverson *et al.* (2003) found that speakers of Japanese were more sensitive to differences between /l/ and /ɹ/ in the F2 dimension and less sensitive to differences in the F3 dimension, while English and German listeners exhibited the opposite pattern. This suggests that Japanese learners of English must learn to attend to F3 in perception and to manipulate this cue to achieve accurate production of the /l/-/ɹ/ contrast in English.

The fact that cue weights differ across languages suggests that they must be learned as part of the developmental process. In fact, several studies have found that young children may not use acoustic cues in the same way as adults in perception (Nittrouer, 2002). Furthermore, these differences across languages may lead to different developmental trajectories. For example, Li *et al.* (2009) reported that in English it is common for young children to produce an error pattern referred to as fronting (e.g. [s] for /ʃ/ substitutions); however, among Japanese children, backing is the more common error pattern in this context (e.g. [ɕ] for /s/ substitutions). We turn now to the topic of perceptual learning in infancy and early childhood.

Perceptual learning among bilingual infants and toddlers

For a long time it was believed that bilingual children treat all language input as part of a single language that they only separate once they begin acquiring a lexicon and syntax (Volterra & Taeschner, 1978). However, modern techniques for testing infants make it possible to assess their ability to discriminate between languages as well as their preference for listening to one language over another, long before the production of first words. It is now known that from birth, bilingual infants recognize their native languages (Byers-Heinlein *et al.*, 2010) and that between 4 and 9 months of age, they are able to separate the two languages being learned (Bosch & Sebastián-Gallés, 1997; Polka *et al.*, 2009). However, despite being able to discriminate languages like monolinguals (for review, see Nazzi & Ramus, 2003), the developmental course of phonetic perception for bilinguals is complex relative to monolinguals. For monolinguals, two major developments occur in perceptual development early in life. During the first year, the infant makes a shift from language-general to language-specific patterns of phonetic perception: specifically, the infant becomes increasingly sensitive to phonetic contrasts that are important in the native language and gradually becomes less sensitive to contrasts that are non-phonemic in the ambient language (Polka *et al.*, 2007). The primary underlying mechanism is a statistical learning mechanism that allows the infant to extract categories from statistical regularities in the distribution of acoustic cues in the variable acoustic-phonetic input (Maye *et al.*, 2008). Furthermore, active engagement by the child with the input appears to be necessary because social interaction rather than passive exposure to the speech input is required in order to prevent loss of responding to a phonetic contrast (Kuhl *et al.*, 2003).

Bilingual infants also show changes in their responses to phonetic contrasts as a consequence of their experience with language input during the first year of life. Bosch and Sebastián-Gallés (2003a) investigated discrimination of Catalan /ɛ–e/ vowels by Catalan, Spanish and bilingual infants aged 4, 8 and 12 months in Barcelona, Spain. All groups discriminated the contrast at 4 months. As expected, attenuation of perception with age was observed for Spanish infants for whom the contrast was non-native, but not for Catalan infants. Interestingly, bilingual infants showed a U-shaped pattern – decline in discrimination between 4 and 8 months, and improved discrimination at 12 months to levels equivalent to Catalan infants. This U-shaped pattern is also present for Spanish-Catalan bilinguals' perception of Catalan /s/-/z/ (Bosch & Sebastián-Gallés, 2003b), and Spanish/Catalan /o/-/u/ (Sebastián-Gallés & Bosch, 2009).

A second important milestone in normal perceptual development is the shift from phonetic perception to phonemic perception during the second year of life. Between 14 and 20 months of age, toddlers learn to use their knowledge of phonetic categories to signal differences in meanings. Initially, they can associate different sounding words (e.g. /nif/ vs. /lɪm/) to new objects, but gradually learn to associate similar sounding words (e.g. /bɪ/ vs. /dɪ/) to novel objects (Werker *et al.*, 2002). The exact phonetic characteristics of the words that bilingual infants hear have an impact on phonemic perception in word-learning tasks at this age. In Vancouver, Canada, Fennell *et al.* (2007) tested 17-month-old English-French bilinguals and English monolinguals' learning of two novel word-object pairings in the Switch task. The novel words /bɪ/ and /dɪ/ were spoken by an English speaker and formed a minimal pair that differed in phonetic realization in English (alveolar) and French (dental). Monolinguals succeeded in word learning, but bilinguals failed. By 20 months, bilinguals succeeded, suggesting that phonetic structures are challenging to access in a single language context and that under these conditions bilinguals take longer to achieve word learning at monolingual levels. A recent study by Mattock *et al.* (2010) conducted in Montreal, Canada, using the Switch task with English, French and bilingual infants, further supports this idea. Bilingual infants, aged 17 months, succeeded at learning novel words /bos/ and /gos/ when they were produced by a bilingual speaker with varied phonetic realizations that matched the infants' bilingual input (e.g. both French-like prevoiced and English-like short-lag tokens). Of note is that monolinguals fail to learn the word-object pairings with mixed language tokens and succeed only when words are produced solely in their native language. Together these findings demonstrate that both monolingual and bilingual infants are sorting out the relevance of the acoustic cues in their environments. At the earliest stages of word learning, like the L2 learner, they may not yet be making robust mappings between sound and meaning. Furthermore, with regard to M.S., they show how mismatch in phonetic realization across languages influences acoustic-phonetic representation and phonemic perception. Importantly for the speech-language pathologist (SLP), these findings also highlight that bilingual language capabilities may not be fully captured by tasks that are designed from the viewpoint of monolingual acquisition.

Clinical implications

The findings presented thus far have implications for the management of children learning a second language by speech-language pathologists (SLPs) and by teachers. We begin with some recommendations for the assessment of the children's perceptual abilities, returning again to M.S. One approach to assessing this child's perceptual knowledge might be for the SLP to ask the child if minimal pair words such as *thin* and *fin* or *they* and *day* sound the same or different. This would *not* be a good strategy because the child's responses do not tell us if she is aware that the differences between the words are phonemically meaningful, only that she has heard the acoustic differences. Second, the procedure does not help us to understand which acoustic-phonetic cues she is attending to when she makes her judgment about the similarities and differences between words. Recall the situation with Japanese learners of English: attending to the F2 transition will sometimes allow the listener to successfully discriminate /l/ from /ɹ/, but the learner cannot achieve accurate production without manipulating the F3 cue.

Meaningful perception testing requires an identification test – in which children are presented with varied productions of a target word that contrast a frequently confused pair of phonemes and are asked to identify them by pointing to printed words or pictures to indicate which word they heard. Research with children with speech delay and L2 learners has systematically varied the important acoustic cues (for review, see Rvachew & Jamieson, 1995), using synthetic speech stimuli to determine exactly which cues the child is attending to when making judgments about the minimal pairs. As this technique is not accessible in the clinical setting, an alternative is to present the child with recorded exemplars from many different talkers. Identification of mispronunciations has been shown to be a valid means of assessing children's phonemic representations for words (McNeill & Hesketh, 2010; Rvachew & Grawburg, 2006). The use of naturally recorded speech will not allow identification of the exact cues that the child is attending to, but it will provide valid assessment of perceptual knowledge of the target phoneme if there are many varied tokens included with the test stimuli. In our example case, it would be helpful to construct stimulus sets to assess the child's perceptual knowledge of each of the voicing, manner and place contrasts that she is having difficulty producing consistently, as shown in Table 8.1.

In order to decide whether the child has a speech delay or whether her difficulties are due to her limited exposure to English, the SLP must seek more information about the child's abilities in Arabic. If the SLP is not proficient in each of the child's languages, the child's parents and/or an interpreter may be consulted. However, Rvachew and Jamieson (1995) argued that L2 learners and children with speech delay alike are essentially uncertain of the acoustic-phonetic characteristics of the phonemes in the language that they are learning; having unclear targets to guide production, they develop inaccurate or inconsistent motor plans for the implementation of these phonemes in their speech. Therefore, barring rare cases of frank motor speech disorders, the intervention strategy should be the same regardless of whether the child's speech difficulties occur in English only or in both languages.

With respect to remediation, this child needs to learn the prototypical combination of acoustic cues that characterize English phoneme categories, such as /t/ vs. /d/, as well as the appropriate placement of the boundaries between these categories. Techniques that are effective for improving the perceptual abilities of children with speech delay should be useful in the L2 learning context. Rvachew (2009) developed a computer-based intervention (SAILS; *Speech Assessment and Interactive Learning System*) for children with moderate or severe speech sound disorder (SSD). Using a mispronunciation detection task, the goal of the intervention is to ensure good perceptual knowledge of the target so that they will be able to compare their own productions against an accurate acoustic-phonetic representation and modify their articulatory gestures to achieve the target phoneme. Three randomized controlled studies and one controlled study without randomization have investigated the efficacy of SAILS to date in English-speaking 4- to 6-year-olds with moderate or severe speech delay (for a review, see Rvachew & Brosseau-Lapré, 2010). The results show that children who received the SAILS intervention made more progress with regard to articulatory accuracy in addition to improving their perceptual knowledge of the target phoneme categories.

Although we believe that a similar approach will be effective with L2 learners, we are not aware of any studies that confirm this experimentally. Furthermore, modifications to the approach will be necessary to ensure linguistically appropriate stimuli when the child is learning an L2 that is not English. Brosseau-Lapré and Rvachew developed a Canadian-French version of SAILS modeled after the English SAILS, targeting phonemes in single-syllable words. The development of a speech perception intervention tool requires in-depth knowledge about typical and atypical phonological development of the language. For instance, whereas incomplete inventories are characteristic of preschool English-speaking children with SSD, French-speaking children with SSD usually have a complete consonant inventory but have difficulties producing more complex syllable structures as well as difficulties perceiving multisyllabic words containing vowels and consonants forming complex syllables (Caravolas & Bruck, 2000). These differences between English and French could be due to differences at the supra-segmental level, French being a syllable-timed language while English is a stress-timed language. Furthermore, French-speaking children with language-impairment have difficulty perceiving mispronunciations that alter the prosodic structure of multisyllabic words (e.g. phoneme deletions and transpositions; Maillart *et al.*, 2004); on the other hand, English-speaking children are more likely to have difficulty with segmental rather than prosodic errors (McNeill & Hesketh, 2010). Modules currently being developed include two-syllable words containing a word-internal coda (e.g. /sɛʁpã/) or a glide in the nucleus (e.g. /pwasɔ̃/) to better reflect the kinds of speech errors that we observe in young French-speaking children.

Another effective technique in our research clinic for francophone children is focused stimulation using live-voice presentation of material that provides repeated exposure to words containing the target phonemes or prosodic structures. Structured listening activities, during which the child is required to make explicit judgments about the SLP's pronunciation of target words, are also valuable in combination with standard minimal pair production activities (Barlow & Gierut, 2002).

The SLP can also offer valuable support to the classroom teacher. The development of speech perception, compared to other language skills, is not a skill that most school teachers would usually notice and work exclusively on with their students. In order to help L2 learners in the classroom, the teacher must gather background information about the students' prior language experience in terms of listening, speaking, reading and writing. The SLP can help the classroom teacher to interpret this information by consulting sources such as McLeod (2007). The teacher may need coaching to introduce focused stimulation and listening activities into the classroom. The SLP is well positioned to provide advice about which words, phonemes and prosodic structures to target during such activities. Teachers also need to understand that there are multiple levels of phonological knowledge: the more basic perceptual and articulatory knowledge of how phonemes should sound and be produced; the higher level of phonological knowledge such as how sounds combine into words; and the social-indexical knowledge of how various pronunciations convey different social identities (Munson *et al.*, 2005). In addition to emphasizing the acoustic and articulatory knowledge of the problematic consonants, the teacher should provide various types of stimuli in words and sentences to maximize the learning opportunities and create a classroom environment that provides high quality and diverse speech input.

Classroom acoustics have been shown to correlate with L2 speech perception (Bovo & Callegari, 2009; Crandell & Smaldino, 1996). If possible, provide students with quality speech input via headphones in a soundproof language laboratory, quiet classroom or even at home via their own computer. Using a microphone in a classroom to deliver material is another option. In addition, arrange students who have more difficulty in perception and production to sit close to the amplifiers or teacher to obtain the best input. In terms of providing diverse speech input to promote speech perception learning, make good use of radio broadcasts, television shows and video clips on the internet to illustrate different dialects and accents from various native speakers.

In conclusion, we have shown that both L1 and L2 learning involves making sense of diverse language input. The L2 learner will be forced to attend to new acoustic-phonetic cues and weight the importance of previously attended cues differently in order to develop a language-specific strategy for processing L2 input. The SLP can help the L2 learner make this transition by structuring the input to focus attention on the critical acoustic cues. The selection of stimuli for such listening tasks should be guided by one's knowledge of the prosodic and segmental characteristics of the target phonology and the typical developmental speech errors that children make when learning the target language. All activities should involve authentic engagement with natural language in meaningful contexts. Well-established perceptual knowledge of the phonological characteristics of the L2 will provide a target to guide the child's acquisition of the articulatory gestures required for accurate production of those phonological structures, facilitating improved speech accuracy and intelligibility over time.

References

Barlow, J.A. and Gierut, J.A. (2002) Minimal pair approaches to phonological remediation. *Seminars in Speech and Language* 23 (1), 57–67.

Best, C.C. (1994) The emergence of native-language phonological influences in infants: A perceptual assimilation model. In H.C. Nusbaum (ed.) *The Development of Speech Perception: The Transition from Speech Sounds to Spoken Words* (pp. 167–224). Cambridge, MA: MIT Press.

Bosch, L. and Sebastián-Gallés, N. (1997) Native-language recognition abilities in 4-month-old infants from monolingual and bilingual environments. *Cognition* 65 (1), 33–69.

Bosch, L. and Sebastián-Gallés, N. (2003a) Simultaneous bilingualism and the perception of a language-specific vowel contrast in the first year of life. *Language and Speech* 46 (2/3), 217–243.

Bosch, L. and Sebastián-Gallés, N. (2003b) Language experience and the perception of a voicing contrast in fricatives: Infant and adult data. Paper presented at the 15th International Conference on Phonetic Sciences, Barcelona, Spain.

Bovo, R. and Callegari, E. (2009) Effects of classroom noise on the speech perception of bilingual children learning in their second language: Preliminary results. *Audiological Medicine* 7, 226–232.

Byers-Heinlein, K., Burns, T.F. and Werker, J.F. (2010) The roots of bilingualism in newborns. *Psychological Science* 21, 343–348.

Canadian Council on Learning (2009) *Effective Literacy Strategies for Immigrant Students.* http://www.ccl-cca.ca/CCL/Reports/LessonsInLearning/LinL20090923Effectivelitera cystrategiesimmigrantstudents.html. Accessed 23.9.09.

Caravolas, M. and Bruck, M. (2000) Vowel categorization skill and its relationship to early literacy skills among first-grade Québec-French children. *Journal of Experimental Child Psychology* 76 (3), 190–221.

Crandell, C.C. and Smaldino, J.J. (1996) Speech perception in noise by children for whom English is a second language. *American Journal of Audiology* 5, 47–51.

Fennell, C.T., Byers-Heinlein, K. and Werker, J.F. (2007) Using speech sounds to guide word learning: The case of bilingual infants. *Child Development* 78, 1510–1525.

Flege, J.E. (1995) Second language speech learning: Theory, findings, and problems. In W. Strange (ed.) *Speech Perception and Linguistic Experience: Issues in Cross-language Research* (pp. 233–277). Timonium, MD: York Press.

Flege, J.E. and Port, R. (1981) Cross-language phonetic interference: Arabic to English. *Language and Speech* 24 (2), 125–146.

Iverson, P., Kuhl, P.K., Akahane-Yamada, R., Diesch, E., Tohkura, Y., Kettermann, A. and Siebert, C. (2003) A perceptual interference account of acquisition difficulties for non-native phonemes. *Cognition* 87 (1), B47–B57.

Khattab, G. (2000) VOT productions in English and Arabic bilingual and monolingual children. *Leeds Working Papers in Linguistics and Phonetics* 8, 95–122.

Kuhl, P.K., Conboy, B.T., Coffey-Corina, S., Padden, D., Rivera-Gaxiola, M. and Nelson, T. (2008) Phonetic learning as a pathway to language: New data and native language magnet theory expanded (NLM-e). *Philosophical Transactions of the Royal Society* 363, 979–1000.

Kuhl, P.K., Tsao, F. and Liu, H. (2003) Foreign-language experience in infancy: Effects of short-term exposure and social interaction on phonetic learning. *Proceedings of the National Academy of Sciences* 100, 9096–9101.

Li, F., Edwards, J. and Beckman, M.E. (2009) Contrast and covert contrast: The phonetic development of voiceless sibilant fricatives in English and Japanese toddlers. *Journal of Phonetics* 37 (1), 111–124.

Maillart, C., Schelstraete, M-A. and Hupet, M. (2004) Phonological representations in children with SLI: A study of French. *Journal of Speech, Language, and Hearing Research* 47, 187–198.

Mattock, K., Polka, L., Rvachew, S. and Krehm, M. (2010) The first steps in word learning are easier when the shoes fit: Comparing monlingual and bilingual infants. *Developmental Science* 13, 229–243.

Maye, J., Weiss, D.J. and Aslin, R.N. (2008) Statistical phonetic learning in infants: Facilitation and feature generalization. *Developmental Science* 11 (1), 122–134.

McLeod, S. (2007) *The International Guide to Speech Acquisition.* Clifton Park, NY: Thomson Delmar Learning.

McNeill, B.C. and Hesketh, A. (2010) Developmental complexity of the stimuli included in mispronunciation detection tasks. *International Journal of Language and Communication Disorders* 45 (1), 72–82.

Munson, B., Edwards, J. and Beckman, M.E. (2005) Phonological knowledge in typical and atypical speech-sound development. *Topics in Language Disorders* 25 (3), 190–206.

Nazzi, T. and Ramus, F. (2003) Perception and acquisition of linguistic rhythm by infants. *Speech Communication* 41 (1), 233–243.

Nittrouer, S. (2002) From ear to cortex: A perspective on what clinicians need to understand about speech perception and language processing. *Language, Speech, and Hearing Services in Schools* 33, 237–252.

Polivanov, E. (1931) La perception des sons d'une langue étrangère [The perception of non-native language sounds]. *Travaux du Cercle Linguistique de Prague* 4, 79–96.

Polka, L., Rvachew, S. and Mattock, K. (2007) Experiential influences on speech perception and speech production in infancy. In E. Hoff and M. Shatz (eds) *Blackwell Handbook of Language Development* (pp. 153–172). Cambridge, MA: Blackwell.

Polka, L., Valji, A. and Mattock, K. (2009) Language preference in monolingual and bilingual infants. *Journal of the Acoustical Society of America* 125, 2772.

Rvachew, S. (2009) Speech assessment and interactive learning system (Ver. 2): [Software]. Available from author by request.

Rvachew, S. and Brosseau-Lapré, F. (2010) Speech perception intervention. In A.L. Williams, S. McLeod and R.J. McCauley (eds) *Interventions for Speech Sound Disorders in Children* (pp. 295–314). Baltimore, MD: Paul Brookes.

Rvachew, S. and Grawburg, M. (2006) Correlates of phonological awareness in preschoolers with speech sound disorders. *Journal of Speech, Language, and Hearing Research* 49, 74–87.

Rvachew, S. and Jamieson, D.G. (1995) Learning new speech contrasts: Evidence from learning a second language and children with speech disorders. In W. Strange (ed.) *Speech Perception and Linguistic Experience* (pp. 411–432). Timonium, MD: York Press.

Sebastián-Gallés, N. and Bosch, L. (2009) Developmental shift in the discrimination of vowel contrasts in bilingual infants: Is the distributional account all there is to it? *Developmental Science* 12, 874–887.

Volterra, V. and Taeschner, T. (1978) The acquisition and development of language by bilingual children. *Journal of Child Language* 5, 311–326.

Werker, J.F., Fennell, C.T., Corcoran, K.M. and Stager, C.L. (2002) Infants' ability to learn phonetically similar words: Effects of age and vocabulary size. *Infancy* 3 (1), 1–30.

Part 2

Multilingual Speech Acquisition

9 A Complexity Theory Account of Canonical Babbling in Young Children

Barbara L. Davis and Sophie Kern

Languages mentioned: Arabic, Dutch, English, French, Korean, Romanian, Turkish

Introduction

The young child's acquisition of phonology lies at the intersection of storing complex knowledge about patterns required for making meanings and progressive mastery of a behavioral repertoire of goal-directed *actions* for using that knowledge. Goal-directed knowledge-action capacities underlying the phonological component of language can be considered as a complex system (Camazine, 2001; Chirotan *et al.*, 2009; Davis & Bedore, in preparation; Kern & Davis, 2009). This complex system can be specified at two levels. Complexity is apparent at the level of the physical and mental capacities in diverse bodily systems that underlie phonological acquisition. It is also apparent in the intertwined dimensions of behavior and knowledge that are observable to others, which define phonology.

The basis for the emergence of phonological complexity at these intertwined levels that define phonological acquisition lies in multiple and heterogeneous interactions among diverse system components. In an emergence view, phonological acquisition does not depend on a single physical or mental system, but on the connectivity across these systems as they support acquiring behavioral and knowledge capacities. At the level of using the system for speaking and listening, phonological acquisition is not founded only on mastery of behavioral patterns or only on mastery of knowledge, but on a confluence of both abilities. This heterogeneous basis for the acquisition of phonology and for the nature of phonological abilities deployed in speaking and listening defines the complex system conceptualization.

An emergence conceptualization for phonology has critical implications for the issues addressed by the authors in this volume relative to acquisition of phonological systems in multilingual speakers. Factors considered as aspects supporting the emergence of phonological complexity, as they will be reviewed here, are the critical dimensions of overall planning for intervention that clinicians must account for in achieving functional and age-appropriate intelligibility outcomes for children who need clinical services. These considerations are applicable in diverse phonological learning environments as clinicians consider the child's ambient language targets that must be remediated, their strengths and challenges in learning those targets, and the cultural values for deployment of the child's phonological system in linguistically based communication. When core sound system properties are considered in isolation from the scaffolding needed to support learning in children with speech sound disorders, regardless of language environment, it may be difficult to achieve age-appropriate speech intelligibility outcomes.

What are the Components of the Complex System Supporting Phonological Acquisition?

From its simplest onset in the first year of life, the *perceptual input-knowledge acquisition-production output* continuum observable in young children illustrates the emergence of a complex system. The child's perception and production of early speech patterns based on maturation of immature physical systems tuned by daily social input is intertwined with emerging neural-cognitive knowledge of phonological distinctions for coding messages. Critically, the young child must also be able to use interaction capacities to maintain consistent contact with persons in her environment. Interaction capacities include joint attention and turn-taking abilities. These abilities are available in rudimentary form at birth (Tomasello, 2003) and grow in complexity across acquisition. Each of these abilities supporting consistent social contact is marshalled in daily experiences with caregivers. These capacities for interaction enable her to learn how to use production system, neural-cognitive and perceptual abilities for linguistic communication.

These physical, mental and social components are necessary to account for acquisition of complex phonological capacities in young children. Crucially, in an emergence view, none of these components of the complex system available to the young child is uniquely causal of the eventual product. While all may be *necessary*, none is *sufficient* to facilitate phonological acquisition. A second basic tenet of an emergence view is the non-language dedicated nature of these components of the complex system. They are available to the young child for acquiring other aspects of language complexity and diverse types of knowledge and behaviour needed to achieve mature levels of independent function in the environment. Thus, each of these abilities is employed in myriad functional situations within the young child's life for gathering general knowledge about the world, not only for acquiring the phonological component of language (Davis & Bedore, in preparation).

Physical systems supporting the child's vocal output (e.g. Boliek *et al.*, 2009; Green *et al.*, 2002) include the respiratory, phonatory and articulatory subsystems. Coordination of these systems supports the vocal forms observed in pre-linguistic vocalizations. They provide a foundation for the increase in complexity of output patterns observed across acquisition, as well as the complexity eventually deployed by mature users of phonological patterns. Perceptual capacities for learning precise phonological character-istics from adult input provide a second avenue for learning phonological regularities. To master the full range of phonological forms in their ambient language(s), children must both perceptually attend to and eventually reproduce complex pattern regularities from their ambient language. By the canonical babbling stage in the second half of their first year, young children have already shown evidence of recognizing precise ambient language regularities available from input (e.g. Saffran *et al.*, 1996; Werker & Curtin, 2005). This early recognition forms a basic foundation for continued learning of the precise requirements of the language(s) the child is learning. Of considerable importance to instantiation of long-term knowledge is the child's growing neural-cognitively instantiated capacities for remembering and storing knowledge. These capacities enable her to begin storing and retrieving vocal forms in the first year of life for later deployment as she begins to acquire spoken language forms.

Each of these physically embodied systems is deployed in consistently occurring social contexts where caregivers talk about objects and activities that are important to the growing child. Interaction capacities for joint attention and turn taking enable the child to sustain these critical social connections. The input from caregivers contains words and utterances that display an array of ambient language forms that the child must learn to perceive, store and reproduce in communication exchanges. Caregivers also demonstrate the cultural requirements for the child in deploying those salient word forms in daily routines and play. From its simplest onset in the first year of life, the input-knowledge-output continuum observable in perception and production and growing knowledge about how early vocal forms may relate to language illustrates the first stages of the emergence of a complex system.

Why Study Babbling for Understanding Phonological Acquisition?

Contrary to Jakobson's assertion (1941) of no relation between babbling and early speech forms, longitudinal investigations of the transition from canonical babbling to speech have shown continuity between phonetic forms in child pre-linguistic vocalizations and earliest speech forms (Locke, 1983; Oller & Steffans, 1993; Vihman *et al.*, 1985, 1986). This continuity supports the importance of considering canonical babbling as a crucial first step in the young child's journey toward mastery of ambient language phonology. With few exceptions, output patterns in canonical babbling correspond to output patterns in first words in sound and syllable type preferences (Kern *et al.*, 2010). Canonical babbling is also characterized by temporal organization that results in perceptually apparent 'syllables' (Dolata *et al.*, 2008; Oller *et al.*, 2001).

Why Study Babbling in Diverse Languages?

Canonical babbling marks a seminal step into production of perceptually speech-like output in infants. Canonical babbling is defined as rhythmic alternations between consonant and vowel-like properties. It gives a percept of rhythmic speech that simulates adult output without conveying meaning (Davis & MacNeilage, 1995; Oller, 2000). These rhythmic consonant and vowel 'syllables' emerge typically at around 8–9 months; in previous stages, infant vocalizations do not exhibit rhythmic syllable-like properties (see Oller, 2000, for a review).

If canonical babbling is considered an early step toward ambient language phonological complexity, a primary question arises. When in their first year of life do young children begin to know and use the precise regularities available from their ambient language input? An additional necessary question concerns the order in which components of vocal output related to ambient language regularities emerge. Do young children produce a wide variety of ambient language sound and syllable types in canonical babbling or are these sound system properties limited to a few dimensions of sound patterning available to young children's production capacities?

To answer these questions, a comparison of children's output patterns in diverse language environments that provide diverse ambient language learning targets is needed. A comparison of child vocalization patterns with phonological patterns in the language/languages they are acquiring illustrates the learning targets that the child must achieve during acquisition. This type of analysis enables the establishment of potentially universal patterns in canonical babbling based on characteristics of the production subsystems common to young children across language environments. It can also highlight the timing and the precise nature of early perceptually based learning from social interactions with adult speakers in an ambient language community.

To the extent that children's vocal output patterns are more diverse within and across languages than they are consistent with one another, perceptual learning and cognitive processes are emphasized as the basis for understanding even the earliest phases of phonological development. By contrast, consistent vocal output trends with little individual variation during canonical babbling implicate patterns based on production system constraints as a starting point for perceptual learning from ambient language input (Saffran *et al.*, 1996). As a result, consideration of common patterns and individual differences in children's earliest phases of acquisition within and across languages provides a critical dimension of inquiry needed for understanding the course of phonological acquisition comprehensively.

Production Output Trends in Canonical Babbling

So what does the available literature targeting this period of development tell us about the phonological characteristics of canonical babbling? Making the case for the appearance of ambient language patterns in young children's earliest output patterns requires corpora that are large enough to reveal vocalization patterns rather than anecdotal instances of a child's vocal output (Kern & Davis, 2009). In addition, in the ideal case, cross-language methodologies and transcription conventions should be consistent. Currently, strongly consistent trends in production patterns as well as preliminary indications about the timing of learning from ambient language input are apparent.

However, empirical investigations of early ambient language learning do not provide strong evidence due to methodological issues. Some studies report results on adult perception of children's patterns (de Boysson-Bardies *et al.*, 1984). Other types of studies report on children's production patterns (e.g. de Boysson-Bardies, 1993). The size of corpora analyzed (Locke, 1983) and the age ranges (Levit & Utman, 1992) of children observed differ as well. Longitudinal (Davis & MacNeilage, 1995) vs. cross-sectional (Kent & Bauer, 1985) data collection methods are employed, complicating comparison of results. All of these diverse considerations about available data complicate strong statements on cross-language commonalities. In addition, the experimental literature targeting the appearance of ambient language regularities is quite narrow relative to the diverse types of sound patterns across languages that young children might display as evidence of ambient language learning (Werker & Lalonde, 1988). Important for the evaluation of the validity of an emergence view for phonological acquisition, studies target core sound system properties in isolation from the nature of naturally occurring parent input as well as considerations of the status of neural-cognitive learning.

To evaluate the emergence of early learning from the ambient language more fully, it must be considered in the context of common production patterns seen across languages. Larger cohorts of children in varied language environments illustrating diverse ambient language targets are necessary. Consistent data collection and analysis procedures are also essential to comprehensively evaluate this question. Based on the available literature to date, strong similarities in sound and utterance type preferences in canonical babbling across different language communities have been documented.

For consonants, the stop, nasal and glide manner of articulation has been most frequently reported across languages (English: Davis & MacNeilage, 1995; Quichua: Gildersleeve-Neumann & Davis, 1998; Korean: Lee *et al.*, 2009; Swedish: Roug *et al.*, 1989). Coronals and labial places of articulation are described, but few dorsals are noted (Locke, 1983; Stoel-Gammon, 1985). Kern and Davis' (2009) recent report on a large-scale longitudinal study of Dutch, Romanian, Turkish, Tunisian Arabic and French children during canonical babbling indicated predominance of the oral stop manner of articulation and coronal followed by labial place of articulation. For place of articulation, however, French children produced more labials and French and Tunisian Arabic-learning children produced a large proportion of the [h] phoneme in contrast to the other language groups. Thus, although the children were largely similar, some cross-language differences were found by language group. These results need to be evaluated statistically relative to the frequency of occurrence of place and manner characteristics in each child's ambient language, as well as individual differences within language groups, to consider the onset and timing of learning from ambient language properties during canonical babbling (Kern & Davis, in preparation).

Vowels from the lower left quadrant of the vowel space (i.e. mid and low, front and central vowels) have most often been observed (Bickley, 1983; Buhr, 1980; Kent & Bauer, 1985; Davis & MacNeilage, 1995; Stoel-Gammon & Harrington, 1990). Kern and Davis (2009) also confirmed that mid and low, front and central vowels account overall for 66% of all vowels produced by children in the Dutch, Romanian, Turkish, Tunisian Arabic and French language environments studied. All other vowel types occurred at low frequencies in any language group.

The phenomenon of serial ordering is one of the most distinctive properties of speech production in languages (Maddieson, 1984). In a typical utterance, consonants and vowels never appear in isolation, but are produced serially. Within and across syllable patterns for consonants and vowels, syllables provide a site for considering the emergence of complexity in utterance structures relative to ambient language targets.

Three preferred within-syllable co-occurrence patterns have been reported in studies of serial properties; coronal (tongue tip closure) consonants with front vowels (e.g. 'di'), dorsal (tongue back closure) consonants with back vowels (e.g. 'ku') and labial (lip closure) consonants with central vowels (e.g. 'ba'). These widely observed serial patterns are predicted by the Frame-Content hypothesis (MacNeilage & Davis, 1990). The Frame-Content hypothesis proposes that the tongue does not move independently of the jaw within syllables, but remains in the same position for the consonant closure and the open or vowel portions of rhythmic cycles. Within-syllable consonant-vowel (CV) characteristics are based on these rhythmic jaw close-open-close cycles without independent movement of articulators independent of the jaw. Evidence for these serial patterns have also been found in analyses of English-learning children (Davis & MacNeilage, 1995), French, Swedish and Japanese infants from the Stanford Child Language database (Davis & MacNeilage, 2000), Brazilian-Portuguese-learning children (Teixiera & Davis, 2002), infants acquiring Quichua (Gildersleeve-Neumann & Davis, 1998) and Korean-learning infants (Lee et al., 2009). Some counterexamples to these CV co-occurrence trends have been reported (de Boysson-Bardies, 1993; Chen & Kent, 2005; Oller & Steffans, 1993; Tyler & Langsdale, 1996; Vihman, 1992). Kern and Davis (2009) found the predicted CV associations in four of the five languages they studied; Dutch infants were the exception to the general pattern observed across the five languages. Thus, the patterns of CV occurrence appear to predominate in production inventories but are not universal.

Vocalization patterns across syllables are also of importance to considering the emergence of vocal complexity. In languages, most words contain varied consonants and vowels across syllables; phonological reduplication, or repetition of the same syllable, is infrequent (Maddieson, 1984). By contrast, two types of canonical babbling in pre-linguistic infants have been described: reduplicated and variegated. Reduplicated or repeated syllables (e.g. 'baba') account for half or more of all vocal patterns in babbling (Davis & MacNeilage, 1995). In variegated forms, infants change vowels and/or consonants in two successive syllables (e.g. 'babi' or 'bada'). Several studies have shown concurrent use of both reduplication and variegation during babbling (Mitchell & Kent, 1990; Smith et al., 1989). In variegated babbling, more manner than place changes for consonants (Davis & MacNeilage, 1995, Davis et al., 2002) and more height than front-back changes for vowels have been shown during babbling (Davis & MacNeilage, 1995). The preference for manner changes for consonants and height changes for vowels is consistent with the Frame-Content hypothesis (MacNeilage & Davis, 1990).

The Kern and Davis (2009) analysis of five additional languages confirmed the prediction for co-occurrence of reduplication and variega-tion. While both reduplication and variegation occurred, infants preferred to repeat the same syllable within utterances more than variegate or produce different consonants and/or vowels. In variegated utterances, infants variegated more in the height than the front-back dimension for vowels. For consonants, manner exceeded place variegation. Both these tendencies indicate a predominance of jaw close-open variegation over tongue movement within utterances.

What about Children in Multilingual Environments?

There is a very small body of research on infants growing up in multilingual environments during the pre-linguistic babbling period. Recent perception studies of infants being raised in bilingual environments suggest that the 10-month time frame asserted for developing focus on native language contrasts for monolinguals (Werker & Tees, 1999) also characterizes infants in bilingual environments (Bosch & Sebastián-Gallés, 2003; Burns *et al.*, 2007; Kovacs & Mehler, 2009; Sundara *et al.*, 2008). Even though these infants receive diverse sound input from more than one language, they are able to focus on the ambient language patterns for each of those languages. Early and adaptable perceptual response by pre-linguistic infants indicates greater flexibility for attuning to all of the language-relevant input they receive rather than limitation and slowed development. Active engagement with the available input from their environment enables these early simultaneously exposed infants to achieve a robust beginning point for the later separation of multilingual input in their language-based listening and speaking experiences.

The literature on production patterns in infants in multilingual environments is sparse. Oller *et al.* (1997) showed similar onset and vocalization patterns during canonical babbling for 17 infants in a Spanish-English bilingual environment compared to their monolingual peers. Poulin-Dubois and Goodz (2001) found that French-English bilingual infants did not babble differently in English or French communication contexts. Zlatic *et al.* (1997) found that twins in an English-Serbian bilingual input environment showed the same vocalization patterns documented for monolingual children (Kern & Davis, 2009). Thus, the small literature available on output patterns in this period suggests that during the pre-linguistic babbling period, infants may exhibit common patterns in output at the same time that they are developing flexible perceptual processing for the languages that they are exposed to.

Early Ambient Language Effects

In the context of strong common patterns across languages in their output systems based on the available research for this period, young children have exhibited abilities to learn rapidly from language input regularities as early as 8–10 months. In contrast to most speech production paradigms, perception results related to narrowing of perceptual responses toward ambient language properties are based on children's responses in experimental laboratory settings (e.g. Saffran *et al.*, 1996; Werker & Lalonde, 1988). Appearance of ambient language influences in production repertoires has been examined for utterance and syllable structures (de Boysson-Bardies, 1993; Kopkalli-Yavuz & Topbaç, 2000), vowel and consonant repertoires and distribution (de Boysson-Bardies *et al.*, 1989, 1992) as well as CV co-occurrence preferences (e.g. Lee *et al.*, 2009).

Some studies of the early appearance of ambient language regularities have focused on adult capacities for perception of differences in children from different language environments. Thevenin *et al.* (1985) failed to find support for adults' ability to discriminate the babbling of 7- to 14-month-old English- and Spanish-learning infants. De Boysson-Bardies *et al.* (1984) presented naïve adults with sequences of early babbling of French, Arabic and Cantonese infants. Adults were able to correctly identify language differences at 6 and 8 months, but not babbling of 10-month-olds.

Other studies targeting the acoustic and phonetic properties of infants' babbling output have provided some support for early ambient language learning. De Boysson-Bardies *et al.* (1989) compared vocalizations of French, English, Cantonese and Algerian 10-month-olds. Based on computation of mean vowels (i.e. mean F1 and F2), they proposed that the acoustic vowel distribution was significantly different for the four language groups. De Boysson-Bardies *et al.* (1992) also suggested an early influence of the language environment on consonants in the four languages. They found significant differences in the distribution of place and manner of articulation across languages. Levitt and Utman (1992) compared one French and one English-learning infant. Each infant's consonant inventory moved toward their own ambient language in composition and frequency; both infants showed a closest match to the ambient frequencies at 5 months. In general, available studies are limited in the size of the databases and number of participants, so conclusions must be considered as needing further confirmation.

Strongly consistent trends in production patterns as well as preliminary indications about the timing of learning from ambient language input are apparent. Appearance of vocalization patterns related to the child's precise ambient language suggests that infants are implementing powerful learning mechanisms in the service of increasing precision relative to ambient language patterns (e.g. Cheor *et al.*, 1998). Available data indicate relatively few clear exemplars of ambient language learning in the context of strong common tendencies across languages (e.g. Kern & Davis, 2009). However, it should be noted that empirical investigations of early ambient language learning do not provide strong evidence because of methodological issues (e.g. adult perceptual studies vs. infant production patterns, amount of data analyzed, age of observation, number of participants, longitudinal vs. cross-sectional data collection and phonetic transcription vs. acoustic analysis). To evaluate the emergence of early learning from the ambient language more fully, it must be considered in the context of common production patterns seen across languages. Larger cohorts of children in varied language environments illustrating diverse ambient language targets are necessary. Consistent data collection and analysis procedures are also essential to comprehensively evaluate this question.

Applications of Complexity Perspectives on Canonical Babbling to Assessment and Intervention for Speech Sound Disorders

Studying canonical babbling is also important insofar as it has been shown that late onset of canonical babbling or atypical babbling may serve as a valid predictor of subsequent speech sound disorder or delay. Oller *et al.* (1999) showed that infants with delayed canonical babbling had smaller production vocabularies at 18, 24 and 30 months than infants in a control group. Moreover, a relatively large group of studies reported late or deviant babbling in language or language-related impaired children. Babbling and first words in children with Down syndrome was shown to emerge later than in children with typical development (Cobo-Lewis *et al.*, 1996). *Late-talkers* are children whose babbling is described as being composed of a restricted phonetic repertoire and simple syllabic structures (e.g. Fasolo *et al.*, 2007). Children with repaired cleft palate produce different vocalization patterns than typically developing children: babbling is less frequent and their phonetic repertoire and syllable combinations are smaller (Salas *et al.*, 2003; Scherer *et al.*, 2008).

Considerations of the course of planning and carrying out assessment and intervention procedures have recently emphasized the importance of considerations of the World Health Organization framework for health and wellness (WHO, 2007). It supports the kind of diverse framework for intervention connoted by the emergence approach to understanding the development of the phonological component of language proposed here. In addition, the preponderance of research evidence over a number of years in widely diverse research disciplines supports the view that speech and language capacities are acquired as a process that includes learning to deploy speech forms to convey intentions to supportive communication partners. Ideally, young children will have multiple interactive opportunities per day that will help them to understand the need and importance of using their vocal systems to get what they want and need. Clearly, phonological acquisition is driven by physical maturation, but equally importantly, it is facilitated by the social and cognitive capacities of the child. Crucially, speech and language acquisition does not proceed via decontextualized 'practice' of component physical abilities. The child must deploy those physical abilities for vocalizations connected with meaning in multiple social interactions with supportive communication partners. To accomplish the social component of communication, the child must have the cognitive capacities for understanding why he wants to communicate and for understanding who to communicate with. In chronologically or developmentally young children who cannot consistently comply with decontextualized drill activities, embedding assessment and intervention protocols in natural communication contexts is crucial to provide the support to optimize their phonological capacities in the context of their general language abilities.

References

Bickley, C. (1983) Acoustic evidence for phonological development of vowels in young infants. Paper presented at the 10th Congress of Phonetic Sciences, Utrecht.

Boliek, C.A., Hixon, T.J., Watson, P.J. and Jones, P.B. (2009) Refinement of speech breathing in healthy 4–6 year old children. *Journal of Speech, Language, and Hearing Research* 52 (4), 990–1007.

Bosch, L. and Sebastián-Gallés, N. (2003) Simultaneous bilingualism and the perception of a language-specific vowel contrast in the first year of life. *Language and Speech* 46 (2), 217–243.

Buhr, R.D. (1980) The emergence of vowels in an infant. *Journal of Speech and Hearing Research* 12, 73–94.

Burns, T.C., Yoshida, K.A., Hill, K. and Werker, J.F. (2007) The development of phonetic representation in bilingual and monolingual infants. *Applied Psycholinguistics* 28 (3), 455–474.

Camazine, S., Deneuborg, J-L., Franks, N.R., Sneyd, J., Theraulaz, G. and Bonabeau, E. (2003) *Self-organization in Biological Systems*. Princeton, NJ: Princeton University Press.

Chen, L-M. and Kent, R.J. (2005) Consonant–vowel co-occurrence patterns in Mandarin-learning infants. *Journal of Child Language* 32, 507–534.

Cheour, M., Ceponiene, R., Lehtokoski, A., Luuk, A., Jüri Allik, J., Kimmo Alho, K. and Näätänen, R. (1998) Development of language-specific phoneme representations in the infant brain. *Nature Neuroscience* 1, 351–353.

Chitoran, I., Coupé, C., Marsico, E. and Pellegrino, F. (2009) *Approaches to Phonological Complexity*. Berlin: Mouton de Gruyter.

Cobo-Lewis, A.B., Oller, D.K., Lynch, M.P. and Levine, S.L. (1996) Relations of motor and vocal milestones in typically developing infants and infants with Down syndrome. *American Journal of Mental Retardation* March (5), 456–467.

Davis, B.L. and Bedore, L. (in preparation) *Knowing and Doing: An Emergence Approach to Speech Acquisition*. New York: Routledge.

Davis, B.L. and MacNeilage, P.F. (1995) The articulatory basis of babbling. *Journal of Speech and Hearing Research* 38, 1199–1211.

Davis, B.L. and MacNeilage, P.F. (2000) An embodiment perspective on the acquisition of speech perception. *Phonetica* 57 (special issue), 229–241.

Davis, B.L., MacNeilage, P.F. and Matyear, C.L. (2002) Acquisition of serial complexity in speech production: A comparison of phonetic and phonological approaches to first word production. *Phonetica* 59, 75–107.

de Boysson-Bardies, B. (1993) Ontogeny of language-specific syllabic production. In B. de Boysson-Bardies, S. de Schoen, P. Jusczyk, P.F. MacNeilage and J. Morton (eds) *Developmental Neurocognition: Speech and Face Processing in the First Year of Life* (pp. 353–363). Dordrecht: Kluwer Academic.

de Boysson-Bardies, B., Halle, P., Sagart, L. and Durand, C. (1989) A cross linguistic investigation of vowel formants in babbling. *Journal of Child Language* 16, 1–17.

de Boysson-Bardies, B., Sagart, L. and Durant, C. (1984) Discernible differences in the babbling of infants according to target language. *Journal of Child Language* 11 (1), 1–15.

de Boysson-Bardies, B., Vihman, M.M., Roug-Hellichius, L., Durand, C., Landberg, I. and Arao, F. (1992) Evidence of infant selection from target language: A cross linguistic phonetic study. In C.A. Ferguson, L. Menn and C. Stoel-Gammon (eds) *Phonological Development: Models, Research, Implications* (pp. 369–392). Monkton, MD: York Press.

Dolata, J.K., Davis, B.L. and MacNeilage, P.F. (2008) Characteristics of the rhythmic organization of babbling: Implications for an amodal linguistic rhythm. *Infant Behavior and Development* 31, 422–431.

Fasolo, M., Majorano, M. and D'Odorico, L. (2007) Babbling and first words in children with slow expressive development. *Clinical Linguistics and Phonetics* 21 (2), 83–94.

Gildersleeve-Neumann, C. and Davis, B.L. (1998) Production versus ambient language influences on speech development in Quichua. Paper presented at the Annual Meeting of the American Speech, Hearing and Language Association, San Antonio, TX.

Green, J.R., Moore, C.A. and Reilly, K.J. (2002) The sequential development of jaw and lip control for speech. *Journal of Speech, Language, and Hearing Research* 45, 66–79.

Jakobson, R. (1941) *Child Language, Aphasia and Phonological Universals*. The Hague: Mouton.

Kent, R.D. and Bauer, H.R. (1985) Vocalizations of one-year olds. *Journal of Child Language* 12, 491–526.

Kern, S. and Davis, B.L. (2009) Emergent complexity in early vocal acquisition: Cross-linguistic comparisons of canonical babbling. In I. Chitoran, C. Coupé, E. Marsico and F. Pellegrino (eds) *Approaches to Phonological Complexity* (pp. 353–376). Berlin: Mouton de Gruyter.

Kern, S. and Davis, B.L. (in preparation) First steps into language complexity: Cross language patterns in canonical babbling. *Monographs of the Society for Research in Child Language*.

Kern, S., Davis, B. and Zink, I. (2010) From babbling to first words in four languages: Common trends, cross language and individual differences. In J.M. Hombert and F. d'Errico (eds) *Becoming Eloquent* (pp. 205–232). Amsterdam: John Benjamins.

Kovacs, A.M. and Mehler, J. (2009) Flexible learning of multiple speech structures in bilingual infants. *Science* 325 (5940), 611–612.

Kopkalli-Yavuz, H. and Topbaş, S. (2000) Infant's preferences in early phonological acquisition: How does it reflect sensitivity to the ambient language? In A. Göksel and C. Kerslake (eds) *Studies on Turkish and Turkic Languages* (pp. 289–295). Wiesbaden: Harrassowitz.

Lee, S., Davis, B.L. and MacNeilage, P.F. (2009) Universal production patterns and ambient language influences in babbling: A cross-linguistic study of Korean- and English-learning infants. *Journal of Child Language* 35, 591–617.

Levitt, A.G. and Utman, J.G.A. (1992) From babbling towards the sound systems of English and French: A longitudinal case study. *Journal of Child Language* 19, 19–49.

Locke, J.L. (1983) *Phonological Acquisition and Change*. New York: Academic Press.

MacNeilage, P.F. and Davis, B.L. (1990) Acquisition of speech production: Frames, then content. In M. Jeannerod (ed.) *Attention and Performance XIII: Motor Representation and Control* (pp. 453–476). Hillsdale, NJ: Lawrence Erlbaum.

Maddieson, I. (1984) *Pattern of Sounds*. Cambridge: Cambridge University Press.

Oller, D.K. (2000) *The Emergence of the Speech Capacity*. Mahwah, NJ: Lawrence Erlbaum.

Oller, D.K. and Steffans, M.L. (1993) Syllables and segments in infant vocalizations and young child speech. In M. Yavaş (ed.) *First and Second Language Phonology* (pp. 45–62). San Diego, CA: Singular Publishing.

Oller, D.K., Eilers, R.E. and Basinger, D. (2001) Intuitive identification of infant vocal sounds by parents. *Developmental Science* 4 (1), 49–60.

Oller, D.K., Eilers, R.E., Neal, A.R. and Schwartz, H.K. (1999) Precursors to speech in infancy: The prediction of speech and language disorders. *Journal of Communication Disorders* 32, 223–245.

Oller, D.K., Eilers, R.E., Urbano, R. and Cobo-Lewis, A.B. (1997) Development of precursors to speech in infants exposed to two languages. *Journal of Child Language* 24 (2), 407–425.

Poulin-Dubois, D. and Goodz, N. (2001) Language differentiation in bilingual infants: Evidence from babbling. In J. Cenoz and F. Genesee (eds) *Trends in Bilingual Acquisition* (pp. 95–106). Amsterdam: John Benjamins.

Roug, L., Landburg, I. and Lundburg, L. (1989) Phonetic development in early infancy: A study of four Swedish infants during the first eighteen months of life. *Journal of Child Language* 17, 19–40.

Saffran, J.R., Aslin, R.N. and Newport, E.L. (1996) Statistical learning by 8-month-old infants. *Science* 274, 1926–1928.

Salas-Provance, M.B., Kuehn, D.P. and Marsh, J.L. (2003) Phonetic repertoire and syllable characteristics of 15-month-old babies with cleft palate. *Journal of Phonetics* 31, 23–38.

Scherer, N.J., Williams, A.L. and Proctor-Williams, K. (2008) Early and later vocalization skills in children with and without cleft palate. *International Journal of Pediatric Otorhinolaryngology* 72, 827–840.

Smith, B.L., Brown-Sweeney, S. and Stoel-Gammon, C. (1989) A quantitative analysis of reduplicated and variegated babbling. *First Language* 17, 147–153.

Stoel-Gammon, C. (1985) Phonetic inventories 15–24 months: A longitudinal study. *Journal of Speech and Hearing Research* 28, 505–512.

Stoel-Gammon, C. and Harrington, P. (1990) Vowel systems of normally developing and phonologically disordered infants. *Clinical Linguistics and Phonetics* 4, 145–160.

Teixeira, E.R. and Davis, B.L. (2002) Early sound patterns in the speech of two Brazilian Portuguese speakers. *Language and Speech* 45 (2), 179–204.

Thevenin, D.M., Eilers, R.E., Oller, D.K. and Lavoie, L. (1985) Where is the drift in babbling? A cross-linguistic study. *Applied Psycholinguistics* 6, 1–15.

Tomasello, M. (2003) *Constructing a Language: A Usage-based Theory of Language Acquisition*. Cambridge, MA: Harvard University Press.

Tyler, A.A. and Langsdale, T.E. (1996) Consonant-vowel interaction in early phonological development. *First Language* 16, 159–191.

Vihman, M.M. (1992) Early syllables and the construction of phonology. In C.A. Ferguson, L. Menn and C. Stoel-Gammon (eds) *Phonological Development: Models, Research, Implications* (pp. 393–422). Monkton, MD: York Press.

Vihman, M.M., Ferguson, C.A. and Elbert, M.F. (1986) Phonological development from babbling to speech: Common tendencies and individual differences. *Applied Psycholinguistics* 7, 3–40.

Vihman, M.M., Macken, M.A., Miller, R., Simmons, H. and Miller, J. (1985) From babbling to speech: A re-assessment to the continuity issue. *Language* 61, 397–445.

Werker, J.F. and Curtin, S. (2005) PRIMR: A developmental framework of infant speech processing, *Language Learning and Development* 1 (2), 197–234.

Werker, J.F. and Lalonde, C.E. (1988) Cross language speech perception: Initial capabilities and developmental change. *Developmental Psychology* 24, 672–683.

Werker, J. and Tees, R. (1999) Influences on infant speech processing: Toward a new synthesis. *Annual Review of Psychology* 50, 509–535.

World Health Organization (2007) *International Classification of Functioning, Disability, and Health: Children and Youth Version*. Geneva: Author.

10 Typical and Atypical Multilingual Speech Acquisition

Brian A. Goldstein and Sharynne McLeod

Languages mentioned: *Arabic, Cantonese, Dutch, English, Farsi, French, German, Gujarati, Hindi, Hungarian, Italian, Maltese, Mirpuri, Norwegian, Pakistani heritage languages, Putonghua, Romanian, Russian, Samoan, Spanish, Swedish, Urdu, Welsh*

> *As SLPs increasingly assess and treat children from varying linguistic backgrounds, knowledge of typical acquisition must expand beyond descriptions of developmental milestones based predominantly on studies of English*
> Davis (2007: 51)

Historically, the focus of studies of speech acquisition in bilingual children was to compare their skills to monolingual children (e.g. Watson, 1991). The finding from these studies was that speech acquisition was slower in both typically developing multilingual children and those with speech sound disorders (SSD)[1] compared with monolingual children. However, recently, the finding of slower speech acquisition in multilingual children has been shown to be both accurate and inaccurate. That is, in comparison to monolingual children, multilingual children exhibit speech sound skills that are less advanced (i.e. negative transfer) and more advanced (i.e. positive transfer) than their monolingual peers. Moreover, results from those studies have indicated that speech sound skills are not simply mirror images of each other in the two languages, but are distributed somewhat differently in each constituent language, owing to the phonotactic properties of the languages being acquired. The purpose of this chapter is to examine positive transfer, negative transfer and cross-linguistic effects during the course of speech sound development and disorders in multilingual children.

Positive Transfer

Positive transfer (i.e. speech sound development that emerges at a faster rate in bilingual children than in monolingual children) is not often associated with speech sound development in multilingual children relative to their monolingual counterparts. However, research exists indicating such an outcome. Such an effect has been found in German-Spanish and Maltese-English bilingual children in comparison to their monolingual peers. Kehoe *et al.* (2001) and Lleó *et al.* (2003) found a higher rate of coda production in the Spanish productions of Spanish-German bilinguals than in those of monolingual Spanish-speaking children. Grech and Dodd (2008) found that 2- to 6-year-olds exposed to Maltese and English at home showed more advanced phonological skills (in terms of consonant accuracy, consistency and fewer number of error patterns) in comparison to monolingual children.

Fabiano-Smith and Goldstein (2010) extended the definition of positive transfer to include findings that 3-year-old bilingual children exhibited speech sound skills that were *similar* (i.e. commensurate), although not identical, to those of monolinguals. The theory behind this extension was that positive transfer should include similar skills in both groups given that multilingual children seemed to acquire multiple speech sound systems in roughly the same amount of time that monolinguals acquired one system. Such examples of this extension of positive transfer are numerous. For example, positive transfer has been noted in that the speech sound skills (as measured by consonant accuracy, vowel accuracy, accuracy of syllable types and whole-word measures) of 3-, 4- and 5-year-old Spanish-English bilingual children did not differ significantly from those of monolingual peers (e.g. Arnold *et al.*, 2004; Fabiano-Smith & Goldstein, 2010; Goldstein & Bunta, in press; Goldstein & Washington, 2001). Moreover, error patterns (percentage-of-occurrence on phonological patterns) (Goldstein & Washington, 2001), substitution types (Goldstein *et al.*, 2005) and syllable-level errors (Gildersleeve-Neumann & Wright, 2009, in Russian-English bilingual children ages 3; 3–5;7) were also found not to differ across bilingual and monolingual children. Studies examining bilingual children with SSD who spoke Spanish-English (Goldstein, 2000), Mirpuri-English, Urdu-English (Holm *et al.*, 1998) and Italian-English (Holm & Dodd, 1999) also generally showed positive transfer. Results showed error patterns (e.g. backing, devoicing, final consonant deletion, stopping and weak syllable deletion) that were exhibited with similar error rates in terms of percentages-of-occurrence across groups.

Negative Transfer

As mentioned previously, researchers and practitioners have expected negative transfer (i.e. speech sound development emerges at a slower rate in multilingual children than in monolingual children) in the speech sound skills of multilingual children. Evidence for such a hypothesis is replete in the literature. In a group of Cantonese-English-speaking bilingual children (ages 26–67 months), Holm and Dodd (2006) found that the phonetic inventories of the majority of bilingual children were not age-appropriate compared to monolinguals, in that their repertoires were not as robust. Results from typically developing Spanish-English bilingual children showed that they exhibited lower accuracy and a higher number of errors than their English and Spanish monolingual counterparts, although there were many similarities in error patterns and phonetic inventory as well (Gildersleeve-Neumann *et al.*, 2008). Goldstein and Washington (2001) found that typically developing Spanish-English bilingual children exhibited significant differences from monolinguals on some sound classes (e.g. spirants, flap and trill), but not on others (e.g. stops, nasals and fricatives). Gildersleeve *et al.* (1996) examined the English speech sound skills of typically developing bilingual (English-Spanish) 3-year-olds. Results indicated that the bilingual children showed an overall lower intelligibility rating, made more consonant and vowel errors and produced more uncommon error patterns than either monolingual English or monolingual Spanish speakers. The bilingual children also exhibited error patterns found in both languages (e.g. cluster reduction) and those that were not exhibited by either monolingual Spanish speakers (e.g. final consonant devoicing) or monolingual English speakers (e.g. initial consonant deletion). Thus, the English speech sound skills of bilingual children were not found to be commensurate with monolingual peers. In Spanish-English bilingual children with SSDs, Goldstein (2000) found that consonant accuracy in Spanish was commensurate with monolingual Spanish norms (Goldstein & Iglesias, 1996); however, consonant accuracy was higher in the English of bilingual children than monolingual English norms (Shriberg & Kwiatkowski, 1994).

Although these studies seem to show negative transfer in the speech sound skills of multilingual children, they are limited in that they are cross-sectional studies. There are few longitudinal studies in this area to show the progression of speech sound skills in this population. That said, Gildersleeve-Neumann and Davis (1998) examined English speech sound skills at the beginning and end of the school year of 27 typically developing 3-year-old bilingual (English-Spanish) children and compared them to the phonological skills of 14 typically developing monolingual 3-year-old English speakers and 6 typically developing 3-year-old monolingual Spanish speakers. The bilingual children exhibited, on average, a higher percentage-of-occurrence for 6 of the 10 error patterns analyzed (cluster reduction, backing, final consonant deletion, final devoicing, initial voicing and stopping) than either the monolingual English or monolingual Spanish speakers. These results indicated that the bilingual children demonstrated different developmental patterns than their monolingual peers and exhibited more errors than monolingual speakers in testing at the beginning of the school year. However, these differences decreased over time, and when they were tested at the end of the school year, again in English, their phonological skills were commensurate with those of their monolingual peers. Holm and Dodd (2006) also found such an effect in the longitudinal study of a Cantonese-English-speaking bilingual child. Thus, speech sound skills measured over time for all three groups were similar, suggesting that all will reach an adult-like system in English with exposure and practice.

In summary, studies examining the speech sound skills of typically developing multilingual children and those with SSD have shown evidence for both positive and negative transfer. Moreover, there is evidence for both types of transfer in the same group of multilingual children (e.g. Fabiano-Smith & Goldstein, 2010). This finding indicates that the speech sound skills of multilingual children are, at the same time, more advanced and less advanced than monolingual children, depending on the specific aspect of the system being investigated. It also argues for taking a multifactorial perspective into account when examining the speech sound skills of multilinguals. That is, it is paramount to examine a variety of speech sound outcomes in these children and compare those outcomes to monolinguals matched on a variety of socio-linguistic variables.

Distributed Skills in Each Language

The studies summarized above indicate that positive and negative transfer occur in the speech sound systems of multilingual children. Research indicating positive or negative transfer does not mean that skills are identical in each of the constituent languages. It is likely that speech sound skills are distributed in each of the two languages. Studies examining typically developing children and those with SSD have found such distributed skills. For example, Holm and Dodd (2006) found that in a group of Cantonese-English bilingual children, consonant accuracy in Cantonese was not significantly different from monolinguals, but was so in English compared to monolinguals. Bunta *et al.* (2009) investigated phonological whole-word measures (pMLU and proximity; Ingram, 2002) and consonant accuracy in 3-year-old typically developing Spanish-English bilingual and monolingual children. Differences were found on each measure (whole-word measures and consonant accuracy) between bilinguals and monolinguals in English; however, in Spanish, only consonant accuracy displayed differences between bilinguals and monolinguals. This finding suggested a distribution of skills across the two languages.

Such a distribution has also been noted in the speech sound skills of children with SSD. Goldstein *et al.* (2008) examined speech sound skills in 18 Spanish-English bilingual children with SSD, ranging in age from 39 to 68 months (mean = 45 months). Results indicated significant differences between languages for vowel accuracy, stop and nasal accuracy, early- and late-developing sounds accuracy, and percentages-of-occurrence for stopping, gliding, final consonant devoicing and fronting. Moreover, across most measures, accuracy tended to be higher in Spanish than in English. Finally, percentages-of-occurrence for phonological patterns were higher for some patterns in English (gliding and final consonant devoicing) and some in Spanish (unstressed syllable deletion, stopping). These results indicate that bilingual children with SSD exhibited distributed phonological skills in their two languages in that their skills are similar, although not identical, in each of the languages, and had skills that conformed to the phonotactic characteristics of the two languages.

Language Experience, Language Ability and Speech Sound Skills

It is well know that there are social and linguistic factors that impinge on speech sound development (see Cruz-Ferreira, Chapter 2). In the case of speech sound development, one such important mitigating factor is language dominance – often defined as 'language of greatest exposure' (Paradis, 2001: 24). A number of studies have examined language dominance in relation to speech sound skills. In examining syllable omissions in French-English bilingual 2-year-olds, Paradis (2001) found that in producing four-syllable target words, English-dominant bilinguals preserved a higher frequency of second syllables than did French-dominant bilinguals. Conversely, French-dominant bilinguals preserved a higher frequency of third syllables than did English-dominant bilinguals. Ball *et al.* (2001) found that the production of the trill /r/ in a group of Welsh-English bilingual children (aged 2;6–5;0) showed different patterns of acquisition depending on language dominance. In their study, Welsh-dominant children acquired the trill earlier than their English-dominant peers.

Such a relationship between language dominance and speech sound skills has not been found in all studies of bilingual children. For example, in a group of simultaneous bilingual Cantonese- and Putonghua-speaking children, aged 2;6–4;11, Law and So (2006) found that Cantonese phonology was acquired earlier than Putonghua phonology regardless of language dominance. However, they also found dominance effect in that Putonghua-dominant children outperformed their Cantonese-dominant peers in Putonghua phonology and Cantonese-dominant children outperformed their Putonghua-dominant peers in Cantonese phonology. In the Goldstein *et al.* (2005) study of 15 typically developing 5-year-old children (five predominantly English speaking, five predominantly Spanish speaking and five Spanish-English bilingual children), there were no significant correlations between language experience as measured by parent report (i.e. frequency of output in each language/how often the children spoke each language) and phonological skills (segmental and syllabic accuracy and percentage-of-occurrence of phonological patterns). Moderate to large effect sizes were found, however, for the effect of language experience on phonological skills. Those effects, however, differed by language. Specifically, there were moderate to large effect sizes of language experience on the accuracy of stops and affricates in English stops and on final voicing in Spanish.

Finally, Goldstein *et al.* (2010) investigated more narrowly defined aspects of language dominance in 50 typically developing Spanish-English bilingual children (mean age = 5;9). Instead of attempting to determine the effect of only one measure, language dominance, on phonological skills, they examined multiple aspects of language experience (parent-reported estimates of frequency of output and language use) and language ability (parent-reported estimates of language proficiency and mean length of utterance-words, MLUw) on phonological skills. Results indicated that the different measures of language experience and language ability had differential effects on segmental accuracy. For example, parent-reported estimates of frequency of output (i.e. the percentage of time the children spoke each language) did not significantly predict segmental accuracy, although parent-reported estimates of language use, parent-reported estimates of language proficiency and MLUw did. Moreover, these effects differed by language. For example, the language experience and language ability variables had an effect on consonant accuracy in Spanish and in English, but only on vowel accuracy in Spanish, and not in English.

Results from these studies indicate that socio-linguistic variables are important to consider in understanding speech sound development in multilingual children. It is likely, however, that these variables will need to extend beyond an omnibus measure of language dominance, as that measure might not be robust enough to account for variation in speech sound development in multilingual children.

Parent report and speech sound skills

One related socio-linguistic variable that has been varied with respect to speech acquisition in multilingual children is parent report. Given that there are relatively few assessment tools standardized on multilingual children (see McLeod, 2007 for a review), parent report of SSD might be at least a valuable tool in making a differential diagnosis of multilingual children with SSD. Studies examining the relationship between parent report and SSD have noted its validity.

Stertzbach and Gildersleeve-Neumann (2005) examined 24 preschool (3- and 4-year-old) Spanish-English children enrolled in Head Start. Results indicated a significant, positive correlation between overall results of the parent survey and vowel ($r = 0.70$) and consonant ($r = 0.69$) accuracy. Moderate and strong correlations were found between specific survey questions and vowel and consonant accuracy. The two questions with the strongest correlations were: *Do other people think your child is hard to understand?* and *Do other people think your child has speech problems?* This result held for all children. This study indicated that parents are sensitive to SSD in their children and that the perception of 'others' was especially critical in identifying SSD.

In another study, Lange *et al.* (2007) investigated the relationship between parental concern and phonological skills in 16 bilingual Spanish-English children (51–84 months). Participants were divided into two groups: experimental (children whose parents expressed concern about their children's speech) and control (children whose parents did not express concern). No significant differences were found between the control and experimental groups in terms of consonant and vowel accuracy, place of articulation and manner of articulation. Effect sizes were negligible or small for all comparisons. Descriptive analyses of error types and phonological error patterns revealed minor differences between groups and across languages. Thus, no clear identifying patterns emerged as diagnostic markers for parent concern. Overall, results from these studies indicated that parents can serve as a valid screener of their bilingual children's SSD as long as parents are asked how people *outside* the family view the child's speech.

Cross-linguistic Effects

One of the hallmarks of speech sound production in multilingual children is cross-linguistic effects, defined as the influence of one system on another (Ellis, 1997). These effects can be segmental and/or suprasegmental. For example, Amastae (1982) noted cross-linguistic effects in his daughter's use of the Spanish spirantization rule in which the voiced stops /b/, /d/ and /g/ become their spirant counterparts [ß], [ð] and [ɣ], respectively. Therefore, in her production of English, for example, she produced /warɚ/ (water) as [waðo]. He found, however, that cross-linguistic effects did not always occur, as exhibited by the production of her own name, *Laura*; '[b]y the time the English [wawa] had developed into [lowa], the Spanish was the correct form [laʷra]' (Amastae, 1982: 8). Children might also exhibit different rates of cross-linguistic effects. Schnitzer and Krasinski found high rates of cross-linguistic effects in one son (1994) but low rates in another son (1996).

It has often been assumed that the frequency of cross-linguistic effects is high. Studies examining phonological cross-linguistic effects seem to show otherwise. Fabiano and Goldstein (2005) examined the frequency and types of phonological cross-linguistic effects that occur over time in bilingual children. Three female, typically developing sequential bilingual Spanish-English-speaking children, aged 5;0, 6;2 and 7;0, participated. There were only eight occurrences of cross-linguistic effects across the three children. In a Farsi-English-speaking child, Keshavarz and Ingram (2002) noted that a few tokens of cross-linguistic effects occurred, but typically in linguistic situations in which only one of the languages dominated (e.g. when both parents spoke in English when having friends over who spoke only English). In a group of 5-year-old typically developing Spanish-English bilingual children, Goldstein *et al.* (2005) found that the frequency of cross-linguistic effects was 0.17% of all consonants produced by the children. Moreover, all of the effects were unidirectional – from English into Spanish. There were no examples in their English productions. Low rates of cross-linguistic effects have been found in other studies as well. In their study of the phonological skills of 3- to 4-year-old Spanish-English bilingual children, Gildersleeve-Neumann *et al.* (2008) found children who produced Spanish phonemes ([x], [ɣ] and [ß]) in their English. Gildersleeve-Neumann and Wright (2009) investigated the English phonological development of 14 Russian-English bilingual children and 28 English children, aged 3;3–5;7, exploring possible influences of Russian on English. Russian-influenced English cross-linguistic effects included palatalized consonants (e.g. /kʲ/) and the trill. The production of the palatalized consonant was relatively common in that at least two such consonants were produced by more than half (57%) of younger children and almost 90% (86%) of older children.

Overall, the results from these studies indicated that the frequency of cross-linguistic effects was largely low. Cross-linguistic effects specific to phonology encompass not only segmental features of a language (i.e. consonants and vowels), but also suprasegmental aspects (i.e. stress, pitch and intonation). For example, placement of stress in English is relatively complex and is determined by factors like syntactic category and weight of the syllable (i.e. whether the vowel is long or short and the number of consonants that follow the vowel) (Goodluck, 1991). Comparatively, stress assignment in Spanish is relatively predictable, most frequently on the penultimate syllable, e.g. *bicicleta* (bicycle). Thus, a native Spanish speaker who applies Spanish stress rules to English may stress words in English using Spanish rules; e.g. *taking* /ˈtekɪŋ/ → [teˈkɪŋ]. In another example, a native Cantonese speaker might produce English words and phrases with relatively equal stress given that syllables in Cantonese are produced with relatively equal stress (So, 2007).

There are few studies examining suprasegmental skills in multilingual children. Ng *et al.* (2010: 230) found that 'speaking F0 and F0 range values were significantly lower in Cantonese than in English. It is speculated that such difference is related to the tonal nature of Cantonese'. Bunta and Ingram (2007) examined speech rhythm in typically developing Spanish-English bilingual children and compared it to that in monolingual English-speaking children, monolingual Spanish-speaking children and Spanish-English bilingual adults. They determined that the children displayed speech rhythm patterns different from monolinguals in English but not in Spanish. However, they noted significant differences in speech rhythm in the English and Spanish of the bilingual children. These findings show further evidence for distributed properties by language in the phonological skills of bilingual children, as was noted previously for segmental characteristics.

Conclusion

Speech acquisition in children is a complex phenomenon, perhaps even more so in children acquiring more than one language. That complexity is related not only to the number and types of languages being acquired, but also to the socio-linguistic environment in which the languages are being learned. Despite those complexities, the extant literature on speech acquisition in multilingual children indicate the possibility of two (or more) highly interactive sound systems in multilingual children, with potential for both positive and negative transfer of information between languages and the possibility of cross-linguistic effects. Such interaction seems to result in overall speech sound development that is similar, but clearly not identical, to that of monolingual children. That similarity is especially clear if taken from a longitudinal perspective. That is, with the ability to hear and use all languages, speech sound development in multilingual children will be commensurate with that of their monolingual peers.

Note

(1) Speech sound disorders refers to both segment- and pattern-based errors

References

Amastae, J. (1982) Aspects of the bilingual acquisition of English and Spanish. *Journal of the Linguistic Association of the Southwest* 5, 5–19.

Arnold, E., Curran, C., Miccio, A. and Hammer, C. (2004, November) Sequential and simultaneous acquisition of Spanish and English consonants. Poster presented at the convention of the American Speech-Language-Hearing Association, Philadelphia, PA.

Ball, M.J., Müller, N. and Munro, S. (2001) The acquisition of rhotic consonants by Welsh-English bilingual children. *International Journal of Bilingualism* 5, 71–86.

Ballard, E. and Farao, S. (2008) The phonological skills of Samoan speaking 4-year-olds. *International Journal of Speech-Language Pathology* 10 (6), 379–391.

Berman, R.A. (1977) Natural phonological processes at the one-word stage. *Lingua* 43, 1–21.

Brice, A.E., Carson, C.K. and Dennis O'Brien, J. (2009) Spanish-English articulation and phonology of 4- and 5-year-old preschool children: An initial investigation. *Communication Disorders Quarterly* 31 (1), 3–14.

Bunta, F., Davidovich, I. and Ingram, D. (2006) The relationship between the phonological complexity of a bilingual child's words and those of the target languages. *International Journal of Bilingualism and Bilingual Education* 10, 71–86.

Bunta, F., Fabiano, L., Ingram, D. and Goldstein, B. (2009) Phonological whole-word measures in three-year-old bilingual children and their monolingual peers. *Clinical Linguistics and Phonetics* 23 (2), 156–175.

Bunta, F. and Ingram, D. (2007) The acquisition of speech rhythm by bilingual Spanish- and English-speaking 4- and 5-year-old children. *Journal of Speech, Language, and Hearing Research* 50, 999–1014.

Cataño, L., Barlow, J.A. and Moyna, M.I. (2009) A retrospective study of phonetic inventory complexity in acquisition of Spanish: Implications for phonological universals. *Clinical Linguistics and Phonetics* 23 (6), 446–472.

Davis, B. (2007) Applications of typical acquisition information to understanding of speech impairment. In S. McLeod (ed.) *The International Guide to Speech Acquisition* (pp. 50–54). Clifton Park, NY: Thomson Delmar Learning.

Dodd, B., So, L. and Li, W. (1996) Symptoms of disorder without impairment: The written and spoken errors of bilinguals. In B. Dodd, R. Campbell and L. Worrall (eds) *Evaluating Theories of Language* (pp. 119–136). London: Whurr.

Ellis, R. (1997) *Second Language Acquisition*. Oxford: Oxford University Press.

Fabiano, L. and Goldstein, B. (2005) Phonological cross-linguistic influence in sequential Spanish-English bilingual children. *Journal of Multilingual Communication Disorders* 3, 56–63.

Fabiano-Smith, L. and Barlow, J.A. (2010) Interaction in bilingual phonological acquisition: Evidence from phonetic inventories. *International Journal of Bilingual Education and Bilingualism* 13, 81–97.

Fabiano-Smith, L. and Goldstein, B.A. (2010) Early-, middle-, and late-developing sounds in monolingual and bilingual children: An exploratory investigation. *American Journal of Speech-Language Pathology* 19 (1), 66–77.

Fabiano-Smith, L. and Goldstein, B. (2010) Phonological acquisition in bilingual Spanish-English speaking children. *Journal of Speech, Language, and Hearing Research* 53, 160–178.

Faingold, E.D. (1996) Variation in the application of natural processes: Language-dependent constraints in the phonological acquisition of bilingual children. *Journal of Psycholinguistic Research* 25, 515–526.

Gildersleeve, C., Davis, B. and Stubbe, E. (1996, November) When monolingual rules don't apply: Speech development in a bilingual environment. Paper presented at the annual convention of the American Speech-Language-Hearing Association, Seattle, WA.

Gildersleeve-Neumann, C. and Davis, B. (1998, November) Learning English in a bilingual preschool environment: Change over time. Paper presented at the annual convention of the American Speech-Language-Hearing Association, San Antonio, TX.

Gildersleeve-Neumann, C., Kester, E., Davis, B. and Peña, E. (2008) English speech sound development in preschool-aged children from bilingual English-Spanish backgrounds. *Language, Speech, and Hearing Services in Schools* 39, 314–328.

Gildersleeve-Neumann, C.E. and Wright, K.E. (2010) English phonological acquisition in 3- to 5-year-old children learning Russian and English. *Language, Speech, and Hearing Services in Schools* 41, 429–444.

Goldstein, B. and Bunta, F. (in press) Positive and negative transfer in the phonological systems of bilingual speakers. *International Journal of Bilingualism*.

Goldstein, B., Bunta, F., Lange, J., Burrows, L., Pont, S. and Bennett, J. (2008, November) Interdependence in the phonological systems of bilingual children with speech sound disorders. Seminar presented at the convention of the American Speech-Language-Hearing Association, Chicago, IL.

Goldstein, B., Bunta, F., Lange, J., Rodriguez, J. and Burrows, L. (2010) The effects of measures of language experience and language ability on segmental accuracy in bilingual children. *American Journal of Speech-Language Pathology* 19, 238–247.

Goldstein, B., Fabiano, L. and Washington, P. (2005) Phonological skills in predominantly English, predominantly Spanish, and Spanish-English bilingual children. *Language, Speech, and Hearing Services in Schools* 36, 201–218.

Goldstein, B. and Iglesias, A. (1996) Phonological patterns in normally developing Spanish-speaking 3- and 4-year-olds of Puerto Rican descent. *Language, Speech, and Hearing Services in Schools* 27, 82–90.

Goldstein, B. and Washington, P. (2001) An initial investigation of phonological patterns in 4-year-old typically developing Spanish-English bilingual children. *Language, Speech, and Hearing Services in Schools* 32, 153–164.

Goodluck, H. (1991) *Language Acquisition: A Linguistic Introduction.* Oxford: Blackwell.

Gould, J. (2009) There is more to communication than tongue placement and 'show and tell': Discussing communication from a speech pathology perspective. *Australian Journal of Linguistics* 29 (1), 59–73.

Grech, H. and Dodd, B. (2008) Phonological acquisition in Malta: A bilingual learning context. *International Journal of Bilingualism* 12, 155–171.

Hochberg, J. (1988) First steps in the acquisition of Spanish stress. *Journal of Child Language* 15, 273–292.

Holm, A. and Dodd, B. (1999a) A longitudinal study of the phonological development of two Cantonese-English bilingual children. *Applied Psycholinguistics* 20, 349–376.

Holm, A. and Dodd, B. (1999b) Differential diagnosis of phonological disorder in two bilingual children acquiring Italian and English. *Clinical Linguistics and Phonetics* 13, 113–129.

Holm, A. and Dodd, B. (2006) Phonological development and disorder of bilingual children acquiring Cantonese and English. In Z. Hua and B. Dodd (eds) *Phonological Development and Disorders in Children: A Multilingual Perspective* (pp. 286–325). Clevedon: Multilingual Matters.

Holm, A., Dodd, B., Stow, C. and Pert, S. (1998) Speech disorder in bilingual children: Four case studies. *Osmania Papers in Linguistics* 22–23, 46–64.

Ingram, D. (2002) The measurement of whole-word productions. *Journal of Child Language* 29, 713–733.

Johnson, C. and Lancaster, P. (1998) The development of more than one phonology: A case study of a Norwegian-English bilingual child. *International Journal of Bilingualism* 2, 265–300.

Keshavarz, M. and Ingram, D. (2002) The early phonological development of a Farsi English bilingual child. *International Journal of Bilingualism* 6, 255–269.

Lange, J., Burrows, L. and Goldstein, B. (2007, February) Parent concern and phonological skills in Spanish-English bilingual children. Poster presented at the Texas Research Symposium on Language Diversity, Austin, TX.

Law, N.C.W. and So, L.K.H. (2010) The relationship of phonological development and language dominance in bilingual Cantonese-Putonghua children. *International Journal of Bilingualism* 10 (4), 405–427.

Lin, L-C. and Johnson, C.J. (2010) Phonological patterns in Mandarin-English bilingual children. *Clinical Linguistics and Phonetics* 24 (4–5), 369–386.

Lleó, C. and Kehoe, M. (2002) On the interaction of phonological systems in child bilingual acquisition. *International Journal of Bilingualism* 6, 233–237.

Lleó, C., Kuchenbrandt, I., Kehoe, M. and Trujillo, C. (2003) Syllable final consonants in Spanish and German monolingual and bilingual acquisition. In N. Müller (ed.) *(In)vulnerable Domains in Multilingualism* (pp. 191–220). Amsterdam: John Benjamins.

McLeod, S. (ed.) (2007) *The International Guide to Speech Acquisition.* Clifton Park, NY: Thomson Delmar Learning.

McLeod, S. (2010) Laying the foundations for multilingual acquisition: An international overview of speech acquisition. In M. Cruz-Ferreira (ed.) *Multilingual Norms* (pp. 53–71). Frankfurt: Peter Lang.

Munro, S., Ball, M.J., Müller, N., Duckworth, M. and Lyddy, F. (2005) The acquisition of Welsh and English phonology in bilingual Welsh-English children. *Journal of Multilingual Communication Disorders* 3, 24–49.

Ng, M., Hsueh, G. and Leung, C.S. (2010) Voice pitch characteristics of Cantonese and English produced by Cantonese-English bilingual children. *International Journal of Speech-Language Pathology* 12 (3), 230–236.

Paradis, J. (2001) Do bilingual two-year-olds have separate phonological systems? *International Journal of Bilingualism* 5 (1), 19–38.

Ray, J. (2002) Treating phonological disorders in a multilingual child: A case study. *American Journal of Speech-Language Pathology* 11 (3), 305–315.

Salameh, E.-K., Nettlebladt, U. and Norlin, K. (2003) Assessing phonologies in bilingual Swedish-Arabic children with and without language impairment. *Child Language Teaching and Therapy* 19, 338–364.

Schnitzer, M. and Krasinski, E. (1994) The development of segmental phonological production in a bilingual child. *Journal of Child Language* 21, 585–622.

Schnitzer, M. and Krasinski, E. (1996) The development of segmental phonological production in a bilingual child: A contrasting second case. *Journal of Child Language* 23, 547–571.

So, L. (2007) Cantonese speech acquisition. In S. McLeod (ed.) *The International Guide to Speech Acquisition* (pp. 313–326). Clifton Park, NY: Thomson Delmar Learning.

Stertzbach, J. and Gildersleeve-Neumann, C.E. (2005, November) Parent report as a screening tool of speech disorders in Spanish-speaking preschool children. Technical presentation presented at the annual convention of the American Speech-Language-Hearing Association, San Diego, CA.

Stow, C. and Pert, S. (2006) Phonological acquisition in bilingual Pakistani heritage children in England. In Zhu Hua and B. Dodd (eds) *Phonological Development and Disorders in Children: A Multilingual Perspective* (pp. 326–345). Clevedon: Multilingual Matters.

Vogel, I. (1975) One system or two: An analysis of a two-year-old Romanian-English bilingual's phonology. *Papers and Reports on Child Language Development* 9, 43–62.

Watson, I. (1991) Phonological processing in two languages. In E. Bialystok (ed.) *Language Processing in Bilingual Children* (pp. 25–48). Cambridge: Cambridge University Press.

Windsor, J., Kohnert, K., Lobitz, K.F. and Pham, G.T. (2010) Cross-language nonword repetition by bilingual and monolingual children. *American Journal of Speech-Language Pathology* 19, 298–310.

Yang, H-Y. and Hua, Z. (2010) The phonological development of a trilingual child: Facts and factors. *International Journal of Bilingualism* 14, 105–126.

Appendix

Studies of speech acquisition by typically developing multilingual children published in English

Languages	Country	Study	No. of children	Age of children
Arabic-Swedish	Sweden	Salameh *et al.* (2003)	20 = 10 typical bilingual children + 10 bilingual children with severe language impairment	3;10–6;7
Cantonese-English	UK	Dodd *et al.* (1996)	16 typical bilingual children	3–5 years
	Australia	Holm and Dodd (1999a)	2 typical bilingual children	2;3–3;1 and 2;9–3;5 years (longitudinal)
	Australia and UK	Holm and Dodd (2006)	56 typical bilingual children	2–5 years
	Canada	Ng *et al.* (2010)	86 typical bilingual children	5–15 years
Cantonese-Putonghua	Hong Kong and Shenzhen, China	Law and So (2006)	100 typical bilingual children	2;6–4;11
Farsi-English	UK and Iran	Keshavarz and Ingram (2002)	1 typical bilingual child	8–20 months
French-English	Canada	Paradis (2001)	53 typical children = 17 French-English bilingual children + 18 French monolingual and 18 English monolingual	23–35 months

German-Spanish	Germany	Lleó et al. (2003)	11 typical children = 3 monolingual German, 3 monolingual Spanish, 5 bilingual German-Spanish children	1;0–3;0
Hebrew-English	Israel	Berman (1977)	1 typical bilingual child	18–23.5 months
Hindi-Gujarati-English	USA	Ray (2002)	1 atypical trilingual child	5 years
Hungarian-English	USA	Bunta et al. (2006)	1 typical bilingual child	2;0
Pakistani heritage languages-English	UK	Stow and Pert (2006)	246 typical bilingual children = 129 Mirpuri + 63 Punjabi + 54 Urdu	1;4–7;11
Maltese-English	Malta	Grech and Dodd (2008)	241 typical children = 93 Maltese-English + 137 Maltese + 11 English	2;0–6;0
Mandarin-English	Taiwan	Lin and Johnson (2010)	48 typical children = 25 bilingual + 23 Mandarin	Bilingual mean = 5;0; monolingual mean = 5;3
Norwegian-English	Canada	Johnson and Lancaster (1998)	1 typical	1;2–1;8 (language); 1;9 (speech)
Romanian-English	USA	Vogel (1975)	1 typical	1;6–2;0

(Continued)

Appendix (*Continued*)

Languages	Country	Study	No. of children	Age of children
Russian-English	USA	Gildersleeve-Neumann and Wright (2010)	42 typical children = 14 Russian-English + 28 English	3;3–5;7
Samoan-English	New Zealand	Ballard and Farao (2008)	20 typical bilingual children	4;0–4;11
Spanish-English	USA	Brice *et al.* (2009)	16 typical Spanish-English children	4- to 5-years
	USA	Bunta *et al.* (2009)	24 typical children = 8 Spanish-English, 8 Spanish and 8 English children	3;0–4;0
	USA	Bunta and Ingram (2007)	30 typical children = 10 Spanish-English + 10 Spanish + 10 English	3;9–5;2
	USA+	Cataño *et al.* (2009)	39 inventories from 16 typical children = 6 Spanish-English + 10 Spanish	0;11–5;1
	USA	Fabiano-Smith and Goldstein (2010)	24 typical children = 8 Spanish-English + 8 English + 8 Spanish	3;0–4;0
	USA	Fabiano-Smith and Barlow (2010)	24 typical children = 8 Spanish-English + 8 English + 8 Spanish	3;0–4;0

Language	Country	Reference	Participants	Age
	USA	Fabiano and Goldstein (2005)	3 typical sequential bilingual Spanish-English-speaking children	5;0, 6;2 and 7;0
	USA	Gildersleeve-Neumann et al. (2008)	33 typical children = 20 bilingual (more English) + 3 bilingual (balanced) + 10 English	3;1–3;10
	USA	Goldstein and Bunta (2010)	30 typical children = 10 Spanish-English + 10 Spanish + 10 English	Mean age 5;10–6;0
	USA	Goldstein et al. (2010)	50 typical bilingual Spanish-English children	4;3–7;1
	USA	Goldstein et al. (2005)	15 typical children = 5 predominantly English speaking + 5 predominantly Spanish speaking + 5 Spanish-English bilinguals	5;0–5;5
	USA	Goldstein and Washington (2001)	12 typical bilingual Spanish-English children	4;0–4;11
Spanish-Mandarin-Taiwanese	Not specified (most likely Paraguay and Taiwan)	Yang and Hua (2010)	1 typical trilingual child	1;3–2;0

(Continued)

Appendix (*Continued*)

Languages	Country	Study	No. of children	Age of children
Spanish-Portuguese-Hebrew	Israel	Faingold (1996)	1 typical trilingual child (longitudinal) contrasted with another similar child	0;11–1;11
Welsh-English	Wales	Munro *et al.* (2005)	83 typical bilingual children	2;6–5;0
	Wales	Ball *et al.* (2001)	83 typical children = 44 Welsh dominant + 39 English dominant	2;6–5;0

11 Translation to Practice: Typical Bidialectal Speech Acquisition in Jamaica

Karla N. Washington

Languages mentioned: Jamaican English, Jamaican Creole

Context

The Jamaican diaspora has resulted in many Jamaicans living outside Jamaica. This exodus has facilitated the introduction of Jamaican culture in the forms of music, cuisine and language to immigrant English-speaking countries such as Canada, the UK and the USA. Jamaican Creole, also known as Patwa (or Patois), is a unique and well-known feature of Jamaican culture (Harry, 2006). Jamaican Creole is spoken by most Jamaicans, and scholars consider it to be one of the major Atlantic English-lexifier creoles used in the Caribbean (Harry, 2006). The aims of this chapter are to: (a) introduce Jamaican Creole, (b) discuss how Jamaican Creole has been recognized recently in Jamaica and (c) discuss what currently happens in Jamaica and other countries for Jamaican Creole-speaking children with speech sound disorders. This chapter will culminate with a brief discussion about the need for research on the acquisition/development of Jamaican Creole.

An Introduction to Jamaican Creole

The language situation in most Caribbean islands (e.g. Belize, Guyana, Jamaica and Trinidad & Tobago) is described as a post-Creole continuum (DeCamp, 1961; Irvine, 2004; Winford, 1997). These continua came about as a natural consequence of 'the historical sociolinguistic contact of speakers of Niger-Congo and speakers of several dialects of English' (Irvine, 2004: 42). Two polar language varieties (i.e. English – the *acrolect*, and Creole – the *basilect*) occur along these continua and are considered by linguistic scholars to be separate linguistic systems connected by middle occurring varieties, the *mesolect* (Winford, 1997). The term *diglossic* is used to characterize these types of language situations due to the high (acrolect) versus low (basilect) status assigned to the polar linguistic systems, each fulfilling specific communicative or social roles (Irvine, 2004).

In Jamaica, Jamaican English and Jamaican Creole are the two polar co-occurring language varieties. Jamaican English is putatively the 'Queen's English', the acrolect, and is used formally both in oral and written forms (Irvine, 2004). Alternately, Jamaican Creole, the basilect, is considered an oral language resulting from multiple etymologies, including English, West African and French languages (Cassidy, 1966), and is used informally (Irvine, 2004, 2008). Jamaicans are typically introduced to Jamaican Creole and Jamaican English from birth (Irvine, 2004; Meade, 2001), making them simultaneous language learners. Jamaican children therefore enter the school system speaking both Jamaican English and Jamaican Creole; however, the language of instruction in schools is Jamaican English (Brown-Blake, 2008; Irvine, 2004).

Jamaican Creole phonology consists of 33 different phonemes, comprising 21 consonants and 12 vowels (Devonish & Harry, 2004; Harry, 2006). Jamaican Creole consonants are similar to Jamaican English consonants having both voiced and voiceless cognates. However, major phonological differences exist between Jamaican Creole and Jamaican English due to specific phonological rules common to Jamaican Creole (Harry, 2006). These rules include /h/ deletion or insertion, palatalization of specific plosives, obstruent neutralization, obstruent weakening and labialization (see Harry, 2006, for a discussion). Jamaican Creole also has 12 phonemic vowels consisting of five short sounds, three long sounds (a combination of short vowels) and four diphthongs (see Devonish & Harry, 2004; Harry, 2006). Examples of sounds (Harry, 2006) present in Jamaican Creole that are not present in Jamaican English include: (a) the long vowel /aa/-/maaga/ for *skinny*; and (b) the long vowel /ua/-/buat/ for *boat*. Table 11.1 provides sample transcriptions for phonological processes common to Jamaican Creole.

Recognizing Jamaican Creole in Jamaica

Jamaican English is the official language spoken in Jamaica; however, most Jamaicans also speak Jamaican Creole (Brown-Blake, 2008). Because Jamaican English and Jamaican Creole are polar language varieties, a breakdown in communication between speakers of either language can occur. As a result of this breakdown, individuals who speak Jamaican Creole may experience discrimination on the basis of language use (Brown-Blake, 2008).

In May 2001, a proposal was made to the Joint Select Committee of the Parliament of Jamaica for the creation of a Charter of Rights (revision to the previous Bill of Rights), which would include protection from discrimination on the basis of language use (Brown-Blake, 2008). To support the right to non-discrimination, the committee recommended that a language planning agency be established to address issues (e.g. the monitoring of state agencies with respect to the non-discriminatory provision of services in Jamaican Creole or Jamaican English, public education on the language issue) related

Table 11.1 Sample transcriptions of phonological rules common to Jamaican Creole

Phonological rules[a]	Target	Broad transcription	Narrow transcription
/h/ deletion[b]: typically observed when /h/ occurs at the onset of the word.	*Hand*	/an/	[an]
/h/ insertion[c]: typically occurs in words beginning with a vowel.	*Eat*	/hiit/	[hiːt]
Palatalization: obstruents (e.g. /k, g, p/) are palatalized as a result of the co-occurrence restriction for a non-low front vowel and back vowel sequence.	*Guard, quarter quart (of rum)*	/giaad/, /kiuu/	[gʲaːd], [kʲuː]
Obstruent neutralization: occurs before a syllabic lateral, thus the contrast between the velar and alveolar stops is neutralized.	*Bottle*	/bakəl/	[bakl]
Obstruent weakening: occurs for voiced stops in word-initial position. Thus, /b, d, g/ become /ɓ, ɗ, ɠ/ particularly when they occur as onsets of 'prominent syllables'.	*Dog*	/dag/	[ɗag]
Labialization: occurs when obstruents precede a back vowel followed by a non-back vowel.	*Boy*	/buai/	[bʷai]

Note. Examples and phonological rules adapted from Harry (2006) and Irvine (2004, 2008).
[a]The status of /h/ in Jamaican Creole is such that it can also be retained (Devonish & Harry, 2004; Harry, 2006).
[b]The term /h/ dropping is also used to describe this phonological rule (Irvine, 2004).
[c]/h/ insertion is also described as hypercorrect use of /h/ and is restricted to word-initial position (Irvine, 2004).

to having two co-existing language varieties in Jamaica. The Jamaican Language Unit took effect in September 2002 as a language planning agency that fosters the examination of Jamaican Creole and Jamaican English in Jamaica.

Speech and Language Services

Government-funded speech-language pathology services are not available in Jamaican schools. Instead, parents of Jamaican Creole-speaking children who have speech sound disorders pay (at times using insurance providers) to access private speech and language services. In Jamaica, these services are offered by registered professionals with a Master's degree in speech therapy or a more advanced degree in speech pathology, who are regulated by the Council for Professions Supplementary to Medicine (Health Access Jamaica, 2010). Currently, no local institutions offer training for either degree (Health Access Jamaica, 2010).

The lack of government-funded services can pose a challenge to parents who do not have the resources to access services and yet have children who require them. Further, the absence of local institutions offering speech therapy programs could result in small numbers of available therapists to provide assessment and intervention services. In other migrant countries, such as Canada, the UK and the USA, however, children with speech sound disorders who speak Jamaican Creole can more readily access government-funded school-based speech and language services. However, they are likely to receive these services in the local variety of English rather than in Jamaican Creole. That said, it should be noted that in some migrant countries, the regulating licensing bodies for the profession of speech-language pathology (e.g. the College of Audiologists and Speech-Language Pathologists of Ontario, Canada) recognize Jamaican Creole as a possible language that speech-language pathologists provide speech and language services.

Research on Jamaican Creole Speech and Language Acquisition

Jamaican Creole is described as an oral language and, as such, there is little known about its acquisition. To date, there is no published peer-reviewed information about the acquisition and development of Jamaican Creole speech or language skills. The paucity of information on Jamaican Creole acquisition hampers the speech-language pathologist's ability to identify children who are typical, delayed or disordered in their development. As such, the provision of services when and where appropriate is negatively impacted, resulting in the inefficient use of available speech-language resources. Thus, research on Jamaican Creole acquisition and development is needed to guide service provision.

Final thoughts on Jamaican Creole

Jamaican Creole is a part of Jamaican culture that helps to distinguish Jamaicans from the rest of the Caribbean and the world. The dearth of information available on Jamaican Creole acquisition has resulted in the need for further investigation of this language and its people.

References

Brown-Blake, C. (2008) The right to linguistic non-discrimiation and creole language situations. *Journal of Pidgin and Creole Languages* 23 (1), 32–74.

Cassidy, F.G. (1966) Multiple etymologies in Jamaican creole. *American Speech* 41 (3), 211–215.

DeCamp, D. (1961) Social and geographic factors in Jamaican dialects. In R. LePage (ed.) *Creole Language Studies* (pp. 61–84). London: Macmillan.

Devonish, H. and Harry, O.G. (2004) Jamaican phonology. In B. Kortman and E.W. Shneider (eds) *A Handbook of Varieties of English,* vol 1: *Phonology* (pp. 441–471). Berlin: Moton De Gruyter.

Harry, O.G. (2006) Jamaican creole. *Journal of the International Phonetic Association* 36 (1), 125–131.

Health Access Jamaica (2010) Health access jamaica your premier health portal. http://www.healthaccessja.com/nmcms.php?content=About Us&show=1&type=about. Accessed 7.9.10.

Irvine, A. (2004) A good command of the English language: Phonological variation in the Jamaican acrolect. *Journal of Pidgin and Creole Languages* 19 (1), 41–76.

Irvine, A. (2008) Contrast and convergence in Standard Jamaican English: The phonological architecture of the Standard in an ideological bidilectal community. *World Englishes* 27 (1), 9–27.

Meade, R. (2001) Acquisition of Jamaican phonology. Unpublished dissertation, Netherlands Graduate School of Linguistics.

Winford, D. (1997) Re-examining Caribbean English creole continua. *World Englishes* 16 (2), 233–279.

12 Translation to Practice: Typical and Atypical Multilingual Speech Acquisition in Iceland

Thóra Másdóttir (Þóra Másdóttir)

Languages mentioned: English, Icelandic, Polish, Tagalog, Thai

In recent years, bilingualism and Icelandic as a second language (ISL) have received some attention (e.g. Arnbjörnsdóttir, 2007, 2008; Thórðardóttir, 2004); however, no studies are available concerning bilingual children needing speech-language pathology services. This chapter will shed light on some of the circumstances faced by children learning ISL. Furthermore, some general issues of speech-language pathology services in Iceland will be discussed.

The Icelandic Language

Icelandic is a North-Germanic language, bearing some similarities with other languages in the same family, such as Norwegian, Swedish, Danish and particularly Faroese. The Icelandic morphological system is more complex than in most other Germanic languages (Barðdal, 2001). Among the segmental and phonological variations that are considered specific to the Icelandic language are the voiceless sonorants (/m̥/, /n̥/, /ŋ̊/, /ɲ̊/, /ç/, /l̥/, /r̥/), and preaspiration (e.g. *dúkka* (doll) /tuhka/, *teppi* (blanket) /tʰɛhpɪ/) and aspiration contrast instead of a voicing contrast for stops (Árnason, 2005; Másdóttir, 2008). Language-specific phonological processes include h-isation (when obstruents are replaced with /h/), deaspiration (/pʰ/ → /p/) in word-initial position and dentalisation (/r/ → [ð]) (Másdóttir, 2008).

Are Icelandic children bilingual?

Prior to 1999, Danish was the first foreign language taught in Icelandic schools (Aðalnámskrá, 1999). Children start learning Danish in seventh grade (age 12). However, children generally are not exposed to Danish in their everyday life as much as they are to English (via television, etc.). Therefore, children are less proficient in Danish compared with English. Since 1999, English has been the first foreign language taught to Icelandic school children. Currently, most children start formal English lessons at the age of 9 or 10 years (Lefever, 2007), sometimes younger. Additionally, since children in Iceland are exposed to English in their daily lives (via television programs, movies), this strengthens their English language skills. When Icelandic children reach the teen years, most are at least 'slightly bilingual', using the definition of bilingualism from Valdés and Figueroa (1994: 115).

Icelandic as a second language

With a population of roughly 317,000 people (Statistics Iceland, 2010), the Icelandic nation is among the smallest in Europe. The population of the Reykjavik area accounts for nearly 60% of the nation's inhabitants. Approximately 35,000 inhabitants are of a 'foreign origin' (Statistics Iceland, 2010). The number of immigrants has increased significantly over the last 10 years, especially with the growing number of immigrants from Poland, which is related to Iceland's participation in the Schengen agreement, activated in 2001. Despite the Icelandic economic crisis over the last two years, the number of immigrants returning to their homelands has been less than anticipated. In the last 10 years, the number of children of foreign origin has increased considerably, from 676 to 2717, from preschool-age children throughout primary/secondary schools (grades 1–10). Although there has been an increase among immigrants in general, the Polish community has grown the most (other common foreign languages in Iceland are English, Tagalog and Thai; see Figures 12.1 and 12.2).

In most schools (1st–10th grade) in Iceland, children who speak ISL make up less than 10% of the students (Jónsson *et al.*, 2010). In around 6% of the schools, the ratio exceeds 20%, and in a few schools, the number

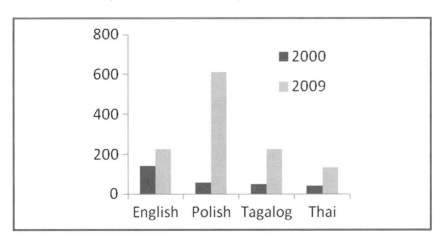

Figure 12.1 The number of preschool children who have Icelandic as a second language (first language: English, Polish, Tagalog and Thai) at two time periods.

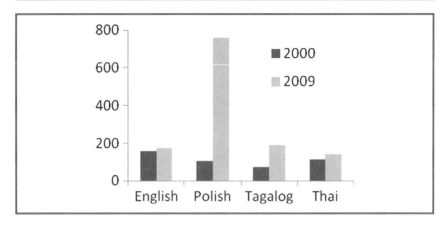

Figure 12.2 The number of school children (1st–10th grade) who have Icelandic as a second language (first language: English, Polish, Tagalog and Thai) at two time periods.

of immigrant children is much higher. In one Reykjavik school serving a large immigrant population (the area of Efra Breiðholt), ISL students comprise nearly 40% of the student population and constitute about 50% of all children referred to the speech-language pathology services (all grades). On the other hand, in another school area with fewer immigrant families (the area of Grafarholt), referrals of ISL children to the school's speech-language pathology were approximately 6%.

Speech-language Pathology Services in Iceland

The Icelandic Association of Speech and Language Pathologists has nearly 60 members, with approximately 40 practicing in the field on a regular basis. Many of them work with children, including bilingual children, either in private practice or in the school system. No official study has been conducted to verify percentages of children with ISL who are referred to speech-language pathology services. However, a recent unofficial survey established that approximately 10% of children referred for speech-language pathology services in the first nine months of 2010 at the National Hearing and Speech Institute of Iceland, were children who spoke ISL. Most of these children were referred because of poor receptive or expressive language skills, not because of speech sound disorders (SSD). The same applies for ISL speakers in Icelandic schools; most of them are not referred because of SSD. However, in the case of SSDs, a child with ISL who needs speech-language pathology services may have problems with both Icelandic sounds that are not found in the child's native language, as well as similar sounds that need treatment in both languages (Holm *et al.*, 2005). For instance, a Polish-speaking child with ISL may have difficulties with /θ/ and /ð/ because these are not found in the Polish phonological system. For the same reason, children may have difficulty producing sounds with preaspiration, or other segments specific to Icelandic (Másdóttir, 1994). Currently, no bilingual speech-language pathologists (SLPs) speak both Polish and Icelandic. Although most SLPs in Iceland could be considered bilingual (usually with English or one of the Scandinavian languages), the large number of Polish-speaking children in Iceland call for SLPs who are also proficient in Polish.

When assessing speech and language skills of a bilingual child, interpreters are called in, if needed. However, problems have emerged when interpreters are not available for the parent's/child's particular language and valuable information may be lost in the translation process (Holm *et al.*, 2005).

Educational Policies and Guidelines in Iceland

A national curriculum for compulsory schools (Aðalnámskrá, 1999, 2006) issues distinct guidelines concerning children with ISL, in that they should be able to maintain their native language as much as possible and should not be judged solely by their proficiency in Icelandic. At the preschool level, teachers are one of the major sources of referrals of children to speech-language pathology services. Many preschools (particularly in areas with many immigrants) use their own guidelines for meeting bilingual children's needs.

Conclusion

In this short documentation of circumstances in Iceland regarding children with ISL and speech-language pathology services, it is clear that a study is warranted to investigate thoroughly the extent and needs of bilingual children in Iceland. Specifically, how many children need speech-language pathology services, what are the primary concerns in terms of speech and language disorders and what are the treatment options for these children.

References

Aðalnámskrá grunnskóla: erlend mál [National Curriculum for Foreign Languages] (1999, 2006) Menntamálaráðuneytið [Ministry of Education]. http://bella.mrn.stjr.is/utgafur/adalnamskra_grsk_erlend_mal.pdf. Accessed 10.10.10.

Arnbjörnsdóttir, B. (2007) English in Iceland: Second language, foreign language, or neither? In B. Arnbjörnsdóttir and H. Ingvarsdóttir (eds) *Teaching and Learning English in Iceland. In Honour of Auður Torfadóttir* (pp. 51–78). Reykjavík: Stofnun Vigdísar Finnbogadóttur/Háskólaútgáfan.

Arnbjörnsdóttir, B. (2008) Tvítyngi, annað mál, erlent mál [Bilingualism, second language, foreign language]. *Málfríður* 24, 17–23.
Árnason, K. (2005) *Íslensk tunga I: Hljóð [Icelandic Language: Sounds]*. Reykjavík: Almenna bókafélagið.
Barðdal, J. (2001) Case in Icelandic: A synchronic, diachronic and comparative approach. *Lundastudier in nordisk språkvetenskap A 57*. Lund: Department of Scandinavian Languages, Lund University.
Holm, A., Stow, C. and Dodd, B. (2005) Bilingual children with phonological disorders: Identification and intervention. In B. Dodd (ed.) *Differential Diagnosis and Treatment of Children with Speech Disorders* (2nd edn; pp. 275–288). West Sussex, UK: Whurr.
Jónsson, A., Sigurðardóttir, H.H. and Daníelsdóttir, H.K. (2010) Nemendur með íslensku sem annað tungumál í grunnskólum – Upplifun skólanna [Students with Icelandic as a second language in primary/secondary schools – The schools' perspective] [in Icelandic]. Report. Reykjavík: Þjónustumiðstöð Miðborgar og Hlíða [The Service Centre for the City Centre and Hlíðar].
Lefever, S. (2007) Putting the cart before the horse. *Málfríður- Tímarit Samtaka tungumálakennara [Icelandic Association of Lauguage Teachers Journal]* 2, 24–28.
Másdóttir, T. (1994) Framburðarþjálfun nýbúa – ágrip af hljóð- og hljóðkerfisfræði [Articulation training for immigrants – Introduction to phonetics and phonology] [in Icelandic]. In I. Hafstað (ed.) *Milli menningarheima – um nám og kennslu nýbúa [Between Cultures – Education and Teaching for Immigrants]* (pp. 74–77). Reykjavík: Námsgagnastofnun.
Másdóttir, T. (2008) Phonological development and disorders in Icelandic-speaking children. Unpublished PhD Thesis, Newcastle University.
Statistics Iceland (2010) Skólamál [Schools] [in Icelandic]. www.hagstofan.is. Accessed 14.10.10.
Thórðardóttir, E. (2004) Tvítyngi er ekkert að óttast [Bilingualism is nothing to be afraid of] [in Icelandic]. *Talfræðingurinn* 18, 5–7.
Valdés, G. and Figueroa, R.A. (1994) *Bilingualism and Testing: A Special Case of Bias*. Norwood, NJ: Ablex.

Part 3

Speech-Language Pathology Practice

13 Multilingual Speech Assessment

Sharynne McLeod

Languages mentioned: Arabic (Egyptian and Jordanian), Cantonese, Dutch, English, Finnish, French, German, Greek, Hungarian, Icelandic, Irish, Israeli Hebrew, Japanese, Korean, Maltese, Mandarin, Mirpuri, Norwegian, Portuguese (Brazilian and European), Punjabi, Putonghua, Russian, Samoan, Spanish, Swedish, Thai, Turkish, Urdu, Welsh, Xhosa, Zulu

Assessing Multilingual Children

The world is multilingual and multicultural. Many children move to different countries where the majority language is not their first and/or are born into multilingual homes. Relocation and international mobility may be initiated because of parental work, curiosity, a family's desire for a different lifestyle, poverty, instability, wars and many other reasons (Weichold, 2010). Children may arrive in a country, for example, with or without their birth parents, as refugees or after international adoption. Even if children are not internationally mobile, many children encounter different languages in their daily lives. Countries such as India, South Africa and Belgium have a number of official languages. For example, in India different languages are used at home, in education, business and religion, necessitating multilingualism in day-to-day contexts. Even in countries that have one official language, such as the USA, many children speak one language at home (e.g. Spanish) and another at school (e.g. English).

Most multilingual children have no difficulty acquiring the languages they speak (see Goldstein & McLeod, Chapter 10). However, some children may have difficulty acquiring all languages (and would benefit from intervention from a speech-language pathologist (SLP)); whereas others may only have difficulty with second and subsequent languages (and would benefit from support from a specialist such as a second language teacher). Differential diagnosis between these two possibilities can be a complex task. A comprehensive assessment is necessary in order to prevent under-diagnosis (describing children with disordered speech as typical), thereby denying children access to appropriate intervention, or over-diagnosis (describing children with typical speech as disordered), thereby extending already over-subscribed SLP resources to children who do not need them. Indeed, 'There is no reason why bilingualism should lead to a greater or lesser need for speech and language therapy (SLT). If there are proportionately more or less bilingual than monolingual children receiving SLT then this difference may be an indication of inequality' (Winter, 2001: 465). SLPs need to compare and contrast children's abilities to speak each of their languages to determine whether these children have a speech sound disorder (SSD), are at risk for one or are developing typically, and if an SSD is identified, to determine appropriate goals and to decide when intervention should conclude. Thus, there are at least five purposes for undertaking an assessment: screening, diagnosis, description, monitoring of progress and determining outcomes of intervention.

The *International Classification of Functioning Disability and Health: Children and Youth Version* (ICF-CY; World Health Organization, WHO, 2007) can be used to inform SLP practice regarding assessment for children with SSD (cf. McLeod & McCormack, 2007). Using the ICF-CY framework, a holistic multilingual assessment should consider children's environmental and personal factors; speech, language, voice and hearing functions; structure and function of the oromusculature; and children's ability to participate in society. One of the reasons for undertaking a holistic diagnostic assessment is because environmental and cultural factors play an important role in children's capacity, functioning and performance in different situations. Additionally, it cannot be assumed that multilingual children, particularly those who were born in a different country, are refugees or who have been adopted internationally, have received routine developmental checks. It is possible that children's speech difficulties may be as a result of an undiagnosed hearing loss, cleft palate (or submucosal cleft), developmental disability, syndrome or cerebral palsy resulting in dysarthria. A holistic assessment can assist with determining whether there is a potential cause.

Preassessment Consideration of Environmental and Personal Factors

Prior to undertaking a face-to-face assessment, it is beneficial to understand children's environmental and personal contexts, including their cultural background and the languages spoken. Each child is unique and their background can provide insight into their speech and language competence and potential. Contextual factors are typically explored during interviews with the child's parents, teachers and the children themselves.

Language proficiency and use

Within multilingual families, languages can be used with different people and in different environmental contexts. In some families, the mother and father may have different first languages from one another and this may be a different language again from the majority language in the country they are living in (e.g. the mother speaks Swedish as her first language, the father speaks German as his first language and they live in England). Often, extended families live together, so the language of the grandparents, aunts, uncles and cousins should also be taken into consideration.

Language proficiency and language use of children and their families provide guidance regarding languages to be included in an SLP assessment and information about possible transfer from one language to the next. For each language spoken by the child, it is useful to map the length of time the language has been spoken, proficiency in the language, its frequency of use and the context the language is used (Stow & Dodd, 2003). A language history of the countries the child has lived in (and, if known, where they intend to live in the near future) also contextualizes language opportunities, proficiency and use. Ascertainment of child, parental and community attitudes toward different languages spoken is also valuable, because some languages may be ascribed higher status than others and some families may choose to use one or multiple languages (Jordaan, 2008). Attitudes toward learning and maintaining different languages can be influenced by a wide variety of factors, including family, friendship, religion, education and employment (Li Wei, 1994), as well as future marriage opportunities (e.g. Gal, 1978). It is important to remember that many families maintain close links with their home countries, through regular visits to and from family and friends. Thus, understanding families' language choice must include a conceptualization of whether migration is permanent or non-permanent because many people have circular migration patterns between countries (Hugo, 2010).

There are a number of ways to quantify language proficiency and use. Many have been developed for adults, including the *Language Experience and Proficiency Questionnaire* (LEAP-Q) (Marian *et al.*, 2007), *History of Bilingualism Questionnaire* (Paradis, 1987), *Language Background Questionnaire* (Rickard Liow & Poon, 1998) and a self-report language dominance questionnaire for Mandarin-English bilinguals validated on 168 participants (Lim *et al.*, 2008). A quick scale validated for Spanish-English bilingual adults is the Bilingual Dominance Scale (Dunn & Fox Tree, 2009). It focuses on 'percent of language use for both languages, age of acquisition and age of comfort for both languages, and restructuring of language fluency due to changes in linguistic environments' (Dunn & Fox Tree, 2009: 273). The *Bilingual Dominance Scale* comprises 12 questions (e.g. 'If you have a foreign accent, which language(s) is it in?') and a scoring system that has been validated on 102 participants.

Children's language proficiency and use has also been explored using different techniques, and two have quantified language proficiency and use of children with SSD. First, Goldstein and Bunta (2010) used a 5-point scale to determine language proficiency ('0 = cannot speak the indicated language to 4 = native-like proficiency with few grammatical errors') and language use ('0 = the child never heard or used the particular language to 4 = the language was heard and used by the child a great deal'). Development of the language proficiency scale was informed by parent and teacher rating scales described in Peña *et al.* (2003). Second, Goldstein *et al.* (2010) asked parents to outline their child's weekly schedule, including activities, language used and conversational partners. Percentage language use for each language was calculated by 'multiplying the number of hours of output of that language by 100 and then dividing that number by the total number of hours of activities reported per week' (Goldstein *et al.,* 2010: 240).

Parent- and teacher-reported concern

Parent- and teacher-reported concern can provide valuable guidance about a child's proficiency in each of the languages spoken. Information can be ascertained in the language of the SLP, or can be asked using an interpreter or questionnaire in the parents' primary language (Roseberry-McKibbin & O'Hanlon, 2005). Two studies identified that parental report of how people *outside* the family view the child's speech can serve as a valid screener for SSD in bilingual children (Lange *et al.*, 2007; Stertzbach & Gildersleeve-Neumann, 2005). Specifically, Stertzbach and Gildersleeve-Neumann (2005) found that the two questions with the strongest correlations were: 'Do *other people* think your child is hard to understand?' and 'Do *other people* think your child has speech problems?'

Restrepo (1998) included two appendices that provide an extensive teacher and parent questionnaire about language use, language concern and family history of education, speech and language difficulties. Restrepo (1998) found that parental report of speech and language problems and family history of speech and language problems were two of four factors that had high sensitivity and specificity for determining Spanish-English children's speech and language status.

The *Alberta Language and Development Questionnaire* (ALDeQ) (see appendix in Paradis *et al.*, 2010) is a psychometrically validated measure of language development that is not specific to a particular language/cultural group. The ALDeQ has been normed on 139 typically developing children and 29 children with language impairment and is a valuable method for quantifying children's early milestones, language use, preferences and family history.

Cultural heritage

When considering a child's language history, language use and language proficiency, it is important to concurrently acknowledge generalized socio-cultural factors alongside individual beliefs and practices, and families' cultural perspectives. Classification systems provide insight into differing cultural perspectives that need to be checked with family perspectives. For example, Ritter (2007) classified differing cultural and temporal attitudes toward children and childhood whereby the child may be seen as a social being, mistrusted agent, object or an optional extra. Additionally, Hofstede and Hofstede (2005) described five dimensions of culture/countries that have been interpreted for use in multilingual SLP contexts by the American Speech-Language-Hearing Association (2010):

(1) Power Distance Index. This extends from *high power distance* where some people have more status/power than others to *low power distance* where people are treated more equally. Hofstede (2010) suggests that this dimension is 'high for Latin, Asian and African countries and smaller for Anglo and Germanic countries'. An example of *high power distance* occurs when children are expected to be obedient to adults, and *low power distance* when adults ask children for their opinions. For example, Johnson and Wong (2002) found that Chinese mothers (high power distance) were less likely to invite personal narratives and talk about non-shared daily events than Western mothers (low power distance).

(2) Individualism vs. Collectivism. People in *individualistic societies* (e.g. 'developed and Western countries', Hofstede, 2010) are expected to care for themselves and their immediate family, whereas *collective societies* (e.g. 'less developed and Eastern countries', Hofstede, 2010) have strong, cohesive groups, often with an emphasis on extended families (uncles, aunts and grandparents).

(3) Masculinity vs. Femininity. In *masculine* societies, men and women are more assertive and competitive, whereas *feminine* societies have modest and caring values. Hofstede (2010) indicates that masculinity is 'high in Japan, in some European countries like Germany, Austria and Switzerland, and moderately high in Anglo countries; it is low in Nordic countries and in the Netherlands and moderately low in some Latin and Asian countries like France, Spain and Thailand'. When considering multilingual families, Lyon (1996) indicated that in some studies the language spoken by the father determined the language spoken in the home, whereas there was cross-gender agreement regarding the language parents wanted their children to learn in Wales.

(4) Uncertainty Avoidance Index. This extends from *high uncertainty avoidance*, where people favor structure and rules to *low uncertainty avoidance*, where people are tolerant of differing opinions and unstructured situations. For example, parents with high uncertainty avoidance may wish to work with the SLP as an expert, whereas parents with low uncertainty avoidance may wish to work in collaboration with SLPs, teachers and community members.

(5) Long-Term Orientation vs. Short-Term Orientation. According to Hofstede (2010), 'Long-term orientation scores are highest in East Asia, moderate in Eastern and Western Europe, and low in the Anglo world, the Muslim world, Latin America and Africa'. Those with *long-term*

orientation are future oriented, respecting perseverance and thrift; e.g. Fung and Roseberry-McKibbin (1999) indicated that Cantonese-speaking parents upheld the importance of academic attainment and an expectation of hard work for their children. Those with *short-term orientation* display respect for tradition; e.g. Maloni *et al.* (2010): 848) described many mothers of children with disability in Bangladesh as reliant on traditional interpretations of disability, including 'possession by ghosts or evil spirits'. In South Africa, Semela (2001) described how parents of 24 Xhosa/Zulu-speaking children with severe learning disability sought traditional and faith healers as 'advisors, therapists, social workers and guides' (Semela, 2001: 130) who were found to be 'helpful and supportive' (Semela, 2001: 132). Semela found that 22 of the 24 children had above average number of incisions/scars, and 21 wore necklaces, strings and bracelets recommended by the healers.

Each of these differing cultural perspectives will impact parent–child interactions, family acknowledgment of disability, access to support services and the role of the child, family and therapist within SLP services. Additionally, SLPs' own cultural competence is enhanced by acknowledgment (self-assessment) of their own cultural perspectives and biases and respectful consideration of the perspectives of children, families and communities (ASHA, 2010).

Assessment of Speech Function

The assessment of speech function includes consideration of production, perception and phonological awareness. Each of these can be considered using formal assessment procedures, informal assessment procedures and dynamic assessment. Within this book, there are separate chapters considering perception (Rvachew, Mattock, Clayards, Chiang and Brosseau-Lapré, Chapter 8) and phonological awareness (Hus, Chapter 28), so this chapter will focus on speech production.

Assessment of speech production using single word tests

Before assessing multilingual children, a decision must be made regarding which languages should be assessed and which others should be considered. The pre-assessment interview will provide guidance. Many SLPs state that they use English speech assessments or informal assessments when assessing multilingual children in English-speaking countries (Caesar & Kohler, 2007; Kritikos, 2003; Skahan *et al.*, 2007; Williams & McLeod, 2011). However, conducting SLP assessments in all languages spoken by children is often recommended as best practice. Assessment of speech production can include children's ability to produce consonants, vowels, phonotactics (including consonant clusters and polysyllabic words), prosody and tones (for tonal languages) for each of the languages that children speak. Elin Thordardottir *et al.* (2006) suggest that at least two factors limit the ability of SLPs to assess children in more than one language. First, there is a lack of systematic, norm-referenced assessment materials in a range of languages with multilingual SLPs to undertake these assessments. Second, there is a lack of guidelines for the interpretation of information about two languages: 'How exactly does one go about taking into consideration knowledge of two different languages within the same child? What are the appropriate developmental expectations for bilingual children?' (Elin Thordardottir *et al.,* 2006: 2). Each of these factors will be discussed in turn.

Availability of speech sound assessments in different languages

Most formal speech assessments assess monolingual competence; that is, they are designed to assess speech production of one language (McLeod, 2007a). The majority of speech assessments for children have been developed in English (the appendix of McLeod and Threats (2008) lists 56 different speech assessments in English). However, there are also a number of speech assessments in languages other than English. Appendix A lists 56 different sampling tools for 18 different languages. Some of these are commercially available standardized tests, while others are word lists published in journal articles (that may or may not be standardized). Each of the sampling tools in Appendix A was designed to assess one language; and generally has been used with or was standardized on monolingual children in a particular country. For example, the *Hong Kong Cantonese Articulation Test* (Cheung *et al.*, 2006) was designed to assess Cantonese spoken by children in Hong Kong. Caution should be taken if using speech assessments outside their original context, particularly if utilizing normative data. There could be differences in the dialect, as well as differences between productions by monolingual and bilingual speakers because of transfer from one language to another (see Goldstein & McLeod, Chapter 10). If an assessment in a language of interest is not listed, then McLeod (Chapter 14) provides guidelines for how to search for additional assessment tools, and how to create an assessment tool if one cannot be located.

Although multilingual assessment of children's speech is documented in the literature (e.g. Holm & Dodd, 1999; Goldstein *et al.*, 2010), there are few sampling tools available for SLPs to use to assess the speech of multilingual children (Carter *et al.*, 2005). Appendix B lists five different multilingual sampling tools designed to assess children who speak Maltese and English, Pakistani heritage languages and English, Spanish and English, Russian and German, and Turkish and German. Different versions of the *Profiling Elements of Prosody in Speech-Communication* (PEPS-C, Peppé *et al.*, 2010; Peppé, Chapter 5) have been designed to assess prosody in a number of different languages. Elin Thordardottir *et al.* (2006) state that an associated limitation to the number of multilingual assessments that are available are the limited number of multilingual SLPs. It is possible, with appropriate training and resources, that SLPs can undertake aspects of assessment in languages that are not their own (e.g. Stow & Pert, 2006).

Interpretation of multilingual speech sound assessment data

When assessing the speech of multilingual children, monolingual assessments in different languages can be administered; however, it is inappropriate to compare multilingual speakers' test results to the mono-lingual reference group (Bedore & Peña, 2008). Due to the lack of normative data for multilingual speakers (see Goldstein & McLeod, Chapter 10), one of the first tasks is to compare the phonemic inventory of languages. A comparative phonemic inventory includes a list of shared sounds and unshared sounds in each of the languages spoken by a child (cf., Fabiano-Smith & Goldstein, 2010). This information should be enhanced by knowledge of differing perception of sounds from each language (see Rvachew *et al.*, Chapter 8). For example, Ha *et al.* (2009) indicated that bilingual Korean-English children will have difficulties with perception and production of the English vowels /ɪ, ɛ, æ/ and English fricatives and affricates, except /s/ and /h/. Next, Yavaş and Goldstein (1998: 58) suggested that SLPs should understand 'common and uncommon phono-logical patterns in first and second language acquisition and bilingual phonology, interference patterns between languages, dialect patterns, and language-specific patterns that are exhibited in one language but not in the other'. Comparisons between many features for 24 languages are summar-ized in McLeod (2007a, 2000b). To continue the example from above, Korean only has three fricatives: /s, s*, h/, so Ha *et al.* (2009) indicated that stopping may be more frequent for Korean-English-speaking children than for English-speaking children. Korean does not use syllable-initial or syllable-final consonant clusters, so in order to preserve the Korean syllable structure, schwa may be produced between consonants within English consonant clusters. Scarpino and Goldstein (Chapter 21) provide additional guidance regarding analysis of multilingual speech samples.

Nonword repetition

Children's ability to repeat nonwords has been found to be a significant clinical marker for difficulties with speech, language and memory (Windsor *et al.*, 2010). Assessments using nonword repetition have occurred across many languages (Crowe *et al.*, 2010). Nonword repetition tasks are rarely language-neutral due to the choice of consonants, vowels and phonotactic structures of languages. Shriberg *et al.* (2009) devised the *Syllable Repetition Task* to include sounds that were typically in the inventories of children with misarticulations: /b/, /d/, /m/ and the vowel /a/. While this task was not specifically designed to assess multilingual children, with accommodations it may be a relevant speech assessment tool for multilingual children since the speech sounds and syllable structures are included in many languages. Recently, Windsor *et al.* (2010) used nonword repetition tasks to assess 187 monolingual and Spanish-English multilingual children's speech. They used the Dollaghan and Campbell (1998) *Nonword Repetition Task* to assess English, and the task created by Ebert *et al.* (2008) to assess Spanish. Windsor *et al.* (2010) concluded that nonword repetition tasks may be a useful 'composite marker' for differentiating first languages and typical vs. impaired language acquisition. They concluded 'NWR [nonword repetition] may be better viewed as a reliable correlate of monolingual groups' speech-language abilities rather than as a diagnostic marker of any particular clinical group with language difficulties' (Windsor *et al.*, 2010: 299).

Assessment of conversational speech production

Many SLPs elicit speech samples from multilingual children using single words (Skahan *et al.*, 2007). Single word tasks have the advantage of being relatively easy to administer, can elicit samples that are representative of the sounds and phonotactic constraints of the ambient languages and are easily glossed given that the SLP knows the intended targets. A conversational speech sample can provide additional information not available from single word sampling. Stockman (1996: 356) identified the 'promises and pitfalls' of conversational speech, or naturalistic language sampling analysis. The promises are that: 'Naturally displayed language behavior brings (a) cultural sensitivity, (b) validity, (c) accessibility, and (d) flexibility to the language assessment task'. The pitfalls are that: 'Naturally displayed behavior creates problems with (a) managing context variation, (b) describing the flow of speech, (c) selecting evaluation parameters, and (d) finding enough time to do the analysis' (Stockman, 1996: 357).

Stockman (1996: 723) recommended that SLPs consider a 'minimal competence core', a criterion-referenced measure collected during connected speech to differentiate between African American preschool children who are typically developing, and those who have difficulty speaking. A phonetic core was subsequently developed and validated on 120 Head Start students aged 3 years (Stockman, 2008). Stockman (2008) recommended that during 75 response turns (approximately 225 words) a minimal core of word-initial consonant clusters plus 13 initial consonant singletons had diagnostic validity. Specifically, to be minimally competent, children should accurately produce word-initial consonant clusters in four different words that minimally span two different consonant sequences (e.g. /pl-/ and /sk-/ as in *play, please, sky, skip*), and they should accurately produce each of the following 13 initial single consonants four times, which minimally span two different words (e.g. *man, man, mom, mom*): /m, n, p, b, t, d, k, g, f, s, h, w, j/. The minimal competence core was developed for children speaking African American English; however, it may be applicable to adapt for children speaking other dialects and languages. For example, Fabiano-Smith and Goldstein (2010) applied the minimal competence core concept when documenting shared and unshared sounds in Spanish-English-speaking children.

Intelligibility, accuracy and acceptability

When assessing a *monolingual* child's speech, a majority of SLPs in the USA indicated that they always estimate intelligibility (Skahan *et al.*, 2007). In the same study, the majority of SLPs indicated they used informal procedures during the assessment of *multilingual* children. It is likely that these SLPs estimated intelligibility during these informal procedures. Intelligibility is 'the degree to which the listener understands what the speaker says when the target is uncertain' (Camarata, 2010: 382). A number of measures have been used to quantify intelligibility. For example, Flipsen (2006) described the Intelligibility Index, whereby a transcriber calculates the number of intelligible words vs. the total number of words in a connected spontaneous speech sample. McLeod *et al.* (2011) described the *Intelligibility in Context Scale*, a parent report measure of children's intelligibility with seven different conversational partners. Both of these measures have psychometric validity with monolingual English-speaking children, and may be applicable for consideration of multilingual children's intelligibility since studies in other languages have described comparable results. For example, Baudonck *et al.* (2009) considered intelligibility of Flemish children and indicated that children aged 4;6–5;0 years were 90% intelligible. Their mothers understood more words than unfamiliar listeners.

Intelligibility is different from speech accuracy: the number of phonemes produced in the same manner as an adult who is a native speaker of the language (and dialect). Speech accuracy is typically calculated using the percentage of consonants correct (PCC) metric (Shriberg *et al.*, 1997). Intelligibility is also different from speech acceptability. Currently, there is no metric for determining speech acceptability; it is context and listener specific. However, determination of speech acceptability is of relevance when assessing multilingual children's speech because transfer of some sounds from one language to another may be acceptable (i.e. not counted as errors and thus are not treated), whereas transference of other sounds may not. Additionally, speech acceptability is an important consideration for children who have craniofacial anomalies (e.g. cleft palate) (Henningsson *et al.*, 2008).

Consideration of dialectal difference vs. disorder

SLPs also assess multi*dialectal* children to differentiate between dialectal speech difference and/or SSD (Ball & Bernhardt, 2008; Goldstein & Iglesias, 2001; McGregor *et al.*, 1997; Toohill *et al.*, 2011; Velleman & Pearson, 2010).

McGregor *et al.* (1997: 52) indicated that the lack of research regarding the acquisition of features in children learning two dialects has resulted in difficulty 'determining the developmental appropriateness of true errors'. Thus, in order to distinguish between true speech errors and dialectal differences, they recommended undertaking a contrastive analysis by comparing children's speech production to two adult targets: one based on the standard dialect, and the other based on the child's home dialect. Seymour (2004) found that children's ability to produce consonant clusters was diagnostically sensitive for 4- to 9-year-old children speaking four different mainstream and non-mainstream US dialects. Goldstein and Iglesias (2001) implemented a contrastive analysis for 4-year-old children with SSD in two dialects of Spanish and reported a 10.1% increase in PCC when the speaker's home dialect was considered. Similarly, Toohill *et al.* (2011) implemented a contrastive analysis for 15 Indigenous Australian 4-year-old children with SSD using both standard Australian English and Australian Aboriginal English. Toohill *et al.* found a 9.26% increase in PCC when the speaker's dialect was considered. Additionally, each of these children had significantly less severe ratings of SSD and one child was no longer identified with an SSD. Toohill *et al.* noted one limitation of contrastive analyses: a number of dialectal differences were also typical of delayed speech (e.g. [f] for /θ/). Overall, contrastive analyses can assist SLPs to analyze and interpret the speech assessment data of children from culturally and linguistically diverse backgrounds in the absence of normative data and standardized tests.

Dynamic assessment

Dynamic assessment is used to consider how children learn when provided with feedback and, generally, has been seen as a valuable protocol for use with children from culturally and linguistically diverse backgrounds (Gutiérrez-Clellen & Peña, 2001). 'When using this kind of assessment, the SLP does not necessarily ask what the student already knows; in other words, language knowledge is not assessed. Rather, he or she asks *how the student learns*. This circumvents the problem seen for so many ELL students: lack of prior knowledge of items presented on standardized tests' (Roseberry-McKibbin & O'Hanlon, 2005: 183). Jacobs and Coufal (2001) developed an example of a dynamic assessment approach for the assessment of language skills in multilingual children. They assessed children's ability to learn grammatical elements of a language (in this case Kiswahili) via a computerized assessment. To date, research regarding dynamic assessment has only been applied to the speech of monolingual children. For example, Glaspey and Stoel-Gammon (2007) presented a protocol for dynamic assessment of monolingual English children's speech, called the Scaffolding Scale of Stimulability. This scale is a formalized and quantified scale for considering how stimulable each English consonant is, using different levels of prompting (e.g. auditory, visual, tactile) in different contexts (e.g. isolation, single word, sentences). There is an opportunity for continued development of dynamic assessment practices for assessing multilingual children's speech production.

Assessment of Language, Voice, Fluency and Hearing Function

A holistic assessment of children's speech must extend beyond consideration of communicative context and speech production to other communicative functions. Thus, language, voice, fluency and hearing will now be considered.

Language function

The assessment of language functioning of multilingual children brings similar challenges to the assessment of speech functioning. There are numerous standardized assessments for monolingual speakers of many languages, but limited standardized assessments for multilingual speakers. Stockman (1996) considered the use of naturalistic language sampling techniques for measuring the language functioning of linguistically and culturally diverse children. An alternative to direct assessment of children's language status is to utilize parent report measures. For example, Elin Thordardottir and Ellis Weismer (1996) developed a parent report measure to screen Icelandic children's language. Additionally, the *MacArthur-Bates Scales*, a parent report tool for children's expressive and receptive language use, has been translated into numerous languages. An example of the development of the *MacArthur-Bates Scales* for Irish-speaking children is provided in O'Toole and Fletcher (2008, 2010). Recent comprehensive review papers provide additional information about the assessment of multilingual children's language abilities (Bedore & Peña, 2008; Caesar & Kohler, 2007; Girolametto & Cleave, 2010; Langdon & Ratner, 2009).

Voice and fluency function

Assessment of voice and fluency may be less constrained by the language spoken (compared with speech and language measures), so best-practice techniques for monolingual children may be applied. The *Universal Parameters for Reporting Speech Outcomes in Individuals With Cleft Palate* (Henningsson *et al.*, 2008) includes a recommendation that five universal speech parameters, most of which describe voice functioning, and the rest speech functioning. Specifically, it is recommended to include the following information should be reported for children with cleft palate (and may also be relevant in a comprehensive assessment of multilingual children): (a) hypernasality, (b) hyponasality, (c) audible nasal air emission and/or nasal turbulence, (d) consonant production errors and (e) voice disorder as well as speech understandability and speech acceptability.

Structure and Function of Oromusculature and Hearing Mechanism

It cannot be assumed that a child who has been born in another country has had prior developmental health checks. Therefore, it is useful to conduct a hearing and oromusculature screening assessment to determine any potential contributing factors to the children's speech production. The oromusculature assessment should include examination of nose, lips, teeth, maxilla, mandible, tongue, hard palate, soft palate, pharynx and uvula. When examining the teeth, consider whether there is evidence of malocclusion, decay or missing teeth. When examining the tongue, consider whether there is ankyloglossia (tongue tie) or short frenulum. When examining the palate, consider whether there is evidence of a cleft (including a bifid uvula or submucosal cleft). SLPs are unable to view the structure of the larynx; however, they should refer to an ear nose and throat specialist if there are concerns about the child's vocal quality. Finally, it may be necessary to also examine swallowing and feeding functioning. Speech motor control is often screened using a diadochokinesis (DDK) task. Normative information exists for a range of languages, including English (Williams & Stackhouse, 2000), Brazilian Portuguese (Wertzner et al., 2008) and Thai (Prathanee et al., 2003).

Activities and Participation

Understanding the impact of SSD on children's ability to participate in daily activities is also an important component of the assessment of multilingual children (WHO, 2007). Parents, teachers and children themselves can provide these insights; however, to date, consideration of activities and participation has primarily occurred for *monolingual* children with SSD. For example, McCormack et al. (2010a) reported that 86 parents of monolingual 4- to 5-year-old children with SSD were concerned about the impact of SSD on their children's verbal communication (e.g. holding a conversation), advanced learning (e.g. learning to read and write), applied learning and general tasks (e.g. handling stress), basic learning (e.g. copying) and interpersonal interactions (e.g. friendships). Next, McCormack et al. (2010b) asked monolingual preschool children with SSD and their significant others about their lives using questions from the *Speech Participation and Activity Assessment of Children* (SPAA-C, McLeod, 2004). A number of children indicated that their conversational partners had trouble with listening/

understanding them; but the children did not mention that they had difficulty speaking. Many of the participants described the frustration caused by breakdown in communication. These insights are likely to be relevant to multilingual children with SSD, although as mentioned previously, some people from *high power distance* cultural groups may not seek children's perspectives on their own lives.

Children's Responses during Speech Assessment

Speech assessment conducted within a clinical setting can impact on children's performance and may not demonstrate children's full capabilities. Children may not respond as anticipated during assessment. For example, Friend and Keplinger (2008) indicated that some children do not touch assessment items because their parents do not allow them to touch items that are not theirs. The formality of the testing situation can impact on dialect density in African American English-speaking children (Seymour & Seymour, 1977; Stockman, 2008) and this may occur for other children as well. Languages such as Samoan have both a formal and colloquial register, and different consonants are produced in each register. The formality of the speech assessment context is congruent with the use of the formal register, so assessment of the colloquial register may be difficult (Ballard & Farao, 2008).

When assessing multilingual children's speech, codeswitching between the languages spoken by the child can occur frequently; particularly if a child does not know all of the lexical items presented within a speech assessment in both languages. Indeed, Pert and Letts (2006: 349) suggested, 'Codeswitched utterances may be the most representative utterances of a bilingual child's expressive potential'. Codeswitching predominantly has been studied during children's language assessments; however, in one speech example, Grech and Dodd (2008) allowed 241 3- to 6-year-old children living in Malta to decide whether they wished to undertake the assessment in Maltese or English or both. The SLP should be aware of the occurrences of codeswitching and their purpose within the assessment process.

Children who are internationally adopted require special consideration for two main reasons. First, many have an 'abrupt switch in language environment' (Pollock, 2007: 107), necessitating becoming 'second first language learners', and second, because the children may have started life in an orphanage and be at risk for other developmental delays. During the first year after adoption, the child's first language is said to decay rapidly, so if assessments are to be conducted in the child's first language, they need to be conducted soon after arrival (Glennen, 2005). Glennen (2005) assessed the language status of 28 children, aged 12–24 months, newly adopted from Eastern Europe. The majority (65%) did not require early intervention, 28% required early intervention and 7% were recommended for follow-up assessments. Roberts *et al.* (2005) found that two years post adoption, few of the 55 children adopted from China had SSD.

SLPs' Assessment Practices

SLPs will never be able to speak all of the languages that are spoken by their clients. During assessment, all SLPs should 'develop sensitivity to their own social interactive styles and cultural biases relative to language sampling variables' (Stockman, 1996: 365). Multilingual SLPs who share a language with their clients should be aware that there may still be cultural and dialectal differences between them. Monolingual SLPs may be able to undertake some aspects of multilingual assessments with training and knowledge of the language and culture of the child (Sell, 2008; Stow & Pert, 2006). High quality audio/video recordings (cf. Vogel & Morgan, 2009) of children's speech should be made in order to check transcriptions and interpretations with SLPs who are competent in the language assessed. Interpreters/translators also may be utilized in assessments for children with SSD (Goldstein & Iglesias, 2009). It is important that professional organizations and academic training programs support SLPs acquisition of languages, and skills to encourage multilingual children within their clinical settings (Caesar & Kohler, 2007; Jordaan, 2008).

Acknowledgements

Preparation of this chapter was supported by an Australian Research Council Future Fellowship (FT0990588).

References

American Speech-Language-Hearing Association, (ASHA, 2010) Cultural competence in professional service delivery. www.asha.org. Accessed 1.11.10.

Ball, J. and Bernhardt, B.M. (2008) First Nations English dialects in Canada: Implications for speech-language pathology. *Clinical Linguistics and Phonetics* 22 (8), 570–588.

Ballard, E. and Farao, S. (2008) The phonological skills of Samoan speaking 4-year-olds. *International Journal of Speech-Language Pathology* 10 (6), 379–391.

Baudonck, N.L.H., Buekers, R., Gillebert, S. and Lierde, K.M.V. (2009) Speech intelligibility of Flemish children as judged by their parents. *Folia Phoniatrica et Logopaedica* 61, 288–295.

Bedore, L.M. and Peña, E.D. (2008) Assessment of bilingual children for identification of language impairment: Current findings and implications for practice. *International Journal of Bilingual Education and Bilingualism* 11 (1), 1–29.

Caesar, L.G. and Kohler, P.D. (2007) The state of school-based bilingual assessment: Actual practice versus recommended guidelines. *Language, Speech, and Hearing Services in Schools* 38 (3), 190–200.

Camarata, S.M. (2010) Naturalistic intervention for speech intelligibility and speech accuracy. In A.L. Williams, S. McLeod and R. J. McCauley (eds) *Interventions for Speech Sound Disorders in Children* (pp. 381–405). Baltimore, MD: Paul H. Brookes.

Carter, J.A., Lees, J.A., Murira, G.M., Gona, J., Neville, B.G.R. and Newton, C.R.J.C. (2005) Issues in the development of cross-cultural assessments of speech and language for children. *International Journal of Language and Communication Disorders* 40 (4), 385–401.

Cheung, P.S.P., Ng, A. and To, C.K.S. (2006) *Hong Kong Cantonese Articulation Test.* Hong Kong: Language Information Sciences Research Centre, City University of Hong Kong.

Crowe, K., McLeod, S. and Ching, T. (2010, May) Nonword repetition: A systematic review of purposes, populations, languages and variables. Poster presentation to Speech Pathology Australia National Conference, Melbourne.

Dollaghan, C. and Campbell, T.F. (1998) Nonword repetition and child language impairment. *Journal of Speech, Language, and Hearing Research* 41, 1136–1146.

Dunn, A.L. and Fox Tree, J.E. (2009) A quick, gradient Bilingual Dominance Scale. *Bilingualism: Language and Cognition* 12 (3), 273–289.

Ebert, K.D., Kalanek, J., Cordero, K.N. and Kohnert, K. (2008) Spanish nonword repetition: Stimuli development and preliminary results. *Communication Disorders Quarterly* 29, 69–74.

Fabiano-Smith, L. and Goldstein, B.A. (2010) Phonological acquisition in bilingual Spanish-English speaking children. *Journal of Speech, Language, and Hearing Research* 53 (1), 160–178.

Flipsen, P., Jr. (2006) Measuring the intelligibility of conversational speech in children. *Clinical Linguistics and Phonetics* 20 (4), 303–312.

Friend, M. and Keplinger, M. (2008) Reliability and validity of the Computerized Comprehension Task (CCT): Data from American English and Mexican Spanish infants. *Journal of Child Language* 35, 77–98.

Fung, F. and Roseberry-McKibbin, C. (1999) Service delivery considerations in working with clients from Cantonese-speaking backgrounds. *American Journal of Speech-Language Pathology* 8, 309–318.

Gal, S. (1978) Peasant men can't get wives: Language change and sex roles in a bilingual community. *Language in Society* 7, 1–16.

Girolametto, L. and Cleave, P.L. (2010) Assessment and intervention of bilingual children with language impairment. *Journal of Communication Disorders* 43 (6), 453–455.

Glaspey, A.M. and Stoel-Gammon, C. (2007) A dynamic approach to phonological assessment. *Advances in Speech-Language Pathology* 9 (4), 286–296.

Glennen, S. (2005) New arrivals: Speech and language assessment for internationally adopted infants and toddlers within the first months home. *Seminars in Speech and Language* 26 (1), 10–21.

Goldstein, B.A. and Bunta, F. (2010, in press) Positive and negative transfer in the phonological systems of bilingual speakers. *International Journal of Bilingualism*.

Goldstein, B.A. and Iglesias, A. (2001) The effect of dialect on phonological analysis: Evidence from Spanish-speaking children. *American Journal of Speech-Language Pathology* 10, 394–406.

Goldstein, B. and Iglesias, A. (2009) Language and dialectal variations. In J. Bernthal and N. Bankson (eds) *Articulation and Phonological Disorders: Speech Sound Disorders in Children* (6th edn; pp. 331–356). Boston, MA: Pearson.

Goldstein, B.A., Bunta, F., Lange, J., Rodriguez, J. and Burrows, L. (2010) The effects of measures of language experience and language ability on segmental accuracy in bilingual children. *American Journal of Speech-Language Pathology* 19 (3), 238–247.

Grech, H. and Dodd, B. (2008) Phonological acquisition in Malta: A bilingual language learning context. *International Journal of Bilingualism*, 12(3), 155–171.

Gutiérrez-Clellen, V. F. and Peña, E. (2001) Dynamic assessment of diverse children: A tutorial. *Language, Speech, and Hearing Services in Schools* 32 (4), 212–224.

Ha, S., Johnson, C.J. and Kuehn, D.P. (2009) Characteristics of Korean phonology: Review, tutorial, and case studies of Korean children speaking English. *Journal of Communication Disorders* 42 (3), 163–179.

Henningsson, G., Kuehn, D.P., Sell, D., Sweeney, T., Trost-Cardamone, J.E. and Whitehill, T.L. (2008) Universal parameters for reporting speech outcomes in individuals with cleft palate. *Cleft Palate-Craniofacial Journal* 45 (1), 1–17.

Hofstede, G. (2010) *Dimensions of national cultures*. http://www.geerthofstede.nl/culture/dimensions-of-national-cultures.aspx. Accessed 2.11.10.

Hofstede, G. and Hofstede, G.J. (2005) *Culture and Organizations: Software of the Mind*. New York: McGraw-Hill.

Holm, A. and Dodd, B. (1999) Differential diagnosis of phonological disorder in two bilingual children acquiring Italian and English. *Clinical Linguistics and Phonetics* 13 (2), 113–129.

Holm, A., Dodd, B., Stow, C. and Pert, S. (1999) Identification and differential diagnosis of phonological disorders in bilingual children. *Language Testing* 16 (3), 271–292.

Hugo, G. (2010) Circularity, reciprocity, and return: An important dimension of contemporary transnationalism. *ISSBD Bulletin* 58 (2), 2–5.

Jacobs, E.L. and Coufal, K.L. (2001) A computerized screening instrument of language learnability. *Communication Disorders Quarterly* 22, 67–76.

Johnston, J.R. and Wong, M-Y.A. (2002) Cultural differences in beliefs and practices concerning talk to children. *Journal of Speech, Language, and Hearing Research* 45, 916–926.

Jordaan, H. (2008) Clinical intervention for bilingual children: An international survey. *Folia Phoniatrica et Logopaedica* 60, 97–105.

Kritikos, E.P. (2003) Speech-language pathologists' beliefs about language assessment of bilingual/bicultural individuals. *American Journal of Speech-Language Pathology* 12 (1), 73–91.

Langdon, H.W. and Ratner, N.B. (2009) Testing bilingual speakers: Challenges and potential solutions. *Seminars in Speech and Language* 30 (4), 217–218.

Lange, J., Burrows, L. and Goldstein, B. (2007, February) Parent concern and phonological skills in Spanish-English bilingual children. Poster presented at the Texas Research Symposium on Language Diversity, Austin, TX.

Li Wei, (1994) *Three Generations, Two Languages, One Family: Language Choice and Language Shift in a Chinese Community in Britain*. Clevedon: Multilingual Matters.

Lim, V.P.C., Liow, S.J.R., Lincoln, M., Chan, Y.H. and Onslow, M. (2008) Determining language dominance in English-Mandarin bilinguals: Development of a self-report classification tool for clinical use. *Applied Psycholinguistics* 29 389–412.

Lyon, J. (1996) *Becoming Bilingual: Language Acquisition in a Bilingual Community*. Clevedon, UK: Multilingual Matters.

Maloni, P.K., Despres, E.R., Habbous, J., Primmer, A.R., Slatten, J.B., Gibson, B.E., Landry, M. D. (2010) Perceptions of disability among mothers of children with disability in Bangladesh: Implications for rehabilitation service delivery. *Disability and Rehabilitation, 32*(10), 845–854.

Marian, V., Blumenfeld, H.K. and Kaushanskaya, M. (2007) The Language Experience and Proficiency Questionnaire (LEAP-Q): Assessing language profiles in bilinguals and multilinguals. *Journal of Speech, Language, and Hearing Research* 50 (4), 940–967.

McCormack, J., McLeod, S., Harrison, L.J. and McAllister, L. (2010a) The impact of speech impairment in early childhood: Investigating parents' and speech-language pathologists' perspectives using the ICF-CY. *Journal of Communication Disorders* 43 (5), 378–396.

McCormack, J., McLeod, S., McAllister, L. and Harrison, L.J. (2010b) My speech problem, your listening problem, and my frustration: The experience of living with childhood speech impairment. *Language, Speech, and Hearing Services in Schools* 41 (4), 379–392.

McGregor, K.K., Williams, D., Hearst, S. and Johnson, A.C. (1997) The use of contrastive analysis in distinguishing difference from disorder: A tutorial. *American Journal of Speech-Language Pathology* 6 (3), 45–56.

McLeod, S. (2004) Speech pathologists' application of the ICF to children with speech impairment. *Advances in Speech-Language Pathology* 6 (1), 75–81.

McLeod, S. (ed.) (2007a) *The International Guide to Speech Acquisition*. Clifton Park, NY: Thomson Delmar Learning.

McLeod, S. (2007b) A comparison of features of speech across 24 languages. *Perspectives on Communication Sciences and Disorders in Culturally and Linguistically Diverse Populations* 14 (1), 12–16. Reprinted in *ACQuiring Knowledge in Speech, Language and Hearing* 9 (2), 74–78.

McLeod, S. and McCormack, J. (2007) Application of the ICF and ICF-Children and Youth in children with speech impairment. *Seminars in Speech and Language* 28, 254–264.

McLeod, S. and Threats, T.T. (2008) The ICF-CY and children with communication disabilities. *International Journal of Speech-Language Pathology* 10 (1), 92–109.

McLeod, S., Harrison, L.J. and McCormack, J. (2011, in press) Intelligibility in Context Scale: Validity and reliability of a subjective rating measure. *Journal of Speech, Language, and Hearing Research.*

O'Toole, C. and Fletcher, P. (2008) Developing assessment tools for bilingual and minority language acquisition. *Journal of Clinical Speech and Language Studies* 16, 12–27.

O'Toole, C. and Fletcher, P. (2010) Validity of a parent report instrument for Irish-speaking toddlers. *First Language* 30 (2), 199–217.

Paradis, J., Emmerzael, K. and Duncan, T.S. (2010) Assessment of English language learners: Using parent report on first language development. *Journal of Communication Disorders* 43 (6), 474–497.

Paradis, M. (1987) *The Assessment of Bilingual Aphasia*. Mahwah, NJ: Erlbaum.

Peña, E.D., Bedore, L. and Rappazzo, C. (2003) Comparison of Spanish, English, and bilingual children's performance across semantic tasks. *Language, Speech, and Hearing Services in Schools* 34, 5–16.

Peppé, S.J.E., Martínez-Castilla, P., Coene, M., Hesling, I., Moen, I. and Gibbon, F. (2010) Assessing prosodic skills in five European languages: Cross-linguistic differences in typical and atypical populations. *International Journal of Speech-Language Pathology* 12 (1), 1–7.

Pert, S. and Letts, C. (2006) Codeswitching in Mirpuri speaking Pakistani heritage preschool children: Bilingual language acquisition. *International Journal of Bilingualism* 10 (3), 349–374.

Pollock, K.E. (2007) Speech acquisition in second first language learners (Children who were adopted internationally). In S. McLeod (ed.) *The International Guide to Speech Acquisition* (pp. 107–113). Clifton Park, NY: Thomson Delmar Learning.

Prathanee, B., Thanaviratananich, S. and Pongjanyakul, A. (2003) Oral diadochokinetic rates for normal Thai children. *International Journal of Language and Communication Disorders* 38, 417–428.

Restrepo, M.A. (1998) Identifiers of predominantly Spanish-speaking children with language impairment. *Journal of Speech, Language, and Hearing Research* 41 (2), 1398–1411.

Rickard Liow, S.J. and Poon, K.K.L. (1998) Phonological awareness in multilingual Chinese children. *Applied Psycholinguistics* 19, 339–362.

Ritter, L. (2007) Historical and international perspectives of childhood. In S. McLeod (ed.) *The International Guide to Speech Acquisition* (pp. 73–77). Clifton Park, NY: Thomson Delmar Learning.

Roberts, J.E., Pollock, K.E., Krakow, R., Price, J., Fulmer, K. and Wang, P. (2005) Language development in preschool children adopted from China. *Journal of Speech, Language, and Hearing Research* 48, 93–107.

Roseberry-McKibbin, C. and O'Hanlon, L. (2005) Nonbiased assessment of English language learners: A tutorial. *Communication Disorders Quarterly* 26 (3), 178–185.

Sell, D. (2008) Speech therapy delivery and cleft lip and palate in the developing world. In M. Mars, A. Habel and D. Sell (eds) *Management of Cleft Lip and Palate in the Developing World* (pp. 193–202). West Sussex, UK: John Wiley & Sons.

Semela, J.J.M. (2001) Significance of cultural variables in assessment and therapy. *Folia Phoniatrica et Logopaedica* 53 (3), 128–134.

Seymour, H.N. (2004) A noncontrastive model for assessment of phonology. *Seminars in Speech and Language* 25, 91–99.

Seymour, H.N. and Seymour, C.M. (1977) A therapeutic model for communicative disorders among Black English speaking children. *Journal of Speech and Hearing Disorders* 42, 247–256.

Shriberg, L.D., Austin, D., Lewis, B.A., McSweeny, J.L. and Wilson, D.L. (1997) The Percentage of Consonants Correct (PCC) metric: Extensions and reliability data. *Journal of Speech, Language and Hearing Research* 40 (4), 708–722.

Shriberg, L.D., Lohmeier, H.L., Campbell, T.F., Dollaghan, C.A., Green, J.R. and Moore, C.A. (2009) A nonword repetition task for speakers with misarticulations: The Syllable Repetition Task (SRT). *Journal of Speech, Language and Hearing Research* 52 (5), 1189–1212.

Skahan, S.M., Watson, M. and Lof, G.L. (2007) Speech-language pathologists' assessment practices for children with suspected speech sound disorders: Results of a national survey. *American Journal of Speech-Language Pathology* 16 (3), 246–259.

Stertzbach, J. and Gildersleeve-Neumann, C.E. (2005, November) Parent report as a screening tool of speech disorders in Spanish-speaking preschool children. Technical presentation presented at the annual convention of the American Speech-Language-Hearing Association, San Diego, CA.

Stockman, I.J. (2006) Evidence for a minimal competence core of consonant sounds in the speech of African American children: A preliminary study. *Clinical Linguistics and Phonetics* 20 (10), 723–749.

Stockman, I.J. (2008) Toward validation of a minimal competence phonetic core for African American children. *Journal of Speech, Language and Hearing Research* 51 (5), 1244–1262.

Stow, C. and Dodd, B. (2003) Providing an equitable service to bilingual children in the UK: A review. *International Journal of Language and Communication Disorders* 38 (4), 351–377.

Stow, C. and Pert, S. (2006) *BiSSS: Bilingual Speech Sound Screen: Pakistani Heritage Languages*. Winslow: Speechmark.

Elin Thordardottir, and Ellis Weismer, S. (1996) Language assessment via parent report: Development of a screening instrument for Icelandic children. *First Language, 16,* 265–285.

Toohill, B., McLeod, S. and McCormack, J. (2011, in press) Effect of dialect on identification and severity of speech impairment in Indigenous Australian children, *Clinical Linguistics and Phonetics*.

Velleman, S.L. and Pearson, B.Z. (2010) Differentiating speech sound disorders from phonological dialect differences: Implications for assessment and intervention. *Topics in Language Disorders* 30 (3), 176–188.

Vogel, A.P. and Morgan, A.T. (2009) Factors affecting the quality of sound recording for speech and voice analysis. *International Journal of Speech-Language Pathology* 11 (6), 431–437.

Weichold, K. (2010) Introduction to mobility, migration, and acculturation. *ISSBD Bulletin* 58 (2), 1.

Wertzner, H.F., Alves, R.R. and de Oliveira Ramos, A.C. (2008) Análise do desenvolvimento das habilidades diadococinéticas orais em crianças normais e com transtorno fonológico [Development of oral diadochokinetic abilities in normal and phonologically disordered children]. *Revista da Sociedade Brasileira de Fonoaudiologia* 31 (2).

Williams, C.J. and McLeod, S. (2011, in press) Speech-language pathologists' assessment and intervention practices with multilingual children. *International Journal of Speech-Language Pathology.*

Williams, P. and Stackhouse, J. (2000) Rate, accuracy and consistency: Diadochokinetic performance of young, normally developing children. *Clinical Linguistics and Phonetics* 14, 267–293.

Windsor, J., Kohnert, K., Lobitz, K.F. and Pham, G.T. (2010) Cross-language nonword repetition by bilingual and monolingual children. *American Journal of Speech-Language Pathology* 19 (4), 298–310.

Winter, K. (2001) Numbers of bilingual children in speech and language therapy: Theory and practice of measuring their representation. *International Journal of Bilingualism* 5 (4), 465–495.

Yavaş, M. and Goldstein, B. (1998) Phonological assessment and treatment of bilingual speakers. *American Journal of Speech-Language Pathology* 7, 49–60.

Appendix

Appendix A Examples of monolingual speech assessments in languages other than English

Language (dialect)	Test/word list*	Name of test	Reference
Arabic (Egyptian)	Word list	Mansoura Arabic Articulation Test (MAAT)	Abou-Elsaad, T., Baz, H. and El-Banna, M. (2009) Developing an articulation test for Arabic-speaking school-age children. *Folia Phoniatrica et Logopaedica* 61 (5), 275–282.
Arabic (Jordanian)	Word list	Amayreh Articulation Test	Amayreh, M.M. and Dyson, A.T. (1998) The acquisition of Arabic consonants. *Journal of Speech, Language, and Hearing Research* 41, 642–653.
	Word list	Amayreh Articulation Test: Modified	Hamdan, J.M. and Amayreh, M.M. (2007) Consonant profile of Arabic-speaking school-age children in Jordan. *Folia Phoniatrica et Logopaedica* 59 (2), 55–64.
Cantonese	Test	Cantonese Phonological Assessment Guideline	So, L.K.H. (1992) *Cantonese Phonological Assessment Guideline*. Hong Kong: Department of Speech and Hearing Sciences, University of Hong Kong.
	Test	Cantonese Segmental Phonology Test	So, L.K.H. (1993) *Cantonese Segmental Phonology Test*. Hong Kong: Bradford Publishing.
	Test	Hong Kong Cantonese Articulation Test	Cheung, P.S.P., Ng, A. and To, C.K.S. (2006) *Hong Kong Cantonese Articulation Test*. Hong Kong: Language Information Sciences Research Centre, City University of Hong Kong.

(Continued)

Appendix A (*Continued*)

Language (dialect)	Test/word list*	Name of test	Reference
	Test	Cantonese Basic Speech Perception Test	Lee, K.Y.S. (2006) *Cantonese Basic Speech Perception Test*. Hong Kong: The Chinese University of Hong Kong.
	Test	Hong Kong Cantonese Tone Identification Test	Lee, K.Y.S. (2011) *Hong Kong Cantonese Tone Identification Test*. Hong Kong: Department of Otorhinolaryngology, Head and Neck Surgery, The Chinese University of Hong Kong.
Dutch	Analysis	Fonologische Analyse van het Nederlands (FAN)	Beers, M. (1995) *The phonology of normally developing and language impaired children*. University of Amsterdam, The Netherlands.
	Test	Logo-art Articulatieonderzoek	Baarda, D., de Boer-Jongsma, N. and Haasjes-Jongsma, W. (2005) *Logo-art Articulatieonderzoek* [in Dutch]. Ternat/Axel: Baert.
	Test	Taaltoets Alle Kinderen	Verhoeven, L. and Vermeer, A. (2001) *Taaltoets Alle Kinderen* [in Dutch]. Arhem: CITO.
	Test	Taaltoets Allochtone Kinderen	Verhoeven, L., Vermeer, A. and van Guchte, C. (1986) *Taaltoets Allochtone Kinderen* [in Dutch]. Tilburg: Zwijsen.
	Test	Utrechts Articulatie Onderzoek	Peddemors-Boon, M., van der Meulen, Sj. and de Vries, K. (1974) *Utrechts Articulatie Onderzoek* [in Dutch]. Tilburg: Zwijsen.

Language	Type	Title	Reference
Finnish	Test	*Artikulaation arviointitehtäviä*	Vainio, L. (1993) *Artikulaation arviointitehtäviä* [in Finnish]. Helsinki: Early Learning.
	Test	*Artikulaatiotesti. Äänteenmukainen sanakuvatesti*	Remes, K. and Ojanen, A.-K. (1996) *Artikulaatiotesti. Äänteenmukainen sanakuvatesti* [in Finnish]. Helsinki: Early Learning Oy.
	Test	*Fonologiatesti*	Kunnari, S., Savinainen-Makkonen, T., & Saaristo-Helin, K. (2012). *Fonologiatesti* [in Finnish]. Jyväskylä, Finland: Niilo Mäki Instituutti.
French	Word list	*Bilan phonologique*	Asselin, C. (n.d.) *Bilan phonologique: Adptation française du Hodson Phonological Process Analysis* [in French]. University of Montreal. http://www.eoa.umontreal.ca/ressources/bilansPhono.htm.
	Word list	*Casse-tête d'Evaluation de la Phonologie* (originally from Auger, 1994)	Macleod, A. A. N., Sutton, A., Trudeau, N., & Thordardottir, E. (2011). The acquisition of consonants in Quebecois French: A cross-sectional study of pre-school aged children. *International Journal of Speech-Language Pathology, 13*(2), 93–109.
German	Test	*ADD – Aachener Dyslalie Diagnostik*	Stiller, U. and Tockuss, C. (2000) *ADD – Aachener Dyslalie Diagnostik – Artikulationsprüfung mit 98 Photos auf CD-Rom* [in German]. Braunschweig: Schubi.
	Test	*AVAK – Analyseverfahren zu Aussprachestörungen bei Kindern*	Hacker, D. and Wilgermein, H. (1999) *Aussprachestörungen bei Kindern* [in German]. München – Basel: Ernst Reinhardt Verlag.

(Continued)

Appendix A (*Continued*)

Language (dialect)	Test/word list*	Name of test	Reference
	Test	*Bilderbuch zur Ausspracheprüfung bei Kindern*	Hild, U. (2002) *Bilderbuch zur Ausspracheprüfung bei Kindern* [in German]. Kassel: Orca.
	Test	*Logo Ausspracheprüfung*	Wagner, I. (1994) *Logo-Ausspracheprüfung* [in German]. Oldenburg: Logo Verlag für Sprachtherapie GbR.
	Test	*PAP – Pyrmonter Ausspracheprüfung*	Babbe, T. (2003) *PAP—Pyrmonter Aussprache Prüfung* [in German]. Köln: Prolog.
	Test	*Patholinguistische Diagnostik von Sprachentwicklungsstörungen*	Kauschke, C. and Siegmüller, J. (2002) *Psycholinguistische Diagnostik von Sprachentwicklungsstörungen* [in German]. München: Urban & Springer.
	Test	*PLAKSS – Psycholinguistische Analyse kindlicher Aussprachestörungen*	Fox, A.V. (2005) *Kindliche Aussprachestörungen—Phonologische Entwicklung, Differentialdiagnostik und Therapie* (3rd edn) [in German]. Idstein: Schultz Kirchner Verlag.
	Test	*Ravensburger Stammler Prüfbogen*	Frank, G. and Grziwotz, P. (1974) *Lautprüfbogen* [in German]. Ravensburg: Ravensburger Sprachheilzentrum Selbstverlag.

Greek	Test (speech and language)	Anomilo 4. Screening Test for Speech and Language Disorders for 4-year-old Children	Panhellenic Association of Logopedists (PAL) (Panellinios Syllogos Logopedikon) [Πανελλήνιος Σύλλογος Λογοπεδικών (ΠΣΛ)] (2005) Anomilo 4. Screening test for speech and language disorders for 4 year old children [in Greek]. Athens: Ellinika Grammata.
	Test	Assessment of Phonetic and Phonological Development	Panhellenic Association of Logopedists (PAL) (Panellinios Syllogos Logopedikon) [Πανελλήνιος Σύλλογος Λογοπεδικών (ΠΣΛ)] (1995) Δοκιμασία Φωνητικής & φωνολογικής Εξέλιξης [Assessment of Phonetic and Phonological Development] [in Greek]. Athens: Author.
Hungarian	Test	GMP Diagnosztika [GMP Diagnostics]	Gósy, M. (1995) GMP Diagnosztika [GMP diagnostics] [in Hungarian]. Budapest: Nikol.
Israeli Hebrew	Test	Articulation and Naming Test	Rosin, D. and Yakir, P. (2000) Pictures for Examining Articulation and Naming of Hebrew-speaking Children in Israel. Rehovot, Israel.
	Test	Goralnik Language Screening Test	Goralnik, E. (1995) Language Screening Test for Hebrew-speaking Preschool Children. Netanya, Israel: Gai Agencies.
Japanese	Test	Kōon Hattatsu Yosoku Kensa	Nagasawa, Y., Fujishima, S. and Oishi, M. (1985) Kōonhattatsu yosoku kensa [in Japanese]. Tokyo: Kokuritsu Tokushu Kyōiku Sōgōkenkyujo.

(Continued)

Appendix A (*Continued*)

Language (dialect)	Test/word list*	Name of test	Reference
	Word list	*Kōon Kensahō* (original reference)	Abe, M., Kato, M., Saito, S., Takeshita, K., Nishimura, B., Funayama, M., Yamashita, S., & Yamashita, Y. (1981) *Kōonkensahō. Onsei Gengo Igaku 22*, 209–217.
	Word list	*Kōon Kensahō*	Funayama, M., Abe, M., Kato, M., Saito, S., Takeshita, K., Nishimura, B., Yamashita, S. & Yamashita, Y. (1989) *Kōonkensahō tsuikahōkoku* [in Japanese]. *Onsei Gengo Igaku 30*, 285–292.
	Test	*Shinteiban Kotoba no Tesuto Ehon*	Taguchi, T. and Ogawaguchi, H. (1992) *Shinteiban kotoba no tesuto ehon – Gengo shōgaiji no senbetsu kensahō* [in Japanese]. Tokyo: Nihon Bunkakagakusha.
Maltese	Test	*Maltese-English Speech Assessment for Children (MESA)*	Grech, H., Dodd, B., & Franklin, S. (2011). *Maltese-English Speech Assessment (MESA)*. Guardamangia, Malta: University of Malta.
Norwegian	Test	*Artikulasjonsprøve*	Backe, L. (n.d.) *Artikulasjonsprøve B [Articulation Test B]* [in Norwegian]. Oslo: Norsk logopedlag.
	Test	*Artikulasjonsprøve for registrering av uttalefeil*	Johnsen, K. (1987) *Artikulasjonsprøve for registrering av uttalefeil [Articulation Test for Registration of Pronunciation Errors]* [in Norwegian]. Jaren, Norway: Vigga forlag.

	Test	*Norsk Fonemtest*	Tingleff, H. and Tingleff, Ø. (2002) *Norsk Fonemtest* [*Norwegian Phoneme Test*] [in Norwegian]. Oslo: Damm forlag.
	Test	*Norsk Logopedlags Språklydsprøve*	Vidsjå, I., Hauglid, J., Kloster-Jensen, M. and Skei, A. (1983) *Norsk Logopedlags Språklydsprøve* [*The Norwegian Association of Speech Therapist's Speech Sound Test*] [in Norwegian]. Oslo: Universitetsforlaget.
Portuguese (Brazilian)	Test	*ABFW – Teste de Linguagem infantile: Nas áreas de fonologia, vocabulário, fluência e pragmática*	Andrade, C.R.F. (2000) *ABFW-Teste de Linguagem infantile: Nas áreas de fonologia, vocabulário, fluência e pragmática* [in Portuguese]. Carapicuiba, SP: Pro-Fono.
	Test	*Avaliação Fonológica da criança* (AFC)	Yavaş, M., Hernandorena, C.L.M. and Lamprecht, R.R. (1991) *Avaliação Fonológica da criança: Reeducação e terapia* [in Portuguese]. Porto Alegre, RS: Artes Medicas.
Portuguese (European)	Test	*Teste Fonético-Fonológico-ALPE* (TFF-ALPE)	Mendes, A.P., Afonso, E., Lousada, M. and Andrade, F. (2009) *Teste Fonético-Fonológico-ALPE (TFF-ALPE)* [*Phonetic-Phonological Test*] [in Portuguese]. Aveiro, PT.
Putonghua	Test	*Putonghua Segmental Phonology Test* (PSPT)	So, L.K.H. and Jing, Z. (2000) *Putonghua Segmental Phonology Test (PSPT)*. Nanjing, China: Nanjing Normal University Press.
	Word list	*Picture-naming task*	Hua, Z. (2002) *Phonological Development in Specific Contexts: Studies of Chinese-speaking Children*. Clevedon Buffalo, NY: Multilingual Matters. (Appendix 1, pp. 201–202)

(Continued)

Appendix A (*Continued*)

Language (dialect)	Test/word list*	Name of test	Reference
Samoan	Word list	*Samoan Word List*	Ballard, E. and Farao, S. (2008) The phonological skills of Samoan speaking 4-year-olds. *International Journal of Speech-Language Pathology* 10 (6), 379–391.
Spanish	Test	*Assessment of Phonological Processes-Spanish*	Hodson, B. (1986) *Assessment of Phonological Processes-Spanish*. San Diego, CA: Los Amigos Research Associates.
	Test	*Assessment of Spanish Phonology – Revised*	Barlow, J.A. (2003) *Assessment of Spanish Phonology-Revised*. San Diego, CA: Phonological Typologies Laboratory, School of Speech, Language, and Hearing Sciences, San Diego State University.
	Test	*Austin Spanish Articulation Test*	Carrow, E. (1974) *Austin Spanish Articulation Test*. Austin, TX: Learning Concepts.
	Word list	*Comprehensive Assessment of Spanish Articulation-Phonology (CASA-P)*	Brice, A.E., Carson, C.K. and Dennis O'Brien, J. (2009) Spanish-English articulation and phonology of 4- and 5-year-old preschool children: An initial investigation. *Communication Disorders Quarterly* 31 (1), 3–14.
	Test	*Contextual Probes of Articulation Competence: Spanish*	Goldstein, B. and Iglesias, A. (2006) *CPACS: Contextual Probes of Articulation Competence: Spanish*. Greenville, SC: Super Duper.

Language			
	Test	*Hodson-Prezas Assessment of Spanish Phonological Patterns*	Hodson, B.W. and Prezas, R.F. (2010) Hodson-Prezas Assessment of Spanish Phonological Patterns. Unpublished test. Wichita State University, KS.
	Test	*Southwest Spanish Articulation Test*	Toronto, A. (1977) *Southwestern Spanish Articulation Test.* Austin, TX: National Education Laboratory Publishers.
	Test	*Spanish Articulation Measures*	Mattes, L.J. (1995) *Spanish Articulation Measures: Revised edition.* Oceanside, CA: Academic Communication Associates.
Swedish	Test	*SVANTE- Svenskt artikulations- och Nasalittets Test [Swedish Articulation and Nasality Test]*	Lohmander, A., Borell, E., Henningsson, G., Havstam, C., Lundeborg, I. and Persson, C. (2005) *SVANTE- Svenskt artikulations- och Nasalittets Test [Swedish Articulation and Nasality Test]* [in Swedish]. Skivarp, Sweden: Pedagogisk Design.
Turkish	Test	*Ankara artikülasyon testi [Ankara Articulation Test]*	Ege, P., Acarlar, F. and Güleryüz, F. (2004) *Ankara artikülasyon testi [Ankara Articulation Test]* [in Turkish]. Ankara: Key Tasarim.
	Test	*Konuşma sorunlu çocukların sesbilgisel çözümleme yöntemi ile değerlendirilmesi [Assessment of Speech Disordered Children by Phonological Analysis]*	Topbaş, S. (1998) *Konuşma sorunlu çocukların sesbilgisel çözümleme yöntemi ile değerlendirilmesi [Assessment of Speech Disordered Children by Phonological Analysis]* [in Turkish]. Eskişehir, Turkey: Anadolu University Press.

(Continued)

Appendix A (*Continued*)

Language (dialect)	Test/word list*	Name of test	Reference
	Test	*Eskişehir Konuşma Değerlendirme Test Takımı [Eskişehir Assessment of Speech Test]*	Özsoy, Y. (1982) *Eskişehir Konuşma Değerlendirme Test Takımı [Eskişehir Assessment of Speech Test]* [in Turkish]. Eskişehir, Turkey: Anadolu University Press.
	Test	*Türkçe Sesletim-Sesbilgisi Testi (SST) [Turkish Articulation and Phonology Test]*	Topbaş, S. (2004/2005) *Türkçe Sesletim-Sesbilgisi Testi (SST) [Turkish Articulation and Phonology Test]* [in Turkish]. Ankara, Turkey: Millî Eğitim Yayınevi 4. Akşam Sanat Okulu.

*Typically, 'tests' are published by a commercial publisher and contain an instructors' manual, pictures, score forms and normative data. 'Word lists' are typically published in an appendix of a journal paper and may or may not have been standardized. Word lists may also be published as tests.

Appendix B Examples of multilingual speech assessments

Language (dialect)	Test vs. published word list*	Name of test	Reference
Maltese-English	Test (speech)	*Maltese-English Speech Assessment (MESA)*	Grech, H., Dodd, B., & Franklin, S. (2011). *Maltese-English Speech Assessment (MESA)*. Guardamangia, Malta: University of Malta.
Pakistani-heritage languages: Mirpuri, Punjabi, Urdu with English	Test (speech)	*BiSSS: Bilingual Speech Sound Screen: Pakistani Heritage Languages*	Stow, C. and Pert, S. (2006) *BiSSS: Bilingual Speech Sound Screen: Pakistani Heritage Languages*. Winslow: Speechmark.
	Test (speech)	*Rochdale Assessment of Mirpuri Phonology with Punjabi, Urdu and English (RAMP)*	Stow, C. and Pert, S. (1998) *Rochdale Assessment of Mirpuri Phonology with Punjabi, Urdu and English: A Speech and Language Therapy Resource for the Phonological Assessment of Bilingual Children*. Rochdale: Pert.
Russian-German Turkish-German	Test (speech)	*Screening der Erstsprachefähigkeit bei Migrantenkindern*	Wagner, L. (2008) *Screemik Version 2. Screening der Erstsprachefähigkeit bei Migrantenkindern: Russisch-Deutsch. Türkisch-Deutsch* [in German]. Eugen: Wagner Verlag.
Spanish-English	Test (speech and language)	*Bilingual English Spanish Assessment (BESA)*	Peña, E.D., Gutiérrez-Clellen, V.F., Iglesias, A., Goldstein, B. and Bedore, L.M. (in development) Bilingual English Spanish Assessment (BESA). Unpublished assessment tool.

14 Translation to Practice: Creating Sampling Tools to Assess Multilingual Children's Speech

Sharynne McLeod

Languages mentioned: Arabic, Cantonese, Greek, Korean, Norwegian, Samoan

The (un)Met Need for Creation of Speech Sampling Tools

Although speech sampling tools are available in a range of languages (see McLeod, Chapter 13), speech-language pathologists (SLPs) around the world often rely on English or informal assessment tools when working with multilingual children (McLeod, 2007; Skahan *et al.*, 2007). For example, when considering assessment of Samoan children, Ballard and Faro (2008): 379) wrote: 'As information about different cultures and languages is limited, few practitioners have the multicultural assessment skills or resources necessary to make such a judgment or a culturally appropriate assessment'. When speech assessments are not available, sampling tools are often created by SLPs themselves. There are at least four situations that may necessitate the creation of speech sampling tools: when no assessment tools have been developed for a particular language (e.g. when working with children from a developing nation); when working with children who speak non-dominant languages (e.g. Stow & Pert, 1998); when assessment tools are available in a particular language, but are difficult to access (e.g. PAL (1995) can be purchased after attending a training workshop in Greece); or when available sampling tools are not appropriate for use in the SLPs' context (e.g. the words are irrelevant for a particular dialect or the accompanying images are culturally inappropriate/insensitive).

Determine whether Suitable Measurement Tools already Exist

Before creating a new tool to assess children's speech, it is important to conduct a thorough search to determine whether suitable tools already exist. There are a number of places to look:

(1) Internet and library databases including: Google scholar, Medline, ERIC and CINAHL. Journal papers can include word lists (sampling tools) as appendices (e.g. a single word test of Samoan is included in the appendix of Ballard and Farao (2008); the *Mansoura Arabic Articulation Test* (MAAT) is included as the appendix in Abou-Elsaad *et al.* (2009); and a single word test for Cantonese tone production is included in Lee *et al.* (2010)).

(2) Professional associations in the countries that speak the language(s) of interest. *The International Directory of Communication Disorders* (IDCD) (Bleile, 2006) provides a list of professional associations around the world. For example, the Panhellenic Association of Logopedists has published a phonology test in Greek (PAL, 1995) and the Norwegian Association of Speech Therapists has published a speech sound test in Norwegian (Vidsjå *et al.*, 1983).

(3) Hospitals, community health centers, schools and universities in countries that speak the language(s) of interest. Within universities, contact linguistic and phonetic departments, teacher education departments (e.g. in Korea, teachers learn the International Phonetic Alphabet), as well as speech-language pathology departments (and try an alternative nomenclature such as speech and language therapy, logopedics and phoniatrics).

(4) Craniofacial/cleft palate medical teams, such as Operation Smile (http://www.operationsmile.org/), Interplast (http://www.intreplast.org) and The Smile Train (http://www.thesmiletrain.org) often include SLPs who assess children's speech.

(5) Non-government organizations (NGOs), charities and mission organizations in countries that speak the language(s) of interest, as well as the office in the home country, to identify SLPs who no longer work in the country. The Summer Institute of Linguistics (www.sil.org) also develops translation tools, including phonetic fonts.

(6) Books and chapters, including the *International Guide to Speech Acquisition* (McLeod, 2007), which lists available assessments in 12 English dialects and 23 languages other than English, and Chapter 13 of the current book, which contains a list of speech assessments in 18 different languages.

Creating a Sampling Tool

If a suitable tool is unavailable, then according to Frytak (2000) there are two steps to creating one: conceptualization and operationalization. Most SLPs who create sampling tools undertake many of the components of the conceptualization step, but few undertake the second step to operationalize the tool.

Conceptualization: Decide on the purpose and scope of the tool

(1) *Purpose*. Will the tool assess one language and/or dialect, or be designed to compare skills in different languages and dialects? Alternatively, will the tool assess a child's ability to learn a language (e.g. Jacobs & Coufal, 2001)? Will the tool be used for screening, diagnostic assessment, describing speech, goal setting for intervention or determination of outcomes? It is unlikely that one tool will be able to achieve each of these purposes.

(2) *Intended population*. Who is the tool designed for? Consider the country, language, dialect and age group(s). Is the test for monolingual or bilingual speakers? What qualifications do the examiners need?

(3) *Target skill*. Will the tool be used to assess production (articulation of speech sounds, phonology, nonword repetition), perception, phonological awareness (emergent literacy skills), stimulability or intelligibility/acceptability? The underlying theoretical construct of the sampling tool should guide this step.

(4) *Scope*. Will the tool assess all or some of the following: consonants, vowels, consonant clusters, onsets, codas, multisyllabic words, prosody, tones (for tonal languages such as Cantonese and Norwegian), phonological processes/patterns and/or phonological awareness?

Guidelines for developing a single word test of consonant production

One of the most common speech sampling tools used throughout the world is the single word test of consonants. This may be (and is typically) the first test that is developed for a language or dialect. The principles provided for developing a single word test of consonants can be applied to the development of other tools.

(1) Prepare an inventory of the consonants that occur within the language and dialect. There are a number of sources to assist with this step, including:
  (a) Handbook of the International Phonetic Alphabet (IPA, 1999), and Illustrations of the IPA in the *Journal of the International Phonetic Alphabet* (http://journals.cambridge.org/action/displayJournal?jid= IPA) (e.g. Bengali is illustrated in Khan (2010) and includes supplementary sound files).
  (b) Books such as *The Sounds of the World's Languages* (Ladefoged & Maddieson, 1996) and *The International Guide to Speech Acquisition* (McLeod, 2007).
  (c) Journal papers and book chapters (e.g. Salameh *et al.* (2003) include inventories of Arabic and Swedish consonants).
  (d) Websites, including the Speech Accent Archive (http://accent. gmu.edu/browse_native.php), American Speech-Language-Hearing

Association (ASHA) Multicultural Affairs and Resources page (http://www.asha.org/practice/multicultural/Phono.htm) and Wikipedia IPA charts (http://en.wikipedia.org/wiki/International_ Phonetic_Alphabet); however, remember that not all websites have undergone rigorous peer review.

(2) Prepare a phonotactic inventory (i.e. sound structure) of the language and dialect. Which sounds occur in all word positions, and which occur only in syllable-initial word-initial, syllable-final within-word, syllable-initial within-word and syllable-final word-final?

(3) Decide on the number of productions of each speech sound to elicit (typically between one and five). Children's speech varies and different phonetic contexts create different co-articulatory situations (e.g. in English, if the only word that is elicited is *yellow* /jɛloʊ/, then it is likely that /j/ will be misarticulated due to co-articulatory effects with /l/).

(4) Decide on the mode, and the phonotactic and morphological context of the words.
   (a) *Mode*. Consonants in single words are typically more accurate than consonants in connected speech; however, different phono-logical processes occur in each mode (Morrison & Shriberg, 1992).
   (b) *Number of syllables*. Consonants in monosyllabic and bisyllabic words are typically more accurate than in polysyllabic words (James *et al.*, 2008) (e.g. *cat* vs. *caterpillar*).
   (c) *Consonant clusters*. Consonants within consonant clusters are typically less accurate than consonants in singleton contexts (Smit *et al.*, 1990) (e.g. *bread* vs. *bed* vs. *red*).
   (d) *Morphophonemes*. Consonants within morphophonemic contexts may be less accurate than consonants in words that do not contain a grammatical morpheme (Song *et al.*, 2009) (e.g. *keys* /kiz/ (plural) vs. buzz /bʌz/). Consequently, a morphophonological context should be avoided so that phonology and morphology are not conflated.

(5) Locate frequently used words for the language and dialect. If possible, this list should comprise words frequently used by *children*. Some word frequency lists on the Internet are taken from compiling words printed in newspapers and will not provide as relevant information for compiling a pediatric assessment tool. The CHILDES database may act as a good reference. An alternative source is children's dictionaries, first word books and early school books.

(6) Select words. The selected words should be:
   (a) Familiar to children, and occur frequently, so that children can produce the word spontaneously, and not rely on imitated productions.

    (b) Culturally sensitive in both word choice and pictures (e.g. the number 4 in Cantonese is considered to be unlucky because it sounds like the word for *death*).

    (c) Picturable. Often this means that the test primarily contains nouns, unless computerized animation is available to demonstrate action verbs. Be aware that languages differ regarding the emphasis on nouns vs. verbs (Peña *et al.*, 2003).

(7) Consider presentation. Words can be presented as objects, pictures, photographs, drawings or computerized images (possibly with animation and an audio example). Clarity and ease of identification is paramount in this step. If pictures are sourced from the Internet, they should be within the public domain (not copyrighted). Try not to mix different illustration styles (e.g. cartoon style drawings vs. line drawings vs. photographs). Color vs. black and white illustrations has been found to effect children's picture-naming ability. For example, Barrow *et al.* (2000) found that when children were less familiar with words, color illustrations were more easily identifiable than black and white illustrations during a picture-naming task.

(8) Consider test administration. Will the tool be administered in a standardized (i.e. static) manner or as a dynamic assessment? Standardized test administration may involve presenting instructions via pre-recorded speech. Dynamic speech assessments typically involve systematic assessment of stimulability (Glaspey & Stoel-Gammon, 2007). Will the children be allowed to code-switch from one language (and/or dialect?) to another during the assessment (e.g. Grech & Dodd, 2008)? Will the tool be administered by a native language speaker? Will testing occur in a formal clinical setting or a more familiar setting where children are more likely to use their home dialect or an informal register (e.g. Ballard & Farao, 2008)?

(9) Consider transcription, scoring, recording and analysis. Document acceptable pronunciations by transcribing 'accurate'/adult-like productions of the words in the chosen dialect(s). Decide whether scoring of the tool will include transcription of consonants only, and/or whole words, and whether broad vs. narrow phonetic transcription will be used (using the International Phonetic Alphabet). Will transcription occur using pen and paper or via a computer program? Will the speech sample be audio- and/or video-recorded for reliability checking and later comparison of outcomes after assessment?

Creating a measurement tool is a fine balance between the need to accurately represent the complexity of speech and a child's capacity to speak, with the realities of children's attention span, SLPs' time and the need to identify and quantify a speech sound disorder.

Operationalization: Testing a test

Once a sampling tool is created, it can then be operationalized and validated. It is useful to work in conjunction with a (bio)statistician or psychometrician to establish the psychometric properties of the tool. Key concepts when operationalizing a sampling tool include determination of:

(4) Reliability: Does the test provide a consistent measure?
   (a) *Internal consistency.* To estimate the extent to which a group of items measure the same overall construct (relevant statistical analyses include: Cronbach's alpha, confirmatory factor analysis). A test may generate one overall score, or a set of subscale scores, depending on the number of domains being assessed.
   (b) *Test-retest reliability.* To estimate the extent to which similar scores would be achieved if the test was readministered under the same circumstances (relevant statistical analyses include: correlation, intra-class correlation).
   (c) *Rater reliability including inter- and intra-rater reliability.* To estimate the extent to which the test results are the same when the test is administered by different people or by the same people at different times. Rater reliability can be affected by training and by provision of external standard comparison measures (relevant statistical analyses include: inter-class correlation, Cohen's kappa).
(2) Validity: Does the test measure what it claims to measure?
   (a) *Content validity.* To consider 'the degree to which the items in the measure cover the domain of interest' (Frytak, 2000: 22). Two common approaches to establishing content validity of a test are: by systematic examination of literature and consultation with experts (Brown, 1985; Chan & Lee, 1999; Millman & Greene, 1993; Thorn & Deitz, 1989). A systematic literature review is important for specifying the initial test content, while expert professional judgments play an integral part in further defining the test areas and evaluating the degree to which the items are relevant and representative to the target construct (AERA, APA, NCME, 1999; Bubela *et al.*, 1990; Haynes *et al.*, 1995). Relevance of test content refers to the appropriateness of the test items for measuring the target construct (Messick, 1993). For example, testing the English phoneme /t/ in the medial position using the word *butter* would be an item with low relevance as the medial /t/ is often realized as [d] or a flap in some dialects of English. Representativeness refers to the extent that test items are proportional to the elements contained in the targeted construct (Nunnally & Bernstein, 1994). A speech sampling tool may have

content validity if there is comprehensive coverage of the phonemes within a language with test items that are appropriately devised (relevant statistical analyses include: correlation).

   (b) *Criterion validity.* To consider the degree of overlap between the test and other standard speech sampling tools that measure the same or similar abilities. Of central importance in criteria-related validity is the choice of criterion measure, which has to be a well-established valid measurement in itself (Gay, 1985; Messick, 1993) (relevant statistical analyses include: correlation).

   (c) *Construct validity.* To demonstrate that the test measures the construct of interest from a number of perspectives and sources of evidence. The central theme is to examine how well the obtained test scores reflect the unobservable attribute. It is the most difficult and yet the most important form of validity to obtain. For test scores to be meaningful, it has to be shown that all the individual test items relate to others in some way so that they are measuring the same rather than diverse dimensions. Intercorrelations among test items, factor analyses and item response theory are often used to determine construct validity (AERA, APA, NCME, 1999; Benson & Clark, 1982; Bubela *et al.*, 1990; Clark & Watson, 1995; Hambelton, 1993; Hasselkus & Safrit, 1976; Nunnally & Bernstein, 1994). Other commonly used approaches to evaluate the strength of the score interpretation include the known groups method, convergence and discrimination (relevant statistical analyses include: correlation, factor analysis, Rasch analysis).

(3) Item analysis. To determine item difficulty and item discrimination scores. James (2001) provided an example of undertaking an item analysis when developing a speech sampling tool and determined that polysyllabic words were better than monosyllabic words for discriminating between English-speaking children.

(4) Sensitivity and specificity. To describe the proportion of cases classified correctly. Measures with high sensitivity are able to accurately identify children with speech sound disorder (indicated as the percent identification of true positives) and measures with high specificity are able to accurately identify typically developing children (indicated as the percent identification of true negatives) (relevant statistical analyses include: linear discriminant function analysis).

(5) Standardization. Testing the sampling tool on a large normative sample (who represent the population of children for whom the test is intended) results in a wide range of raw scores. These scores can be converted into percentiles or standard scores to construct a normal distribution or test norms. Typical and unusual error patterns can also be

documented. Identification accuracy can be increased if the normative sample only includes typically developing children (Peña *et al.*, 2006).

The often-cited paper by McCauley and Swisher (1984) discusses the importance of establishing psychometric properties for speech and language assessments. The *Contextual Probes of Articulation Competence – Spanish* (Goldstein & Iglesias, 2009) provides an example of how to use McCauley and Swisher's guidelines when operationalizing a speech sampling tool and Friberg (2010) provides an updated version of these criteria.

Finally, Stockman (1996: 355) offers the following words of caution 'an adequate assessment is not insured simply by creating new norm-referenced standardized tests'. Assessment using a speech sampling tool should be complemented by other techniques, including criterion-referenced tools and dynamic assessment, as well as listening carefully to the children, their parents and teachers (see McLeod, Chapter 13).

Acknowledgements

Preparation of this chapter was supported by an Australian Research Council Future Fellowship (FT0990588) and helpful insights from Kathy Yuet Sheung Lee are also acknowledged.

References

Abou-Elsaad, T., Baz, H. and El-Banna, M. (2009). Developing an articulation test for Arabic-speaking school-age children. *Folia Phoniatrica et Logopaedica* 61 (5), 275–282.

American Educational Research Association, American Psychological Association and National Council on Measurement in Education (AERA, APA, NCME) (1999) *Standards for Educational and Psychological Testing*. Washington, DC: American Educational Research Association.

Ballard, E. and Farao, S. (2008) The phonological skills of Samoan speaking 4-year-olds. *International Journal of Speech-Language Pathology* 10 (6), 379–391.

Barrow, I.M., Holbert, D. and Rastatter, M.P. (2000) Effect of color on developmental picture-vocabulary naming of 4-, 6-, and 8-year-old children. *American Journal of Speech-Language Pathology* 9 (4), 310–318.

Benson, J. and Clark, F. (1982) A guide for instrument development and validation. *American Journal of Occupational Therapy* 36 (12), 789–800.

Bleile, K. (2006) *International Directory of Communication Disorders* (IDCD). San Diego, CA: Plural Publishing. http://www.comdisinternational.com/agreement.html. Accessed 26.10.10.

Brown, S. (1985) *What Do They Know? A Review of Criterion-referenced Assessment*. Scottish Education Department, Edinburgh: Her Majesty's Stationery Office.

Bubela, N., Galloway, S., McCay, E., McKibbon, A., Nagle, L., Pringle, D., Ross, E. and Shamian, J. (1990) The patient learning needs scale: Reliability and validity. *Journal of Advanced Nursing* 15, 1181–1187.

Chan, C.C.H. and Lee, T.M.C. (1999) Clinical evaluation: From validation to practice. In K.N. Anchor and T.C. Felicetti (eds) *Disability Analysis in Practice: Framework for an Interdisciplinary Science* (pp. 357–375). Dubuque, IO: Kendall/Hunt Publishing.

Clark, L.A. and Watson, D. (1995) Construction validity: Basic issues in objective scale development. *Psychological Assessment* 7 (3), 309–319.

Friberg, J.C. (2010) Considerations for test selection: How do validity and reliability impact diagnostic decisions? *Child Language Teaching and Therapy* 26 (1), 77–92.

Frytak, J. (2000) Measurement. *Journal of Rehabilitation Outcomes* 4 (1), 15–31.

Gay, L.R. (1985) *Educational Evaluation and Measurement: Competencies for Analysis and Application* (2nd edn). Cleveland, OH: Charles E. Merrill.

Glaspey, A.M. and Stoel-Gammon, C. (2007). A dynamic approach to phonological assessment. *International Journal of Speech-Language Pathology* 9 (4), 286–296.

Goldstein, B. and Iglesias, A. (2009) *CPACS: Contextual Probes of Articulation Competence: Spanish. Normative Data Manual*. Greenville, SC: Super Duper.

Grech, H. and Dodd, B. (2008) Phonological acquisition in Malta: A bilingual language learning context. *International Journal of Bilingualism* 12 (3), 155–171.

Hambleton, R.K. (1993) Principles and selected applications of item response theory. In R.L. Linn (ed.) *Educational Measurement* (3rd edn; pp.147–200). Phoenix, AZ: Oryx Press.

Hasselkus, B.R. and Safrit, M.J. (1976) Measurement in occupational therapy. *American Journal of Occupational Therapy* 30 (7), 429–436.

Haynes, S.N., Richard, D.C.S. and Kubany, E.S. (1995) Content validity in psychological assessment: A functional approach to concepts and methods. *Psychological Assessment* 7 (3), 238–247.

Jacobs, E.L. and Coufal, K.L. (2001) A computerized screening instrument of language learnability. *Communication Disorders Quarterly* 22, 67–76.

James, D.G.H. (2001) An item analysis of Australian English words for an articulation and phonological test for children aged 2 to 7 years. *Clinical Linguistics and Phonetics* 15, 457–485.

James, D.G.H., van Doorn, J. and McLeod, S. (2008) The contribution of polysyllabic words in clinical decision making about children's speech. *Clinical Linguistics and Phonetics* 22 (4), 345–353.

Khan, S.U.D. (2010) Bengali (Bangladeshi Standard). *Journal of the International Phonetic Association* 40, 221–225.

Ladefoged, P. and Maddieson, I. (1996) *The Sounds of the World's Languages*. Oxford: Blackwell.

Lee, K.Y.S., van Hasselt, C.A. and Tong, M.C.F. (2010) Age sensitivity in the acquisition of lexical tone production: An evidence from children with profound congenital hearing impairment. *Annals of Otology, Rhinology and Laryngology* 119 (4), 258–261.

McCauley, R.J. and Swisher, L. (1984) Use and misuse of norm referenced tests in clinical assessment: A hypothetical case. *Journal of Speech and Hearing Disorders* 49, 338–348.

Messick, S. (1993) Validity. In R.L. Linn (ed.) *Educational Measurement* (3rd edn; pp. 13–103). Phoenix, AZ: Oryx Press.

Millman, J. and Greene, J. (1993) The specification and development of tests of achievement and ability. In R.L. Linn (ed.) *Educational Measurement* (3rd edn) (pp. 335–366). Phoenix, AZ: Oryx Press.

Morrison, J.A. and Shriberg, L.D. (1992) Articulation testing versus conversational speech sampling. *Journal of Speech and Hearing Research* 35, 259–273.

Nunnally, J.C. and Bernstein, I.H. (1994) *Psychometric Theory*. New York: McGraw-Hill.

Panhellenic Association of Logopedists (PAL) (1995) Δοκιμασία Φωνητικής & φωνολογικής Εξέλιξης *[Assessment of Phonetic and Phonological Development]* [in Greek]. Athens, Greece: author.

Peña, E.D., Bedore, L. and Rappazzo, C. (2003) Comparison of Spanish, English, and bilingual children's performance across semantic tasks. *Language, Speech, and Hearing Services in Schools* 34, 5–16.

Peña, E.D., Spaulding, T.J. and Plante, E. (2006) The composition of normative groups and diagnostic decision making: Shooting ourselves in the foot. *American Journal of Speech-Language Pathology* 15, 247–254.

Salameh, E-K., Nettelbladt, U. and Norlin, K. (2003) Assessing phonologies in bilingual Swedish-Arabic children with and without language impairment. *Child Language Teaching and Therapy* 19, 338–364.

Smit, A.B., Hand, L., Freilinger, J.J., Bernthal, J.E. and Bird, A. (1990) The Iowa articulation norms project and its Nebraska replication. *Journal of Speech and Hearing Disorders* 55, 779–798.

Song, J.Y., Sundara, M. and Demuth, K. (2009) Effects of phonology on children's production of English 3rd person singular –s. *Journal of Speech, Language, and Hearing Research* 52 (3), 623–642.

Stockman, I.J. (1996) The promises and pitfalls of language sample analysis as an assessment tool for linguistic minority children. *Language, Speech, and Hearing Services in Schools* 27 (4), 355–366.

Stow, C. and Pert, S. (1998) The development of a bilingual phonology assessment. *International Journal of Language and Communication Disorders* 33 (Supplement), 338–343.

Thorn, D.W. and Deitz, J.C. (1989) Examining content validity through the use of content experts. *Occupational Therapy Journal of Research* 9 (6), 334–346.

Vidsjå, I., Hauglid, J., Kloster-Jensen, M. and Skei, A. (1983) *Norsk Logopedlags Språklydsprøve [The Norwegian Association of Speech Therapist's Speech Sound Test]* [in Norwegian]. Oslo: Universitetsforlaget.

15 Translation to Practice: Assessment of the Speech of Multilingual Children in Turkey

Seyhun Topbaş

Languages mentioned: Arabic, Armenian, Bulgarian, Greek, Kurdish, Persian, Turkish

Context

Turkey, historically, has cultural variety. A multilingual milieu consisting of Turkish, Arabic, Persian and other European languages, such as Greek, Bulgarian and Armenian, have been spoken since the time of the Seljuk and Ottoman Empires. After the foundation of the Turkish Republic, the members of each speech community had been determined on the basis of 'language(s)' they speak (Karahan, 2005). Notwithstanding, government policy is to keep the national identity under one nation and one official language, namely, Turkish. International immigration and mobility have also been changing the structure of the society. Consequently, there are many speech communities in Turkey whose first language (L1) is not Turkish. A recent national poll entitled *Who Are We?* has shown that Turkish is the mother tongue for 84.54% of the inhabitants, Kurdish is the second with 12.98% (Kurmanji and Zaza dialects) and Arabic is the third with 1.38%, followed by other languages with 1.11% (KONDA, 2006). Although the multicultural aspects of these communities are preserved, the use of these first languages is officially not allowed. The focus of this chapter will be on the largest bilingual population of these minority languages, namely, Kurdish-Turkish.

Brief characteristics of Turkish and Kurdish

Turkish, belonging to the *Altaic* linguistic family, is an agglutinating language. The neutral word order is subject-object-verb (SOV). Turkish contains 29 letters in the orthography; 8 short vowels /i, y, ɯ, u, ɛ, ø, a, o/ and 21 consonants /p, b, t, d, k, g, f, v, s, z, ʃ, ʒ, h, m, n, ɾ, l, j, tʃ, ʤ/. For the letter ğ, the so-called 'soft-g', the IPA symbol it represents is a controversial issue. Usually, it functions to lengthen the preceding vowel or occurs in borrowed vocabulary (see Kopkallı-Yavuz, 2010). The canonical syllable type is CV, allowing syllable structures as (C)V(C)(C), in that the vowel nucleus is the only obligatory element. There are no onset clusters; only certain cluster codas consisting of not more than two consonants are permitted (Göksel & Kerslake, 2005; Yavaş, 2010).

The Kurdish language belongs to the Indo-European family, forming a dialectal continuum. In Turkey, the Northern Kurdish/Kurmanchi dialect and Dimili/Zaza dialect are mostly spoken in southeast and eastern Turkey. It is an inflecting language, possessing a morphological ergativity. Like Turkish, Kurdish is based on the Latin alphabet with 8 vowels /i, e, æ, î, u, ə, a, o/ and 23 consonants /p, b, t, d, k, g, f, v, s, z, ʃ, ʒ, m, n, ɾ, l, j, tʃ, ʤ, x, q, w, ɣ, ħ/ (http://classweb.gmu.edu/accent/nl-ipa/kurdishipa.html) where the letter-sound-correspondence is predictable, although there are allophonic variations. The canonical word order is SOV, but shows variations (Aygen, 2007; Thackston, 2006).

Cultural, Linguistic and Educational Aspects

Kurdish is widespread, especially among the old, women and those who live in rural areas. The older generation, especially women, cannot speak Turkish very well and the literacy rate is very low (Gürsel et al., 2009). According to a poll conducted in six cities in southeast Turkey, 65% of the residents in this region speak Kurdish at home; outside the home, 52% speak a language mixture of Kurdish-Turkish and 21% only speak Kurdish (Yıldız & Düzgören, 2007). Consequently, this pattern of language use causes a great barrier for those who move to large cities where it is important to speak Turkish. For reasons such as seeking jobs, earning money, education, having equal rights with and being accepted by other groups, Kurds find speaking Turkish very important. However, for interactions with their friends and being considered a member of their community, Kurds find their mother tongue as important as Turkish. Depending on their strong ethnic relations with their groups, Kurds continue to use their mother tongue but in limited domains, such as in the home (Çoban, 2005; Karahan, 2005; Polat, 2007).

Kurdish children must acquire a high level of competency in Turkish in order to receive an education and survive in the community (Polat, 2007). Although the demographic data are not clear enough to indicate the extent to which Kurdish people are bilingual in Kurdish and Turkish, most Kurdish children living in particular regions in Turkey learn Kurdish as their mother tongue. Compared to studies in Turkish as L1, there is no documentation on the language development of Kurdish-Turkish speaking bilingual children (either the age when Turkish is typically introduced as the children's L2 or age of acquisition norms for Kurdish as an L1) (Topbaş, 2007). Kurdish children generally learn Kurdish at home and begin learning Turkish as their L2 via the media at home and outside and/or formally at age 7 when they go to school (Derince, 2010). Currently, there are vast regional disparities, where the lowest enrolment rates in pre-primary and primary education are observed in southeastern and eastern Anatolian provinces. Those children whose mother tongue is not Turkish do not receive necessary formal (both nursery and primary) additional support in either language. It can be inferred that these Kurdish-Turkish-speaking children do not fully fit the definition of either simultaneous or sequential bilinguals.

Because Kurdish is not allowed as the medium of instruction in primary schools, a mismatch occurs between the language spoken at home and the medium of instruction at school. That is, in the school context, children have to learn literacy skills and the instructional content of science and mathematics in Turkish, which may lead to some reading and writing problems, and academic learning difficulties in the L2 (i.e. Turkish). As an example, in the southeastern region, the majority of students are Kurdish and are listed as underachieving in all the national examinations, undertaken in Turkish, conducted yearly by the Ministry of Education. Both teachers and families attributed this underachievement to the children's low level of Turkish because most children speak Kurdish at home. Many teachers recommend that families should not speak Kurdish at home and many families agree; however, they do not speak Turkish fluently. Additionally, most teachers in Turkey do not speak Kurdish, therefore they cannot use Kurdish to support children's learning at school. Aksu-Koç *et al.*'s (2002) study, carried out in three provinces (İstanbul, Diyarbakır and Van) with 5- to 6-year-olds and 1st and 2nd graders, showed that the highest proportions of bilingual speakers, mainly Kurdish-Turkish, were found in Diyarbakır, followed by Van and a very small percentage in Istanbul. The teachers stated that these children's linguistic skills in Turkish were very low. Additionally, the fact that these provinces have the highest proportion of uneducated mothers and the least accessible early childhood education services constitute some of the factors that contribute negatively to the level of linguistic development in children (Aksu-Koç *et al.*, 2002), perhaps in both languages. Consequently, this may result in subtractive bilingualism or monolingualism that may be characterised as having less than native-like proficiency in one or both languages (Derince, 2010). Ayan-Ceyhan and Koçbaş (2009) suggested that one of the main reasons for underachievement among the Kurdish-speaking students might be the fact that their L1 Kurdish is disregarded in school settings. Hence, the switch in home-school language in submersion programmes may lead to poor academic achievement and an inadequate command of both the L1 and L2.

Speech assessment

A brief description of two Kurdish-Turkish bilingual children's speech is presented here to show the importance of assessing children's speech in two languages.

Helin is a 6 year, 7-month-old girl and *Yunus*, her brother, is 3 years and 4 months. They are Kurdish-Turkish bilinguals living in a suburb of Eskişehir where the socio-economic level is low. The family migrated from Van, in eastern Turkey, three months ago. The children's father is a construction worker. The mother mainly speaks Kurdish and is not proficient in Turkish.

The children were assessed by using the *Turkish Articulation-Phonology Test* (SST; Topbaş, 2004/2005) and a non-word repetition test (Topbaş *et al.*, in preparation). The non-word repetition performance of both Helin and Yunus was lower than that of typical children, but better than children with specific language impairment (SLI) at the same age. Helin's speech intelligibility was good in both Kurdish and Turkish; however, there were a number of errors in both languages (Percentage of Consonants Correct (Topbaş, 2004/5) 84% in Turkish and 88% in Kurdish). As an example, the velar sounds /k, g/ of Turkish were typically pronounced as velar fricatives or [x, χ] or glottal [q] and uvular stops [ʔ].

Yunus's phonological patterns seemed developmentally appropriate in Kurdish when compared with the target adult patterns. His skills in Turkish were lower than would be expected for typically developing children, and Kurdish interference could easily be observed; that is, there was some transfer of sounds from the L1 into L2. As can be seen from the examples below, the target /k, g/ consonants of Turkish were pronounced as uvular consonants or velar fricatives. A person who is not a speech-language pathologist (SLP) may interpret such a difference as a disorder; however, either the place or manner of articulation were preserved in most of the words, resembling a dialectal difference.

Target Turkish	*Child*	
/jatʌk/	[jataχ]	(bed)
/kulak/	[qulaχ]	(ear)
/gazetɛ/	[xæstə]	(newspaper)
/kɯz/	[quʃ]	(girl)
/kaʃuk/	[qæʃîx]	(spoon)
/koɫtuk/	[qotɯχ]	(armchair)

Conclusions and Implications for Children with Speech Sound Disorders

Many Kurdish-Turkish bilingual children, as outlined above, are often among those who are least well prepared for school life where the language of instruction is Turkish. Developing bilinguals, when compared to monolinguals, may show evidence of different linguistic representations and/or difficulties related to the amount of exposure to each language. It is also likely that they may experience increased difficulty in coping both academically and socially. The danger is that this situation may lead to disadvantage and stigmatisation of being language impaired. Due to the reduced input in both languages the language characteristics of many Kurdish-Turkish bilingual children may superficially resemble children with specific language impairments since it is often difficult to differentiate language impairments at the early phases of sequential bilingualism. For example, phonological processes are often claimed to be impaired in children with SLI, but they should be intact in bilingual children. Languages in contact may influence each other in phonology (Pena & Bedore, 2009) and language transfer may lead to a mixed knowledge of the phonological system, which may lead to misevaluation of a child as speech impaired.

Information about the speech and language development of children with varied language backgrounds is essential for SLP services to interpret the performance of these children and assess their development. Moreover, it is important to identify these difficulties in languages in order to understand whether the difficulty is stemming from a lack of exposure to either language or is specific to impairment, and if so, what intervention or remedial approaches are needed. Thus, phonology allows one of the promising assessment domains, generally tested by non-word repetition tasks (Kohnert, 2007), for disentangling the two (language impairment and difficulty due to lack of exposure in bilingual development) and how speech impairment may be manifested. Currently, there are no tools to assess the speech and language performance of Kurdish children. As shown in this chapter, an SLP can analyse the differences and similarities from the speech samples in the two languages and can demonstrate whether the differences are due to impairment or not. Additionally, there is a need for interpreters/ translators in children's first languages. Hence, an important contribution may be to conduct research in the acquisition of L1 and bilingual Kurdish-Turkish at the early phases, compare the performances and develop tests in Kurdish to assess children's performance for intervention purposes.

Recent research using more reliable methodology has shown that development in the L1 has positive effects on the L2 and that both languages nurture each other when the educational environment permits children access to both languages (Cummins, 2000). Recent research undertaken by Derince (2010) showed that learning L1 Kurdish is not an obstacle to school success; on the contrary, enhancing L1 language development before and during schooling is an essential predictor of higher proficiency in both L2 Turkish as well as L3 English. Derince further suggests that Kurdish-speaking parents should not refrain from speaking Kurdish to their children; on the contrary, they need to explicitly enforce the mother tongue development of their children for more effective multilingualism to occur. As Cummins (2000) proposed, bi/multilingual education programmes that take the role of the mother tongue as a central part of the education process is generally the best method of achieving long-term school success of bi/multilingual minority students and attaining language development both in the L1 and in subsequently learned languages (cf. Derince, 2010). Thus, educational policies should encourage development of the mother tongue and bi/multilingualism, and support organisations such as The Mother Child Education Foundation (ACEV) of Turkey, which has taken serious interest in contributing to the improvement of the social and linguistic development of children in eastern and southeastern Turkey. Services may be provided by SLPs and other educators to enrich speech, language, reading and writing skills for children who are at risk for academic performance.

Acknowledgements

The author is grateful to the family for their permission and insights during data collection and to Dilber Kaçar, MSc student in SLT, for collecting and transcribing the speech sample and to Dr. Özcan Karaaslan for support as the Kurdish-Turkish translator.

References

Aksu-Koç, A., Erguvanlı-Taylan, E. and Bekman, S. (2002) Need assessment in early childhood education and an evaluation of children's level of linguistic competence in three provinces of Turkey. Research Report No. 00R101. Boğaziçi University and Mother Child Education Foundation, İstanbul, Turkey.

Ayan-Ceyhan, M. and Koçbaş, D. (2009) *Çiftdillilik ve Eğitim* [*Multilingualism and Education*]. Eğitimde Haklar II Projesi. Istanbul: SabancI University Education Initiative Report.

Aygen, G. (2007) *Kurmanji Kurdish Grammar.* Munchen: Lincom Europa.

Cummins, J. (2000) *Language, Power and Pedagogy: Bilingual Children in the Crossfire.* Clevedon: Multilingual Matters.

Çoban, S. (2005) *Azınlıklar ve Dil* [*Minorities and Language*]. Istanbul: Su Yayınları.

Derince, M.ş. (2010) The role of first language (Kurdish) development in acquisition of a second language (Turkish) and a third language (English). Unpublished Master's thesis, Boğaziçi University.

Göksel, A. and Kerslake, C. (2005) *Turkish: A Comprehensive Grammar.* London: Routledge.

Gürsel, S., Uysal-Kolaşin, G. and ve Altındağ, O. (2009) *Anadili Türkçe nüfus ile Kürtçe nüfus arasInda eğitim uçurumu var* [*Educational gulf between Turkish and Kurdish population*] [in Turkish]. http://www.betam.bahcesehir.edu.tr/UserFiles/File/ArastirmaNotu49. pdf. Accessed 30.10.10.

Karahan, F. (2005) Bilingualism in Turkey. In J. Cohen, K.T. McAlister, K. Rolstad and J. MacSwan (eds) *Proceedings of the 4th International Symposium on Bilingualism* (pp. 1152–1166). Somerville, MA: Cascadilla Press.

Kohnert, K. (2007) *Language Disorders in Bilingual Children and Adults.* San Diego, CA: Plural Publishing.

KONDA (2006) Who are we? Social structure research. http://www.konda.com.tr/html/ dosyalar/ttya_tr.pdf. Accessed 1.11.10.

Kopkallı-Yavuz, H. (2010) The sound inventory of Turkish: Consonants and vowels. In S. Topbaş and M. Yavaş (eds) *Communication Disorders in Turkish* (pp. 27–48). Bristol: Multilingual Matters.

Peña, E.D. and Bedore, L.M. (2009) Bilingualism in child language disorders. In R.G. Schwartz (ed.) *Handbook of Child Language Disorders* (pp. 281–308). New York: Psychology Press.

Polat, N. (2007) Linking social networks and attainment in an L2 accent: Kurds acquiring Turkish. *Texas Linguistic Forum* 51, 144–153.

Thackston, W.M. (2006) *Kurmanji Kurdish: A Reference Grammar with Selected Readings.* On WWW at www.fas.harvard.edu/~iranian/Kurmanji/index.html. Accessed 2.11.10.

Topbaş, S. (2004/2005) *Türkçe Sesletim-Sesbilgisi Testi [Turkish Articulation and Phonology Test].* Ankara: Milli EğitimYayınevi 4. Akşam Sanat Okulu.

Topbaş, S. (2006) A Turkish perspective on communicative disorders. *Logopedics, Phoniatrics and Vocology* 31 (2), 76–89.

Topbaş, S. (2007) Turkish speech acquisition. In S. McLeod (ed.) *The International Guide to Speech Acquisition* (pp. 566–579). Clifton Park, NY: Thomson Delmar.

Topbaş, S., Kopkallı-Yavuz, H., Kaçar, D. and Aksoy, E., (in preparation). *Development of Non-Word Repetition Test for Turkish Children* (In: Ongoing Project supported by TÜBİTAK-Scientific and Technological Research Council of Turkey, No: 109K001). Eskişehir: Anadolu University.

Yavaş, M. (2010) Some structural characteristics of Turkish. In S. Topbaş and M. Yavaş (eds) *Communication Disorders in Turkish* (pp. 48–64). Bristol: Multilingual Matters.

Yıldız, K. and Düzgören, K. (2007) Denial of a language: Rights of Kurdish language in Turkey. In M. Erbey (ed.) *The Obstacles to Use Kurdish Language in the Public Sphere* (pp. 30–100). Brussels: Institute for International Assistance and Solidarity (IFIAS).

16 Translation to Practice: Assessment of the Speech of Spanish-English Bilingual Children in the USA

Raúl F. Prezas and Raúl Rojas

Languages mentioned: English, Spanish

Context

Children in the United States (US) are becoming more linguistically diverse. Although the majority of the US population speaks English at home (80%), speakers of other languages are steadily increasing (Shin & Kominski, 2010). The number of bilingual children classified as English Language Learners (ELLs; children learning English as a second language) in US schools has more than doubled (from 1990 to 2005), with 75% of ELLs being native Spanish-speaking bilingual children (Shatz & Wilkinson, 2010; Swanson, 2009). The larger population of bilingual children has heightened demand for bilingual speech-language services, as speech-language pathologists (SLPs) work with more culturally and linguistically diverse caseloads.

Overview of Assessment Practices in the USA

The American Speech-Language-Hearing Association (ASHA, 2010a) and the Individuals with Disabilities Education Act (IDEA, 2004) have provided recommendations for accurate, non-biased assessment practices for all US children (including bilingual children). For example, legal mandates and ASHA guidelines state that school-based SLPs should assess the native language of bilingual children 'unless it is clearly not feasible to do so' (IDEA, Sections 300.304(c)(1)(ii) and 614(b)(3)(A)(ii). Although most SLPs in the USA work with at least one bilingual student (Kritikos, 2003), practitioners primarily rely on formal English assessments to determine bilingual children's abilities (Skahan *et al.*, 2007). Therefore, clinical decisions are often made without a complete inventory of the speech sounds and word structures in children's native language, leading to over- or under-identification (Goldstein, 2004).

Bilingual Speech Assessment

Children with speech sound disorders (SSDs) comprise the largest number of individuals on clinical caseloads in US schools (ASHA, 2010b). Although developmental milestones and numerous assessment protocols are available for diagnosing SSDs in monolingual English-speaking children, assessment data based on bilingual children are scarce (Skahan *et al.*, 2007). Apart from conducting language, hearing and oral peripheral examinations, the following are recommended practices for assessing SSDs in bilingual children (see Goldstein, 2004): (a) collecting background information (e.g. family concerns, dialect/s), including the child's language history (e.g. use, proficiency); (b) use of support personnel, if needed (e.g. interpreter); and (c) testing phonological skills in both languages (e.g. single word test, connected speech sample).

In order to adequately assess SSDs in bilingual children, consideration of dialectal information is important. Whereas vowels distinguish the differences between English dialects, Spanish dialects are primarily differentiated by consonant differences. For instance, substitutions of /l/ for /r/ in coda position and final consonant /s/ deletion are common in the Puerto Rican dialect of Spanish, but not in the Mexican dialect. Determining the phonological skills in both languages is critical. Fabiano (2007) provides an outline for evidence-based phonological assessment of bilingual children, including the importance of performing: (a) an independent analysis; (b) a relational analysis; (c) an error analysis; and (d) a phonological pattern analysis. Single word and connected speech samples are recommended for independent analysis to obtain a phonetic inventory of phonological strengths and weaknesses in both languages. Spanish single word assessments include the *Contextual Probes of Articulation Competence – Spanish* (Goldstein & Iglesias, 2006), *Hodson-Prezas Assessment of Spanish Phonological Patterns* (Hodson & Prezas, 2010) and the *Spanish Articulation Measures* (Mattes, 1995). Connected speech samples should be analyzed to yield percentage estimates of intelligibility in known and unknown contexts. Information regarding consonant and vowel accuracy, including the accuracy of shared (e.g. /p/ in both languages) and unshared (e.g. Spanish trill /r/; English /v/) consonants, is recommended for relational analysis. Ruling out cross-linguistic effects via an error analysis (substitution of the liquid /ɹ/ in place of Spanish flap /ɾ/ and trill /r/) is necessary to prevent counting typical substitution differences that transfer from one language to the other, as errors. Phonological pattern analysis, which is a means of making language comparisons of common patterns (cluster reduction) and uncommon patterns (initial consonant deletion) in each language, aids in determining the overall severity of the disorder. Together, these analyses inform decisions related to prognosis and direction for intervention.

Other Assessment Recommendations

Over- and under-identification of SSDs in bilingual children can be reduced via: (a) metaphonological assessment; (b) differentiation of deviation types; and (c) collaborations with bilingual personnel. Children with SSDs often have concomitant difficulties with skills related to literacy (Rvachew & Grawberg, 2006). Therefore, diagnostic evaluations can include some measure of a child's phonemic awareness skills (segmentation, blending, rhyming). Differentiating deviation types (omission, substitution, distortion) is critical, especially for children with highly unintelligible speech (Hodson, 2007). Distortions (e.g. lisp) should not be weighted equally as omissions and substitutions, as the latter impact intelligibility more negatively. Otherwise, a child may receive the same score for a pre- and post-treatment analysis if an omission or substitution has been replaced with a distortion. Moreover, children with differing levels of severity may receive similar scores during post-treatment measures. Finally, collaboration with bilingual personnel via a team approach is recommended (Langdon & Cheng, 2002). For instance, monolingual SLPs can work with interpreters and translators, as well as with bilingual SLPs. Many US school districts are appointing bilingual SLPs as lead diagnosticians and using collaboration in order to better accommodate and serve the growing bilingual population.

References

American Speech-Language-Hearing Association (2010a) Roles and responsibilities of speech-language pathologists in schools [Professional issues statement]. http://www.asha.org/docs/pdf/PI2010-00317.pdf. Accessed 2.8.10.

American Speech-Language-Hearing Association (2010b) Schools survey report: SLP caseload characteristics trends 1995–2010. On WWW at http://www.asha.org/uploadedFiles/Schools10CaseloadTrends.pdf. Accessed 2.8.10.

Fabiano, L.C. (2007) Evidence-based phonological assessment of bilingual children. *Communication Disorders and Sciences in Culturally and Linguistically Diverse Populations* 14 (2), 21–23.

Goldstein, B.A. (2004) Phonological development and disorders. In B.A. Goldstein (ed.) *Bilingual Language Development and Disorders in Spanish-English Speakers* (pp. 259–286). Baltimore, MD: Paul H. Brookes.

Goldstein, B.A. and Iglesias, A. (2006) *Contextual Probes of Articulation Competence – Spanish*. Greenville, SC: Super Duper Publications.

Hodson, B.W. (2007) *Evaluating and Enhancing Children's Phonological Systems: Research and Theory to Practice*. Wichita, KS: Phonocomp.

Hodson, B.W. and Prezas, R.F. (2010) Hodson-Prezas assessment of Spanish phonological patterns. Unpublished manuscript, Wichita State University.

IDEA (2004) Individuals with Disabilities Education Act of 2004, [Final Regulations] http://idea.ed.gov/explore/view/p/,root,regs, Accessed 2.8.10.

Kritikos, E.P. (2003) Speech-language pathologists' beliefs about language assessment of bilingual/bicultural individuals. *American Journal of Speech-Language Pathology* 12, 73–91.

Langdon, H.W. and Cheng, L.L. (2002) *Collaborating with Interpreters and Translators*. Eau Claire, WI: Thinking Publications.

Mattes, L.J. (1995) *Spanish Articulation Measures: Revised Edition*. Oceanside, CA: Academic Communication Associates.

Rvachew, S. and Grawberg, M. (2006) Correlates of phonological awareness in preschoolers with speech-sound disorders. *Journal of Speech, Language, and Hearing Research* 49, 74–87.

Shatz, M. and Wilkinson, L.C. (2010) Introduction. In M. Shatz and L.C. Wilkinson (eds) *The Education of English Language Learners: Research to Practice* (pp. 1–22). New York: The Guildford Press.

Shin, H.B. and Kominski, R.A. (2010) *Language Use in the United States: 2007*. American Community Survey Reports, ACS-12. U.S. Census Bureau, Washington, DC.

Skahan, S.M., Watson, M. and Lof, G.L. (2007) Speech-language pathologists' assessment practices for children with suspected speech sound disorders: Results of a national survey. *American Journal of Speech-Language Pathology* 16, 246–259.

Swanson, C.B. (2009) *Perspectives on a Population: English-language Learners in American Schools*. Bethesda, MD: Editorial Projects in Education.

17 Translation to Practice: Assessment of Children's Speech Sound Production in Hong Kong

Carol Kit Sum To and Pamela Sau Ping Cheung

Languages mentioned: Cantonese, English, Putonghua

Language Context in Hong Kong

With a land area of just 1104 km^2, Hong Kong Special Administrative Region (HKSAR) is home to 7 million people. While over 95% of Hong Kong people are ethnic Chinese, 90.9% of the total population speaks Cantonese as their usual language (Census and Statistics, Hong Kong, 2007). During the British colonial rule, English was the official language; however, in 1974, Chinese also became an official language. Modern Standard Chinese (MSC) was employed as the official written form, while standard Cantonese was used as the *de facto* spoken dialect of Chinese. Since the handover of Hong Kong to China in 1997, the government of HKSAR has promoted the policy of being 'biliterate (English and MSC as the written languages) and trilingual (English, Cantonese and Putonghua as the spoken forms)'. Putonghua, the national language of China and the spoken form of MSC, is widely taught in schools.

From a language-learning perspective, most young children in Hong Kong are mainly exposed to Cantonese in their toddler years. At kindergarten entry, English and Putonghua are taught as second languages. In school years, the majority of schools teach English and Putonghua as subjects in the school curriculum, while some schools opt to use these two languages as the medium of instruction, e.g. teaching Mathematics in English and Chinese Language in Putonghua. However, outside class, Cantonese remains the dominant language in daily communication.

Speech-language Pathology Services in Hong Kong

In the 1980s, speech-language pathology services started to appear in Hong Kong, provided by speech-language pathologists (SLPs) trained overseas. With the urgent demands for this service in society, the Department of Speech and Hearing Sciences was founded at The University of Hong Kong in 1988. The department provides a four-year degree program that is recognized by the Royal College of Speech and Language Therapists in the UK. Since then, about 30–40 SLPs have been trained locally every year. SLP services have expanded dramatically to serve both pediatric and geriatric clients with communication and swallowing disorders. They cover the rehabilitation settings of hospitals, child assessment and intervention clinics, special schools, private clinics and training centers, and recently mainstream schools. SLPs work on the native or usual language of a client and Cantonese is the main language used within their clinics. Cantonese standardized speech and language assessment tools normed on the local population have been developed and used widely (see Appendix). Currently, there are no local assessment tools standardized for clients speaking English or Putonghua.

Cantonese Sound System

Cantonese has a relatively simple syllable structure of (C)V/C$_{syllabic}$(C). Standard Cantonese is based on the Cantonese spoken in Guangzhou. In the system, there are 19 initial-consonants, 6 final-consonants, 8 vowels and 10 diphthongs (Wong, 1941). For initial-consonants, the five pairs of voiceless aspirated and unaspirated plosives/affricates are /p-, p^h-, t-, t^h-, k-, k^h-, k^w-, k^{wh}-, ts-/ and /ts^h-/. There are three fricatives /f-, s-/ and /h-/, two approximants /j-/ and /w-/, one lateral approximant /l-/ and three nasals /m-, n-/ and /ŋ-/. The final-consonants are three nasals /-m, -n/ and /-ŋ/ and three unreleased plosives /-p, -t/ and /-k/. The nasals /m/ and /ŋ/ can also behave as syllabic segments. There are seven long vowels, namely, /i, y, ɛ, œ, a, ɔ/ and /u/, and one short vowel /ɐ/. The 10 diphthongs are /ai, ɐi, au, ɐu, ei, ɵy, ɔi, ui, iu/ and /ou/, and the colloquial diphthong /ɛu/ has recently been added (Zee, 1999). As a tone language, Cantonese uses pitch changes to indicate lexical meaning. There are nine contrastive tones in Cantonese distinguished by tone height and contour. For example, the syllable /ji/ can combine with the six level and contour tones to form different words, namely, 衣 *clothes* /ji1/, 椅 *chair* /ji2/, 意 *meaning* /ji3/, 兒 *son* /ji4/, 耳 *ear* /ji5/ and 二 *two* /ji6/.

Sound Changes and Implications for Assessment

Sound changes have been noted in Hong Kong Cantonese (HKC) and the realizations started to appear some decades ago. For example, local speakers generally use [l-] for /n-/ (e.g. 男 *male* /nam/ → [lam]), interchange zero initial Ø- and /ŋ-/ (e.g. 牛 *ox* /ŋau/ → [au] and 屋 *house* /ɔk/ → [ŋɔk]), dissimilate /k^w/- to [k-] before /ɔ/ (e.g. 果 *fruit* /k^{w}ɔ / → [kɔ]), and replace syllabic /ŋ/ by [m] (e.g. 五 *five* /ŋ/ → [m]). There are also ongoing changes in final consonants /-ŋ/ to [-n] (e.g. 橙 *orange* /tsʰaŋ/ → [tsʰan]), /-n/ to [-ŋ] (e.g. 乾 *dry* /kɔ n/ → [kɔŋ]), /-k/ to [-t] (e.g. 腳 *leg* /kœk/ → [kœt]) and -t to [-k] (e.g. 渴 *thirsty* /hɔt/ → [hɔk]). A number of reasons contribute to these changes, e.g. language or dialect contact and internal linguistic factors (To *et al.*, 2010).

These sound changes and variations have raised significant debate about reviving standard pronunciations of HKC. People, such as educators, advocate standard pronunciations in school children, while some socio-linguists believe that sound change is a natural process and should not be stopped. Clinically, SLPs need to have clear differentiation between sound changes and speech sound disorders. An updated reference on the phonological system of a particular speech community is crucial to a least-biased evaluation. 'Popular' realizations need to be considered as free variants rather than speech sound errors. For example, if a child produces initial /n-/ as /t/, this is not a substitution error and no therapeutic intervention is indicated because most adults produce /n-/ in that manner. However, caution is needed in managing the recent changes of alveolarization and velarization of finals /-ŋ, -n, -t/ and /-k/. For example, given that these variations in final consonants are vowel specific, if a client shows alveolarization of /-ŋ/ in all vowel contexts, the SLP may need to determine if a client has real difficulties in producing velar consonants or if the change is a free variation. Such a clear differentiation not only helps in making accurate clinical judgments, but also allows for the remediation of true speech sound errors.

References

Census and Statistics, Hong Kong (2007) *2006 Population by-census: Hong Kong resident population by duration of residence in HK, ethnicity and usual language.* http://www.bycensus2006.gov.hk/en/data/data3/statistical_tables/index.htm#A1. Accessed 19.10.10.

Cheung, P.S.P., Ng, A. and To, C.K.S. (2006) *Hong Kong Cantonese Articulation Test.* Hong Kong: Language Information Sciences Research Centre, City University of Hong Kong.

Hong Kong Education and Manpower Bureau (2006) *Cantonese Expressive Language Scales.* Hong Kong: Education and Manpower Bureau (Speech Therapy Services Section), Government of Hong Kong SAR.

Lee, K.Y.S. (2006) *Cantonese Basic Speech Perception Test.* Hong Kong: The Chinese University of Hong Kong.

Lee, K.Y.S. (in press) *Hong Kong Cantonese Tone Identification Test.* Hong Kong: Department of Otorhinolaryngology, Head and Neck Surgery, Chinese University of Hong Kong.

Lee, K.Y.S., Lee, L.W.T. and Cheung, P.S.P. (1996) *Hong Kong Cantonese Receptive Vocabulary Test.* Hong Kong: Hong Kong Society for Child Health and Development.

Leung, M-T., Cheng-Lai, A. and Kwan, S.M.E. (2008) *Hong Kong Graded Character Naming Test.* Hong Kong: Centre or Communication Disorders, The University of Hong Kong.

PLK District-based Speech Therapy Team (2008) *Cantonese Oral Language Deficiency Early Identification Test for Pre-primary Children.* Hong Kong: Education Bureau.

Reynell, J. and Huntley, M. (1985) *Reynell Developmental Language Scales – Cantonese version.* Windsor: NFER-Nelson.

So, L.K.H. (1993) *Cantonese Segmental Phonology Test.* Hong Kong: Bradford.

Tardif, T., Fletcher, P., Liang, W. and Kaciroti, N. (2008) *Chinese Communicative Developmental Inventories.* Beijing: Peking University Medical Press.

T'sou, B., Lee, T.H.-T., Tung, P., Chan, A.W.K., Man, Y. and To, C.K.S. (2006) *Hong Kong Cantonese Oral Language Assessment Scale.* Hong Kong: Language Information Sciences Research Centre, City University of Hong Kong.

To, C.K.S., Cheung, P.S.P. and McLeod, S. (2011) *Sound change in Hong Kong Cantonese and implications for the assessment of sound production.* Manuscript in submission.

Wong, S.L. (1941) *A Chinese Syllabary Pronounced According to the Cantonese Dialect.* Hong Kong: Chung Hwa Book Co.

Yiu, E.M.L. (1992) Linguistic assessment of Chinese-speaking aphasics: Development of a Cantonese aphasia battery. *Journal of Neurolinguistic* 7 (4), 379–424.

Zee, E. (1999) Change and variation in the syllable-initial and syllable-final consonants in Hong Kong Cantonese. *Journal of Chinese Linguistics* 27 (1), 120–167.

Appendix

Summary of speech and language assessment for Cantonese speakers developed in Hong Kong

Areas	Tools	Available age range of normative data
Language	*Chinese Communicative Developmental Inventories* (Tardif *et al.*, 2008)	0;8–2;6
	Reynell Developmental Language Scales – Cantonese version (Reynell & Huntley, 1985)	1;0–7;0
	Cantonese Oral Language Deficiency Early Identification Test for Pre-primary Children (PLK District-based Speech Therapy Team, 2008)	2;0–6;0
	Hong Kong Cantonese Receptive Vocabulary Test (Lee *et al.*, 1996)	2;0–6;1
	Cantonese Expressive Language Scales (Hong Kong Education and Manpower Bureau, 2006)	6;0–12;0
	Hong Kong Cantonese Oral Language Assessment Scale (T'sou *et al.*, 2006)	5;0–12;0
	Cantonese Aphasia Battery (Yiu, 1992)	Adults

Table (*Continued*)

Areas	Tools	Available age range of normative data
Speech sound production	*Cantonese Segmental Phonology Test* (So, 1993)	2;0–6;0
	Hong Kong Cantonese Articulation Test (Cheung *et al.*, 2006)	2;6 to adults
Speech sound perception	*Cantonese Basic Speech Perception Test* (Lee, 2006)	3;0–4;9
	Hong Kong Cantonese Tone Identification Test (Lee, in press)	3;0 to adults
Reading	*Hong Kong Graded Character Naming Test* (Leung *et al.*, 2008)	Grades 1–6

18 Transcription of the Speech of Multilingual Children with Speech Sound Disorders

Jan Edwards and Benjamin Munson

Languages mentioned: English, Greek, Japanese, Spanish

It goes without saying that our assessments of and interventions for children with speech sound disorder rest on the reliability and validity of our transcriptions of their speech. An examination of the literature on multilingual phonological acquisition makes it clear that there is a need for research to develop evidence-based best practices for phonetic transcription of multilingual children with typical development and those with speech sound disorders. The most common practice is for a bilingual speaker to phonetically transcribe children's productions in both languages (e.g. Fabiano-Smith & Goldstein, 2010; Faingold, 1996; Goldstein *et al.*, 2005; Holm & Dodd, 1999; Holm *et al.*, 1999; Paradis, 2001; Vihman, 2002). All of the studies on multilingual phonological acquisition make several assumptions. They assume that transcription alone is adequate to describe the speech sound system of bilingual children and they assume that differences in children's phonological systems across languages can be described in terms of International Phonetic Alphabet (IPA) phoneme categories. The purpose of this chapter is first, to question these assumptions based on the cross-linguistic research literature on first language phonological acquisition, and then to consider the clinical implications of these assumptions.

Phonemes are not Platonic Ideals, or an /s/ by the Same Name is not really the Same

The first problem with the methodology described above is that there are cross-linguistic differences in the denotational values of the transcription system itself. That is, the same symbol does not necessarily denote the same sound across languages. We tend to think of IPA symbols as a universal denotational system – as if the same symbol reliably denotes the same sound across languages. After all, IPA does stand for the *International Phonetic Alphabet*, doesn't it? However, the same symbol does not always stand for the same sound across different languages. The voicing contrast for stops is probably the best-known example of this. Researchers have known for more than 40 years that there are three basic voicing categories for word-initial stop consonants that can be defined primarily in terms of voice onset time (VOT; Lisker & Abramson, 1964). These three categories are prevoiced stops (voicing begins prior to the stop release), short-lag stops (voicing begins at or almost immediately after the stop release) and voiceless aspirated stops (voicing begins considerably after the stop release, with a period of aspiration between the stop release and the onset of voicing). Languages with a two-way voicing contrast generally use two of these three categories – typically either prevoiced vs. short lag (e.g. European French (Allen, 1985), Spanish (Macken & Barton, 1980b)) or short lag vs. voiceless unaspirated (e.g. English (Macken & Barton, 1980a), Cantonese (Clumeck *et al.*, 1981)). In languages that contrast prevoiced vs. short-lag stops, the symbols /b, d, g/ are used to represent the prevoiced stops and the symbols /p, t, k/ are used to represent the short-lag stops. In languages that contrast short-lag vs. voiceless aspirated stops, the symbols /b, d, g/ can be used to represent the short-lag stops and the symbols /p, t, k/ represent the aspirated stops, to avoid the awkwardness of the aspiration diacritic. Thus, the short-lag stops can be represented by the symbols /b, d, g/ in one set of languages and by the symbols /p, t, k/ in another set of languages. This can lead to confusion for English speakers learning a second language, such as the 10-year-old American boy living in France who decided that the French word for (the game of) *tag* was *douche* (shower) instead of *touche* (touch). This confusion arose because the boy heard French people saying /tuʃ/, and associated the initial voiceless unaspirated sound /t/ with English 'd', and hence with the French word spelled *douche*.

We have also known for some time that these cross-language differences in the phonetics of the voicing contrast explain seemingly contradictory acquisition patterns across languages. Short-lag stops are acquired earliest across languages, regardless of whether they are the /b, d, g/ of English or the /p, t, k/ of Spanish (e.g. Macken & Barton, 1980a, 1980b). Voiceless unaspirated stops are acquired next, and prevoiced stops are acquired last (e.g. Allen, 1985; Davis, 1995; Gandour *et al.*, 1986; Macken & Barton, 1980a, 1980b). As Kewley-Port and Preston (1974) point out, these acquisition patterns can be explained in terms of the relative difficulty of satisfying aerodynamic requirements for the different stop types. The buildup of oral air pressure during stop closure inhibits voicing even when the vocal folds are adducted, so producing prevoiced stops requires the child to perform other maneuvers, such as expanding the pharynx. The production of voiceless aspirated stops is not as complex, but it does require the child to keep the glottis open exactly long enough after the release of the oral closure to create an audible interval of aspiration during the first part of the following vowel.

If cross-linguistic phonetic differences were as simple as we have described thus far, then it would be relatively easy to capture them within the IPA using the standard IPA conventions for differentiating *narrow* phonetic transcription from *broad* phonemic transcription. That is, [b, d, g] could be used to denote voiced stops, [p, t, k] could denote voiceless unaspirated stops and [p^h, t^h, k^h] could denote voiceless aspirated stops, even if the phonemic transcription uses only the unadorned /b, d, g/ vs. /p, t, k/. In fact, many phoneticians already use 'narrow' transcription in this way. However, the phonetic differences are actually more complicated than this. For example, Canadian French is different from European French in having shifted the voiced-voiceless distinction slightly, but not completely, in the direction of the English one (Caramazza & Yeni-Komshian, 1974). Riney *et al.* (2007) show that VOT values for Japanese voiceless stops are similar to those in Canadian French, and Kong (2009) provides data showing that VOT is necessary but not sufficient to describe the two-way voicing contrast in Japanese. While VOT alone correctly categorizes 94% of the stop consonants produced by 2- to 5-year-old English-speaking children, it correctly categorizes only 80% of the stop consonants produced by Japanese-speaking children in the same age range. Adding H1-H2 of the following vowel at vowel onset (the amplitude difference between the first and second harmonic, an acoustic measure of breathiness of the onset of the vowel) is needed to improve classification for the productions of the Japanese-speaking children.

The results of a recent series of cross-linguistic studies of the acquisition of lingual obstruents reinforce the suggestion that differences in the production of what are ostensibly the *same* sounds across different languages (Cantonese, English, Greek, Japanese, Korean and Mandarin) are both much more pervasive and much more complex than has been described previously (Arbisi-Kelm *et al.*, 2009; Edwards & Beckman, 2008a, 2008b; Li *et al.*, 2009; Kong *et al.*, 2007). We will illustrate this with two examples from the παιδολογος (Paidologos) database (http://www.ling.ohio-state.edu/~edwards). This database consists of single word productions of familiar words and nonwords from at least 20 adults and 100 children, aged 2 through 5 years, for each of the six languages. The productions were elicited by a combination of a picture and an auditory prompt. All words and nonwords contain word-initial lingual obstruents followed by one of the five vowels (/i, e, a, o, u/) and were transcribed by an adult native speaker who was also a trained phonetician.

One example of the complexity of these cross-linguistic differences is exactly the contrast that we have already discussed, the voicing contrast. Kong *et al.* (2007) observed that children acquiring Greek correctly produced prevoiced stops at a much younger age than had been described in the literature for children learning other languages with a contrast between prevoiced and short-lag stops. On investigating this phenomenon further, Kong found that the word-initial prevoiced stops in Greek are optionally prenasalized in adult productions. This prenasalization essentially solves the problem of maintaining voicing during closure because the speaker can vent air through the nasal cavity. Thus, prevoiced stops are acquired earlier in Greek than in French because Greek-acquiring children have the option of prenasalization and French-acquiring children do not. Similarly, voiceless unaspirated stop allophones of phonemically voiced stops are acquired later in Japanese than in English because Japanese-speaking children have to learn to control two parameters (VOT and degree of breathiness as measured by H1-H2), while English-speaking children only have to learn to control VOT (Kong *et al.*, 2009).

Another example of a cross-linguistic difference in sound production concerns the most commonly occurring fricative in the world's languages, /s/. Typical descriptions of English /s/ are that it has a relatively long interval of aperiodic noise, with a concentration of energy in the higher frequencies. Cross-linguistic differences in the acoustic characteristics of /s/ were the subject of a recent study by Li *et al.* (2009). Li *et al.* examined Japanese- and English-speaking adult and children's productions of /s/ and the corresponding post-alveolar fricative. In descriptions of Japanese /s/ in the English-language literature, it is typical to equate the two post-alveolar sounds as well as the alveolar/dental sounds, reflecting the cross-language assimilation patterns that we have already noted in loan words such as *sushi*, although the Japanese post-alveolar fricative has a higher second-formant frequency at vowel onset than the English /ʃ/, as well as a concentration of energy in the higher frequencies overall than /ʃ/ (Li *et al.*, 2009). Somewhat surprisingly, Li *et al.* also found that the acoustics of /s/ differed across the two languages. The /s/ of English was much louder and had a more compact spectrum than Japanese /s/. Li *et al.* showed that the two fricatives in the adult English speakers could be discriminated with high accuracy using just one parameter, centroid frequency. In Japanese, two parameters were needed: centroid and the frequency of the second formant at the onset of the following vowel.

Again, these cross-linguistic differences appear to explain a cross-language asymmetry. English- and Japanese-acquiring 2- and 3-year-old children produce /s/ with very different accuracy rates. As described by Li *et al.* (2009), Japanese-acquiring 2-year-old children produced /s/ with an accuracy rate of just over 30%, while English-acquiring children produced it with over 70% accuracy rates. More surprisingly, however, the two posterior fricatives, whose articulatory characteristics differ much more sharply across these languages, were produced with very similar accuracy rates. To examine why this is so, Li *et al.* (2011) conducted a cross-linguistic perception study in which English listeners (tested in Minneapolis, USA) and Japanese listeners (tested in Tokyo, Japan) were presented with children's productions and asked to determine in one block whether they were instances of correct /s/, and in the other block whether they were instances of correct /ʃ/ (for English listeners). Responses were pooled over the listeners and were categorized as either instances of /s/, /ʃ/ or neither (a category for sounds that reliably received 'no' answers in both blocks of questions). The fricatives labeled as /s/ by the English-speaking adult listeners covered a larger part of the two-dimensional centroid-by-onset-F2 space than did the fricatives labeled as /s/ by the Japanese adults. Similarly, the fricatives labeled as /ʃ/ by English adults occupied a smaller area in the two-dimensional space than did those labeled as /ʃ/ by the Japanese adults, although this difference was smaller than the difference in /s/. This finding suggests that the cross-linguistic difference in acquisition is the result, in part, of the greater willingness to label an ambiguous sound as /s/ on the part of the English listeners vs. as /ʃ/ on the part of the Japanese listeners.

Critically, Li *et al.* show that cross-language differences in order of acquisition of phonemes may not be explained solely by the children's productions and the articulatory-motor demands of particular sounds (e.g. Kewley-Port & Preston, 1974). Rather, differences may also be related to the different ways that listeners in the ambient language perceive children's productions. Such a finding is potentially very powerful, as it suggests that something as seemingly objective as the perception of sounds that are ostensibly shared by languages might not be as objective as it seems.

Intermediate Productions, Multilingualism and Speech Sound Disorders

Another problem with relying solely on transcription is that it assumes that children proceed directly and categorically from incorrect productions to correct productions. Both researchers and clinicians have known for many years that this assumption is not correct. As early as 1980, Macken and Barton described the existence of covert contrast, a subphonemic difference between two phoneme categories that can be observed acoustically. In a longitudinal study of three children, Macken and Barton (1980a) found evidence of a covert contrast in voicing for stop consonants. While the VOTs for the target voiceless stop consonants produced by these children were systematically longer than the VOTs for the voiced stop consonants, all VOTs were within the voiced range and so all consonants were transcribed as voiced. Since then, covert contrast has been observed for many contrasts, including place of articulation for stops (Forrest & Rockman, 1988), place of articulation for fricatives (Baum & McNutt, 1990; Li *et al.*, 2009) and voicing for stops (Gierut & Dinnsen, 1986; Macken & Barton, 1980a; Maxwell & Weismer, 1982). Covert contrast has been observed in children with typical development and children with speech sound disorders (e.g. Forrest *et al.*, 1994; Hewlett, 1988) and in children learning languages other than English (e.g. Li *et al.*, 2009). Tyler *et al.* (1993) found that covert contrast was clinically significant. Children who produced a covert contrast made faster progress in therapy than children who produced no contrast at all.

In our own research, we have found that covert contrast is even more widespread than had been shown in previous studies and that even naïve adults can identify covert contrast, given the appropriate task. The παιδολογος database was transcribed by trained native-speaker phoneticians for each language. In addition to coding initial consonant productions as correct or incorrect, the transcribers were trained to code clear substitutions, distortions and intermediate productions (Stoel-Gammon, 2001). For example, 's:θ' means ambiguous between [s] and [θ] but closer to [s]. We then asked naïve adult native speakers of English to rate children's productions of target /s/ and /θ/ using visual analog scaling (VAS). In VAS rating tasks, participants are asked to scale a psychophysical parameter by indicating their percept on an idealized visual display, as shown in Figure 18.1 (e.g. Urberg-Carlson *et al.*, 2009). In one experiment (Schellinger *et al.*, 2010), the stimuli were initial /s/-vowel and /θ/-vowel sequences extracted from English-speaking children's productions from the παιδολογος database. The stimuli included roughly equal numbers of tokens from six transcription categories: correct productions of 's' for target [s] to correct productions of 'θ' for target [θ], with substitutions of 's' for target [θ], the two intermediate categories and substitutions of 'θ' for target [s] in between. The naïve listeners' task was to rate the stimuli along a scale from 'the "th" sound' at one end to 'the "s" sound' at the other. We found significant differences between mean VAS ratings for each of the six transcription

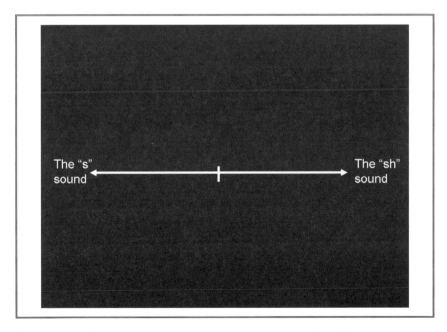

Figure 18.1 Illustration of the visual analogue scale (VAS) display

categories. In other words, naïve listeners even rate substitutions as less close to the target than correct productions. This result suggests that covert contrast is not an isolated phenomenon observed in a few research studies using acoustic analyses. Rather, covert contrast is pervasive and can be measured in native speaker responses.

To our knowledge, there is no research on the existence of covert contrast in multilingual children with or without speech sound disorders. In fact, there are no systematic studies of whether covert contrast, as measured perceptually by VAS, is more widespread in monolingual children with speech sound disorders relative to monolingual children with typical speech development. We might predict, however, that children with speech sound disorders will have more intermediate productions because their speech is generally transcribed as having more substitution errors and more protracted development than children with typical development. Are intermediate productions also more prevalent in the productions of young multilingual children? One might expect this to be the case if young children learning two or more languages have non-autonomous phonological systems, as Paradis (2001) suggested, but we do not yet have enough data to make a strong prediction either way.

Problems with Transcription and Clinical Practice

In this final section, we present several clinical stories that describe how these problems with phonetic transcription described above may influence clinical practice for speech sound disorders with bilingual children. We also describe some alternative strategies that clinicians may take.

Story 1

The setting is Marysville, OH, home of the first Honda plant in the USA. A 4-year-old boy, Tetsuo, speaks Japanese at home and English at preschool. His father is fluent in both English and Japanese, while his mother relies primarily on Japanese. The parents bring their son, Tetsuo, to the speech-language-hearing clinic at Ohio State University in Columbus, OH. The mother is very concerned that her son does not produce some sounds correctly at the age of 4, while his older sister, Kiyoko, had 'perfect speech' at the same age. The clinician decides to test Tetsuo in English, as he speaks both languages well and she does not speak Japanese. She gives him the *Goldman-Fristoe Test of Articulation-2* (Goldman & Fristoe, 2000) and also analyzes his phoneme production in a 50-utterance language sample. She finds that he scores above the mean on the GFTA-2 and has only a few errors on late-developing sounds (/r/, /l/, /z/, /ð/) on both the standardized test and the language sample. When she looks up the sound system of Japanese on Wikipedia, she realizes that Tetsuo's errors on /l/ and /ð/ may be because these sounds do not exist in Japanese. However, when she explains her findings to the father (who then translates for the mother), the mother is upset and insists that her son has difficulty on other sounds also, such as the consonant in the first syllable of *sushi*. The clinician then asks the father to elicit some Japanese /s/-initial words from Tetsuo, thinking that perhaps he produces /s/ correctly in English, but not in Japanese. However, when she transcribes the Japanese words, she also codes Tetsuo's productions of /s/ as correct.

What is going on here?

Japanese speakers have a smaller acoustic space for /s/ as compared to English speakers (Li *et al.*, 2010). Thus, when the Japanese-speaking mother and the English-speaking clinician are listening to the *same* productions, the English speaker hears correct /s/ and the Japanese speaker hears [ʃ] for /s/ substitutions.

What could this clinician do?

Tetsuo does not make enough speech sound errors to warrant a diagnosis of speech sound disorder by most clinical criteria. However, the fact that his mother has expressed concern about his Japanese abilities indicates that it is of great cultural importance for him to produce /s/ with articulatory and acoustic characteristics that are appropriate for Japanese. This clinician has two invaluable resources at her disposal: an aware and engaged mother, and a sibling to serve as a peer model. The clinician could train the mother on the differences between English and Japanese /s/, and could enlist Tetsuo's sister Kiyoko to model the Japanese and English /s/ tokens. The clinician could provide Tetsuo's mother with lists of cognate words like *sushi*, *sport* and *soccer* so that he can practice producing different types of /s/ in words that are otherwise similar in form.

Story 2

Two Spanish-English bilingual boys are 5 years old. They are best friends and they both have velar fronting (e.g. [d] for /g/and [t] for /k/). Both boys are enrolled in speech therapy at their dual-immersion elementary school in Madison, WI, with two different bilingual therapists. José is in therapy for two months with Juanita and the problem resolves completely. Pedro is in therapy for three months with María and he is just beginning to produce alveolar stops in isolation. Pedro's mother demands that he start seeing Juanita instead of María. However, even after Pedro has worked with Juanita for two months, he is only starting to produce alveolar stops consistently at the word level.

What is going on here?

It is quite likely that Pedro and José had very different amounts of knowledge of alveolar stops when they begin therapy. It may be the case that José had a covert contrast between velar and alveolar stops before therapy began, but that Pedro did not.

What could the clinicians do?

Juanita and María have several options. First, they could do a more fine-grained transcription by including intermediate categories such as 'in between /t/ and /k/'. Juanita and María could also use VAS to rate their clients' productions to determine if Pedro and José were producing a covert contrast. This information is critical for therapy, both for prognosis and for planning treatment. If Jose has a covert contrast between velar and alveolar stops, then he needs a different approach to treatment than Pedro, who is neutralizing the contrast and may not even be able to perceive the difference between /t/ and /k/.

Story 3

The last scenario takes place in your own place of employment, and is a scenario that you have probably encountered many times before. You have been working with Evan, a 4-year-old boy with a severe speech sound disorder for three months. You are using the cycles approach (Hodson & Paden, 1991) because Evan's speech was transcribed to have numerous substitution and deletion patterns resulting in similar sounding words (i.e. velar fronting, making *tea* and *key* sound similar; depalatalization, making *ship* and *sip* sound similar; final consonant deletion, making *keep* and *key* sound similar; and combinations like final consonant deletion and velar fronting, making *keep* and *key* and *teach* and *tea* sound similar). As is so often the case with children with multiple speech sound errors and numerous neutralizations, Evan's progress is slow. Your transcription of probe words shows no changes from baseline. Evan's parents perceive his speech as improving – extended family members and other caregivers report impressionistically that he's slightly more intelligible – but this is not reflected in your assessments. You are worried that he will not make the progress needed to continue on in therapy. You begin to worry that your approach to therapy is not the best for him, and wonder whether you should use another, less-tested therapy, like non-speech oral-motor exercises.

What do you do?

Before you make a big change in Evan's therapy plan, you need to make sure that you are using the right assessment to measure his abilities. You remember from your graduate school coursework articles – including many referenced in this chapter – illustrating that speech sound acquisition is gradual. You wonder whether Evan is demonstrating the kind of gradual acquisition that is often obscured by transcriptions. You decide to measure his progress by taking pairs of productions that you transcribe as the same (like *tea* and *key*, or *sip* and *ship*), and rate the productions using a VAS scale similar to that used by Schellinger *et al.* (2010) and Urberg-Carlson *et al.* (2009). After doing this for three weeks (which ends up being six data points, as you see him twice a week), you see that indeed his productions are moving closer to the end-points of the VAS scale. You record some more productions and this time have another rater, a fellow clinician, do the VAS task. Your predictions are confirmed – he is making gradual progress toward the /t/, /k/, /s/ and /ʃ/ endpoints. You continue with therapy, and as you would predict, his productions soon become distinct enough that your transcriptions reflect the progress seen in VAS and noted by his family and caregivers. You are happy that you have saved Evan from the potential setback of changing the way you go about therapy. As you continue along in your therapy, you begin to incorporate VAS more and more, and find that it is very useful for demonstrating the small but the nonetheless important differences that are sometimes present across different dialects or different languages, like the differences between /t/ and /k/ that you encountered in bilingual Spanish-English-acquiring children during a job you once had in Madison, WI, or the differences between Japanese and English /s/ that you encountered in a job in Columbus, OH.

Conclusion

To conclude, it is clear that the assumptions that clinicians and researchers make regarding phonetic transcription are problematic even for typically developing children learning only one first language. Transcription as the sole analysis tool is even more problematic when we are analyzing the speech of multilingual children or the speech of children with speech sound disorders, let along the speech of children with speech sound disorders who speak more than one language. The fine phonetic detail of a single sound based on IPA transcription differs from language to language. Furthermore, children do not proceed directly and categorically from incorrect to correct productions. These problems with transcription have real-life consequences for clinical assessment and treatment. We have suggested a few supplements to transcription that should be relatively easy for clinicians to implement and that should greatly improve their ability to describe the speech of multilingual children with speech sound disorders.

Acknowledgements

This research was supported by NIH grant R01 DC02932 and NSF grant BCS0729140 to Jan Edwards and by NSF grant BCS0729277 to Benjamin

Munson. We generously thank Mary E. Beckman for her long-time collaboration on issues related to this work, as well as Sarah Schellinger and Kari Urberg-Carlson for their instrumental roles in developing alternative measures of children's speech production accuracy.

References

Allen, G.D. (1985) How the young French child avoids the pre-voicing problem for word-initial voiced stops. *Journal of Child Language* 12, 37–46.

Arbisi-Kelm, T., Beckman, M.E., Kong, E. and Edwards, J. (2009, January) Psychoacoustic measures of spectral properties of Cantonese, Greek, English, Japanese lingual stop bursts. Paper presented at the 2009 Linguistics Society of America Convention, San Francisco.

Baum, S.R. and McNutt, J.C. (1990) An acoustic analysis of frontal misarticulation on /s/ in children. *Journal of Phonetics* 18, 51–63.

Caramazza, A. and Yeni-Komshian, G.H. (1974) Voice onset time in two French dialects. *Journal of Phonetics* 2, 239–245.

Clumeck, H., Barton, D., Macken, M.A. and Huntington, D.A. (1981) The aspiration contrast in Cantonese word-initial stops: Data from children and adults. *Journal of Chinese Linguistics* 9, 210–224.

Davis, K. (1995) Phonetic and phonological contrasts in the acquisition of voicing: Voice onset time production in Hindi and English. *Journal of Child Language* 22, 275–305.

Edwards J. and Beckman, M.E. (2008a) Methodological questions in studying consonant acquisition. *Clinical Linguistics and Phonetics* 22, 937–956.

Edwards, J. and Beckman, M.E. (2008b) Some cross-linguistic evidence for modulation of implicational universals by language-specific frequency effects in phonological development. *Language, Learning, and Development* 4, 122–156.

Fabiano-Smith, L. and Goldstein, B.A. (2010) Early-, middle-, and late-developing sounds in monolingual and bilingual children: An exploratory investigation. *American Journal of Speech-Language Pathology* 19, 66–77.

Faingold, E.D. (1996) Variation in the application of natural processes: Language-dependent constraints in the phonological acquisition of bilingual children. *Journal of Psycholinguistic Research* 25, 515–526.

Forrest, K. and Rockman, B. K. (1988) Acoustic and perceptual analyses of word-initial stop consonants in phonologically disordered children. *Journal of Speech and Hearing Research* 31, 449–459.

Forrest, K., Weismer, G., Hodge, M., Dinnsen, D.A. and Elbert, M. (1990) Statistical analysis of word-initial /k/ and /t/ produced by normal and phonologically disordered children. *Clinical Linguistics and Phonetics* 4, 327–340.

Gandour, J.H., Petty, S.H., Dardarananda, R., Dechongkit, S. and Munkongoen, S. (1986) The acquisition of the voicing contrast in Thai: A study of voice onset time in word-initial stop consonants. *Journal of Child Language* 13, 561–572.

Gierut, J.A. and Dinnsen, D. (1986) On word-initial voicing: Converging sources of evidence in phonologically disordered speech. *Language and Speech* 29, 97–114.

Goldman, R. and Fristoe, M. (2000) *The Goldman-Fristoe Test of Articulation* (2nd edn). Circle Pines, MN: American Guidance Services.

Goldstein, B.A., Fabiano, L. and Washington, P.S. (2005) Phonological skills in predominantly English-speaking, predominantly Spanish-speaking, and Spanish-English bilingual children. *Language, Speech, and Hearing Services in Schools* 36, 201–218.

Hewlett, N. (1988) Acoustic properties of /k/ and /t/ in normal and phonologically disordered speech. *Clinical Linguistics and Phonetics* 2, 29–45.

Hodson, B.W. and Paden, E.P. (1991) *Targeting Intelligible Speech: A Phonological Approach to Remediation*. Austin, TX: Pro-Ed.

Holm, A. and Dodd, B. (1999) An intervention case study of a bilingual child with a phonological disorder. *Child Language Teaching and Therapy* 15, 139–158.

Holm, A., Dodd, B., Stow, C. and Pert, S. (1999) Identification and differential diagnosis of phonological disorder in bilingual children. *Language Testing* 16, 271–292.

Kewley-Port, D. and Preston, M.S. (1974) Early apical stop production: A voice onset time analysis. *Journal of Phonetics* 2, 195–210.

Kong, E. (2009) The development of phonation-type contrasts in plosives: Cross-linguistic perspectives. Unpublished PhD dissertation, Ohio State University.

Kong, E., Beckman, M.E. and Edwards, J. (2007, August) Fine-grained phonetics and acquisition of Greek voiced stops. Proceedings of the XVIth International Congress of Phonetic Sciences, Saarbruecken, Germany.

Kong, E., Beckman, M.E. and Edwards, J. (2009, January) VOT is necessary but not sufficient for describing the voicing contrast in Japanese. Paper presented at the 2009 Linguistics Society of America Convention, San Francisco.

Li, F., Edwards, J. and Beckman, M.E. (2009) Contrast and covert contrast: The phonetic development of voiceless sibilant fricatives in English and Japanese toddlers. *Journal of Phonetics* 37, 111–124.

Li, F., Munson, B., Edwards, J., Yoneyama, K. and Hall, K.C. (2011) Language specificity in the perception of voiceless sibilant fricatives in Japanese and English: Implications for cross-language differences in speech-sound development. *Journal of the Acoustical Society of America*, 129, 999–1011.

Lisker, L. and Abramson, A. (1964) A cross-language study of voicing in initial stops: Acoustical measurements. *Word* 20, 384–422.

Macken, M. and Barton, D. (1980a) The acquisition of the voicing contrast in English: A study of voice onset time in word-initial stop consonants. *Journal of Child Language* 7, 41–74.

Macken, M. and Barton, D. (1980b) The acquisition of the voicing contrast in Spanish: A phonetic and phonological study of word-initial stop consonants. *Journal of Child Language* 7, 433–458.

Maxwell, E.M. and Weismer, G. (1982) The contribution of phonological, acoustic and perceptual techniques to the characterization of a misarticulating child's voice contrast for stops. *Applied Psycholinguistics* 3, 29–43.

Paradis, J. (2001) Do bilingual two-year-olds have separate phonological systems? *International Journal of Bilingualism* 5, 19–38.

Riney, T.J., Takagi, N., Ota, K. and Uchida, Y. (2007) The intermediate degree of VOT in Japanese initial voiceless stops. *Journal of Phonetics* 35, 439–443.

Schellinger, S., Edwards, J. and Munson, B. (2010) The role of intermediate productions and listener expectations on the perception of children's speech. Manuscript in submission.

Stoel-Gammon, C. (2001) Transcribing the speech of young children. *Topics in Language Disorders* 21, 12–21.

Tyler, A.A., Figurskl, G.R. and Langdale, T. (1993) Relationships between acoustically determined knowledge of stop place and voicing contrasts and phonological treatment progress. *Journal of Speech and Hearing Research* 36, 746–759.

Urberg-Carlson, K., Munson, B. and Kaiser, E. (2009, May) Gradient measures of children's speech production: Visual analog scale and equal appearing interval scale measures of fricative goodness. Poster presented at the spring 2009 meeting of the Acoustical Society of America, Seattle, WA.

Vihman, M.M. (2002) Getting started without a system: From phonetics to phonology in bilingual development. *International Journal of Bilingualism* 6, 239–254.

19 Translation to Practice: Transcription of the Speech of Multilingual Children

B. May Bernhardt and Joseph P. Stemberger

Languages mentioned: Chinese, English, French, Spanish

Speech-language pathologists (SLPs) in many areas now require skills in multilingual, multidialectal phonological assessment. As the number of regional home languages or dialects increases, differentiation of accent from impairment becomes more difficult. Within-language/dialect testing can facilitate this differentiation. Hack *et al.* (2010) tested Chinese-English bilingual children in both Chinese and English and found that they had age-appropriate speech in Chinese, but Chinese-influenced 'misarticulations' in English (i.e. accents, not impairments). The question remains whether non-native speakers of a language can reliably transcribe speech samples from that language. This chapter discusses enhancement of phonetic transcription reliability in the multilingual context, addressing (a) basic sampling considerations and orthographic transcription; (b) phonetic symbol use; (c) perceptual biases, assumptions and transcriber training; and (d) acoustic analysis support.

Basic Sampling Considerations and Orthographic Targets

Reliable transcriptions begin with good quality audio-recordings of speech samples. Lapel microphones and quiet environments will enhance the signal-to-noise ratio. Video-recordings can help distinguish referents for orthographic targets and provide phonetic transcription support through observation of articulators. Single-word elicitation (using a set of pictures or toys) can also enhance orthographic transcription reliability because referents are likely to be identifiable. As noted in the introduction, assessment within all of the child's languages is crucial to understanding whether their pronunciations of the ambient language are accented or 'disordered'. Having a native or near-native speaker help the SLP conduct the elicitation will both encourage the client to speak the intended language and help with determination of orthographic targets. The SLP can demonstrate elicitation procedures to the elicitation partner (whether it be a speech-language assistant, an interpreter or a family member) before the actual session begins (perhaps at a pre-assessment appointment). In some cases, if the child attempts to use the ambient rather than the home language during elicitation (because of the context and the SLP's involvement), the SLP may need to step out of the room for the recording session. During elicitation, the native speaker can check off a list of words as they are pronounced and/or indicate words 'mispronounced'. For later transcription, it will be important to have a recording of the words by an adult native speaker of the language.

Phonetic Symbols

In terms of phonetic transcription, the International Phonetic Alphabet (IPA; International Phonetic Association, 1999) and the Extensions to the IPA for disordered speech (Duckworth *et al.*, 1990) are useful for multilingual assessment because they include symbols for all world languages and aspects of speech disorders. However, it is important to note that each IPA consonant and vowel symbol represents a (narrow) range of pronunciations. For example, Spanish /tʃ/ is actually closer to IPA [tɕ]; that is, it is less grooved and more forward than English [tʃ], yet is still [tʃ]. Languages and dialects differ in their 'phonetic settings', in terms of exact tongue position, grooving, rounding, nasalization, etc. (Laver, 1994). A [tɕ] used in English by a native Spanish speaker is a Spanish-influenced /tʃ/ (i.e. an accented pronunciation). IPA diacritics provide a way to describe such details of transcription. A caveat is that narrow transcription has been reported to have relatively low reliability in speech-language pathology literature (Shriberg & Lof, 1991).

Perceptual Biases, Assumptions and Transcriber Training

In general, listeners have developed perceptual biases to their own language by 12 months of age (Werker & Tees, 1984). Perception, however, is not a static phenomenon, but changes through training and experience (Kraljcic & Samuel, 2006). Everyday listeners can adjust to an initially unintelligible speaker and, over time, understand more from that speaker, assuming that words in the language are known (Bradlow & Bent, 2003). Training and practice can therefore help increase transcription competency (Knight, 2010), with two crucial components being: (a) training for the entire IPA and (b) information on language-specific perceptual biases. Two people with the same language and training background may transcribe something the same way, but both may be 'inaccurate' because of their language-specific category boundaries or assumptions about what is important. Perceptual boundaries even vary from speaker to speaker within a language. The boundaries between IPA categories are thus likely to vary immensely for speakers of languages without the contrast. As noted above, the mean articulation for various IPA symbols varies across languages (de Boysson-Bardies *et al.*, 1989). Articulation of a single native-language category may straddle several IPA categories across or within speakers. For example, in English, /b/ may be prevoiced or short lag, depending on the speaker or moment; in Japanese or Arabic voiceless stops, voice onset time (VOT) is often intermediate between aspirated and unaspirated; in Spanish and Icelandic, some voiced consonants may be neither clearly approximant nor fricative between vowels. Native speakers are rarely aware of this, and we have little information on how it affects boundaries in phonetically trained individuals. One probable effect is that native speakers might perceive a given token as an acceptable member of a category, unless it is extremely different. This is a reasonable interpretation of the findings of Edwards and Beckman's (2008) observations about the differences between native and non-native transcribers, and their generalization that the perceptions of native-speaker transcribers have greater validity for the phoneme categories of that language. On the other hand, non-native listeners may be able to detect important effects (e.g. short vs. long consonants in child pronunciations of the English word *donkey* [dɑki] vs. [dɑkːi]) that are overlooked by native speakers unused to such differences.

There is another aspect to learning about the phonology of non-native language(s). Not all aspects of pronunciation matter in terms of phonological analysis. Thus, within Spanish, the vowel /i/ is [+tense] in adult speech, but it does not really matter if a child produces /i/ as [ɪ], because even phonetically trained adults often do not notice the difference. However, for English, it matters whether the vowels in *fish* and *feet* are produced as tense [i] or lax [ɪ] because the contrast is meaningful. In a current cross-linguistic study of phonological development, transcription convention documents are being created to describe what is important to take into account for the purposes of reliability and for phonological analysis in that language (Bernhardt & Stemberger, 2010).[1] (See the appendix for an example of Canadian French, Manitoba.)

For multilingual or multidialectal assessment, the SLP first needs to become familiar with the sound system of the client's language or dialect (with attention to at least major allophones), and become aware of his or her own perceptual biases in transcription. A basic starting point is McLeod's (2007) *The International Guide to Speech Acquisition*. There are also websites concerning the phonology of various languages. Phonetics websites provide sound files illustrating unfamiliar symbols (International Phonetic Association, 1999: http://web.uvic.ca/ling/resources/ipa/charts/IPAlab/IPAlab.htm; Ladefoged, 2006).

As noted earlier, the non-native speaker can verify the general accuracy of the transcriptions with native speakers (e.g. the client's family members or interpreters). Untrained listeners, however, with minimal awareness of their own perceptual biases, may miss some nuances of pronunciation. Over time, the SLP may need to trust his or her own transcriptions, given that she or he has paid attention to language-specific perceptual biases. For English native-speaker transcribers, this means learning to distinguish differences between: (a) voiceless unaspirated and voiced stops word-initially, (b) true voicing in codas and (c) glottal stop presence. For Spanish native-speaker transcribers transcribing English, this means learning to identify (a) tense vs. lax vowels, (b) voiceless unaspirated vs. aspirated stops, (c) low-amplitude voiced fricatives vs. approximants and (d) glottal stops.

Acoustic Analysis Support

Finally, digital acoustic analysis programs, including free programs such as PRAAT (Boersma, & Weenink, 2009) and Audacity (http://audacity.source forge.net/), provide waveform and spectral analyses that can help make decisions about difficult transcription targets. These programs provide a playback device that allows the listener to easily listen to a given word multiple times, while zooming in on the waveform or spectrogram, which can confirm the presence or absence of segments (including glottal stop), VOT, pitch contours, etc., increasing not only agreement across transcribers, but also the accuracy of the transcription.

Conclusion

Phonetic transcription is a crucial component of phonological assess-ment. Partnership with native speakers, transcriber training and acoustic analysis are three factors that can enhance the reliability of the phonetic transcription component in a multilingual, multidialectal context.

Note

(1) Transcription convention documents available from the authors.

References

Audacity. http://audacity.sourceforge.net/. Accessed 31.10.10.
Bernhardt, B.M. and Stemberger, J.P. (2010) Language-specific transcription conventions for a crosslinguistic investigation of protracted phonological development in diverse languages. Unpublished manuscript.
Boersma, P. and Weenink, D. (2009) *Praat: Doing phonetics by computer.* http://www.fon. hum.uva.nl/praat/. Accessed 31.10.10.

Bradlow, A.R. and Bent, T. (2003) Listener adaptation to foreign accented English. In M.J. Sole, D. Recasens and J. Romero (eds) *Proceedings of the XVth International Congress of Phonetic Sciences* (pp. 2881–2884). Barcelona: Futurgraphic.

de Boysson-Bardies, B., Halle, P., Sagart, L. and Durand, C. (1989) A crosslinguistic investigation of vowel formants in babbling. *Journal of Child Language* 16, 1–17.

Duckworth, M., Allen, G., Hardcastle, W. and Ball, M. (1990) Extensions to the International Phonetic Alphabet for the transcription of atypical speech. *Clinical Linguistics and Phonetics* 4, 273–280. (2002 revision. http://www.langsci.ucl.ac.uk/ipa/sounds.html. Accessed 31.10.10.)

Edwards, J. and Beckman, M.E. (2008) Methodological questions in studying consonant acquisition. *Clinical Linguistics and Phonetics* 22, 937–956.

Hack, J., Marinova-Todd, S. and Bernhardt, B.M. (2010). Accent or impairment: Speech assessment of Chinese-English bilingual children. Unpublished manuscript.

International Phonetic Association (1999) *Handbook of the International Phonetic Association: A Guide to the Use of the International Phonetic Alphabet*. Cambridge: Cambridge University Press. (2005 revision. http://www.langsci.ucl.ac.uk/ipa/ipachart.html. Accessed 31.10.10.)

Knight, R.-A. (2010) Transcribing nonsense words: The effects of numbers of voices and repetitions. *Clinical Linguistics and Phonetics* 24, 473–484.

Kraljic, T. and Samuel, A.G. (2006) Generalization in perceptual learning for speech. *Psychonomic Bulletin and Review* 13, 262–268.

Ladefoged, P. (2006) A course in phonetics. http://www.phonetics.ucla.edu/course/chapter1/chapter1.html. Accessed 31.10.10.

Laver, J. (1994) *Principles of Phonetics*. Cambridge: Cambridge University Press.

McLeod, S. (2007) *The International Guide to Speech Acquisition*. Clifton Park, NY: Thomson Delmar Learning.

Shriberg, L.D. and Lof, L. (1991) Reliability studies in broad and narrow phonetic transcription. *Clinical Linguistics and Phonetics* 5, 225–279.

Werker, J.F. and Tees, R.C. (1984) Cross-language speech perception: Evidence for perceptual reorganization during the first year of life. *Infant Behavior and Development* 7, 49–63.

Appendix

Transcription considerations for Canadian French (Province of Manitoba) in the cross-linguistic study of protracted phonological development

B.M. Bernhardt, J.P. Stemberger, D. Bérubé (Manitoba French speaker), R. Girard (Quebec French speaker), M. Ly (Parisian and Montreal French), 2010

Category	Important: consider for reliability/data entry	Less important: do not consider for reliability/data entry
Articles: *Un, une, la, le, l'*	Transcribe if used	
CONSONANTS		
● Place differences	Labial: bilabial, labiodental Coronal: dento-alveolar, alveopalatal, palatoalveolar, palatal Dorsal: velar, uvular	
● Manner differences	Stop/fricative/nasal/lateral/glide/glottal	
● Voicing differences	Voiced/voiceless in onset	Partial devoicing vs. complete devoicing for fricatives and rhotic
Dentalization (as placement, not as lack of stridency or grooving)		Dentalization (place of articulation) of (strident) grooved /s/, /z/ or /t/, /d/, /n/, /l/ unless verified visually

(Continued)

Appendix (*Continued*)

Category	Important: consider for reliability/data entry	Less important: do not consider for reliability/data entry
Grooving vs. lack of grooving (stridency) for coronal sibilants	Grooved, strident [s], [z], [ʃ], [ʒ] vs. ungrooved [θ], [ð], [sθ], [zθ], [ðs], [ðz], [ç(θ)], [z(ð)]ᵃ (with visual information and acoustic stridency)	[sθ] vs. [θs] or [çθ] or [zθ] vs. [ðz] or [ʑθ]
Slight fronting/backing		Slight fronting or backing of sibilants, i.e. [ʃ<] (fronted [ʃ]) vs. backed [s>]
STOPS		
Release		Unreleased
Aspiration		Not unless highly aspirated and frequent by child (aspiration occurs in Manitoba adult French)
STOP CLUSTERS		
/l/	Light /l/ in syllable-initial and word-final positions	Aspiration of stops in clusters
Manitoba French 'R'	Word-initial 'R' is often a trill but elsewhere a fricative and often at least partially devoiced. Indicate voicing or lack of it	Variants as indicated on the left for adult Manitoba French will not be considered mismatches
	English /ɹ/ or apical trills are sometimes used in Canadian French. Transcribe if heard	

Labiodentals		Labiodental nasal when before /f/ or /v/
LENGTHENING	When exceptionally long and especially if a long consonant replaces a cluster consonant	When used for emphasis/playfulness
Glottal Stop	Glottal stop, syllable-initial. It is not a necessary feature of French but should be transcribed if perceptible	• Glottal stop, word-final unless it is used frequently by a child to replace other word-final consonants • Creaky voice as variant of glottal stop
VOWELS		
Place/height/rounding differences	Back/front; high/mid/low; round/unround, tense/lax except for vowels to right	/ʌ/ vs. /ɔ/ (weakly rounded) [ɛ] vs. [ẽ] vs. [ɛ̃]
Schwa	Schwa vs. other vowels except for vowels to right	[ə] vs. [œ] vs. [ɶ]
Diphthongs		Light diphthongization for mid front vowels
VOICING/DEVOICING	Devoicing of vowels	
LENGTHENING OR SHORTENING	If excessive and appearing in contexts where a consonant is missing	When used for emphasis/playfulness/in rapid speech
NASALIZATION	Nasalization of non-nasal vowels or denasalization of nasal vowels	

(Continued)

Appendix (*Continued*)

Category	Important: consider for reliability/data entry	Less important: do not consider for reliability/data entry
STRESS	Stress. Agreement on primary stressed syllable	
SYLLABLE ADDITION	When used for phonological reasons (e.g. codas impossible)	When used for emphasis/playfulness
SYLLABLE DELETION	Deletion of syllables where adults never delete syllables	Deletion of syllables where adults delete syllables (transcribed but not considered mismatch)
TRANSITIONS		Transitions between /ʃ/ and /u/ as in [ʃju]

[a]Superscripts indicate an intermediate phone between a grooved and ungrooved sibilant. If there is a primary percept of /s/ and a secondary percept of lack of grooving, the superscript is the ungrooved component and vice versa. This differs from the dental diacritic, which indicates actual place of articulation (on the teeth), but does not indicate lack of grooving.

20 Translation to Practice: Transcription of the Speech and Sign of Bimodal Children with Hearing Loss

Kathryn Crowe

Languages mentioned: American Sign Language, Australian English, Australian Sign Language (Auslan), British Sign Language

Context

Children with hearing loss may use more than one oral and/or sign language to communicate, and may also present with speech sound disorders. Children with hearing loss who use more than one spoken language can be described as *oral multilingual* and children who use a sign language and a spoken language can be described as *bimodal multilingual*. Speech-language pathologists (SLPs) working with children with hearing loss who speak and sign may need to transcribe their client's speech and signs. This translation chapter will provide a beginning guide to speech and sign transcription for SLPs working with children with hearing loss.

Speech Transcription

The International Phonetic Alphabet (IPA; International Phonetic Association, 1999, see Appendix), the Extension IPA (extIPA; Duckworth *et al.*, 1990, see Appendix) and the Voice Quality Symbols (VoQS; Ball *et al.*, 1995, see Appendix) are valuable tools available to SLPs to examine the speech of bimodal children. Hearing loss affects the ability to access all aspects of the acoustic signal (i.e. volume, quality and timing). In addition to this, the digitisation of speech through hearing aids and cochlear implants further alters the acoustic signal. This can be further complicated if the child has speech production difficulties related to a craniofacial anomaly, speech sound disorder or motor speech disorder. Together, these factors may necessitate the use of detailed transcription and acoustic analysis to accurately describe these children's speech.

A brief description and transcription of the speech of three children with hearing loss is presented to show how detailed transcription can be used to accurately describe their speech. The focus is on four areas of speech production: (a) sounds outside the phonetic inventory of the target language; (b) suprasegmentals (including resonance, stress, pitch and volume); (c) unclear phoneme production; and (d) voice quality.

Karina is a 4-year-old bimodal multilingual girl with a unilateral cochlear implant. Her speech intelligibility is affected by her use of typical and atypical phonological patterns, atypical stress and intonation, and non-standard Australian-English pronunciations of sounds in some contexts (Percentage of Consonants Correct (PCC) 46%, Percentage of Vowels Correct (PVC) 83%; Dodd *et al.* (2002)) (Table 20.1).

Kelli is a bimodal multilingual three-and-a-half-year-old girl with Treacher-Collin's syndrome. She has bilateral atresia resulting in a permanent conductive hearing loss, micrognathia and an unrepaired cleft palate. She had a tracheostomy *in situ* from birth until 3 years of age. Following jaw lengthening surgery and tracheostomy removal at 3 years, she has been speaking for 6 months (PCC 17%, PVC 91%). Her non-standard and unclear articulation and nasal resonance and voice quality means that detailed transcription is needed to accurately describe her speech. It is interesting to note that post-surgery, Kelli is now making a variety of articulatory gestures for consonants; however, she is producing glottal stops in place of most consonants. This means that acoustic analysis of her speech provides a different perspective to visual analysis (Table 20.2).

Matthew is a bimodal multilingual 6-year-old boy with a severe bilateral sensorineural hearing loss. He uses binaural hearing aids. His speech intelligibility in connected speech is lower than would be expected given

Table 20.1 Transcription of Karina's speech

Gloss	*The giraffe got a long neck A crab at the beach*
Target	/ðə dʒəɹaf gɒt ə lɒŋ nɛk ʌ kɹæb æt ðə bitʃ/
Transcription (broad)	[tə tʃəwaf gō̃ nō̃ nei əx wa ɑth ðə beitʃ]
Transcription (narrow)	[ˌtə ˈtʃə.ẃaf gō̃ nō̃: ˌnéi: əx ˈwa: {_allegro_ɑth ðə ˈbeĩtʃ_allegro_}]

Table 20.2 Transcription of Kelli's speech

Gloss	*A sheep is pushing a pram* (stroller) *with a strawberry on it*
Target	/ʌ ʃip ɪz puʃɪŋ ʌ pɹæm wɪð ʌ stɹɔbəɹi ɒn ət/
Transcription (broad)	[ʌ̃ ĩʔ ĩ ʔõ̃ʔ æ̃ gwẽn ĩ ʌ̃ ɪɔ̃ʔõ̃keĩ ɒ̃ ẽʔ]
Transcription (narrow)	[{₅V̰ ʌ̃ ˈĩʔ ĩ ʔõ̃.ʔ æ̃ ˈgw̃ẽn ĩ ˈʌ̃ ɪɔ̃.ʔõ̃.kĩ̃ ɒ̃ ˌẽʔ₅V̰}]

Table 20.3 Transcription of Matthew's speech

Gloss	*Can I take it off and find the dinosaur?*
Target	/kæn aɪ teɪk ɪt ɒf ænd faɪnd ðə daɪnəsɔ/
Transcription (broad)	[kən aɪ teɪk ɪd ɒ ən faɪn də daɪnəθɔ]
Transcription (narrow)	[{₇Ṽ {ᵣkən ˌaɪ teɪk íd ɒ ˌənꜰ} {ₙˈfaɪːnd˥ də ˌdaɪ.nɔ̄.θɔ̄ꜰ} ₇Ṽ}]

his performance on single word tests (PCC 78%, PVC 96%) due to exaggerated volume, atypical stress patterns and nasal resonance. Detailed transcription of his connected speech is necessary to capture these elements of his speech production (Table 20.3).

Sign Transcription

Sign languages are neither universal nor bound to the spoken languages with which they co-occur. While Australian Sign Language (Auslan) and British Sign Language (BSL) are very similar, Auslan and American Sign Language (ASL) are very different and mutually unintelligible. Sign languages have phonological, morphological, semantic and syntactic rules, which differ between languages. SLPs should always consider information relating to clients' sign language/s.

Transcription systems such as Stokoe notation (Stokoe *et al.*, 1976) and the Hamburg Notation System (HamNoSys; Prillwitz *et al.*, 1989) provide detailed information on sign parameters. Stokoe notation was the first notation system developed for sign languages, specifically for ASL; however, HamNoSys is now more widely used around the world as it can be used to describe all sign languages. HamNoSys, like the IPA, has symbols to represent each element, which can comprise a parameter and variations within these. For example, ○ represents a flat handshape with thumb parallel to the index finger and ○ represents a flat handshape with the thumb perpendicular to the index finger. However, these transcription systems are inaccessible to SLPs without specific training in these methods.

SLPs are able to create meaningful sign transcriptions without learning these notation systems, by representing signs through a description of their Handshape, Orientation, Location, Movement (HOLM) parameters (Schembri, 1996). The HOLM parameters are similar to describing speech sounds by their place, manner and voicing. The use of HOLM parameters is especially useful when an explanation of signs is required by an audience without expertise in this area, such as parents or teachers. Table 20.4 contains examples of Auslan signs with HOLM and HamNoSys transcriptions.

Table 20.4 Transcription of four Auslan signs using HOLM and HamNoSys

	THANK YOU	BALLET	3-OF-US	ORANGE
Handshape Dominant Subordinate	Flat	Middle Flat	Three	Fist
Orientation Dominant Subordinate	Palm to body	Palm down Palm down	Palm to body	Palm inward
Location Dominant Subordinate	Chin	Back of hand Neutral space	Neutral space	Jaw
Movement – Primary – Secondary	Away from signer	Up Twisting	Elliptical	Squeezing
HamNoSys	⌐⌐·⊙∪ˠᴵˣ	⊙ˠ⊙⫙³⌐³·ˣˣ	⫙5ˠ⊙ᴰ·⊙⁺	⫙⋀⊙)(ᶜ⧉⊙⁺

Detailed transcription of the speech of bimodal multilingual children with hearing loss gives SLPs a method of recording and viewing all aspects of their speech, which may impact on their intelligibility. Transcription of the sign of bimodal multilingual children with hearing loss gives SLPs a method of recording children's signs for their own records and for communicating information about a child's signs to others.

References

Ball, M.J., Esling, J. and Dickson, C. (1995) The VoQS System for the transcription of voice quality. *Journal of the International Phonetics Association* 25 (2), 71–80.

Dodd, B., Hua, Z., Crosbie, S., Holm, A. and Ozanne, A. (2002) *Diagnostic Evaluation of Articulation and Phonology*. London: Psychological Corporation.

Duckworth, M., Allen, G., Hardcastle, W. and Ball, M.J. (1990) Extensions to the International Phonetic Alphabet for the transcription of atypical speech. *Clinical Linguistics and Phonetics* 4 (4), 273–280.

International Phonetic Association (1999) *Handbook of the International Phonetic Association: A Guide to the Use of the International Phonetic Alphabet*. Cambridge: Cambridge University Press.

Prillwitz, S., Leven, R., Zienert, H., Hanke, T. and Henning, J. (1989) *Hamburg Notation System for Sign Language: An Introductory Guide*. Hamburg: Signum Press.

Schembri, A. (1996) *The Structure and Formation of Signs in Auslan (Australian Sign Language)*. North Rocks, Australia: North Rocks Press.

Stokoe, W.C., Casterline, D.C. and Croneberg, C.G. (1976) *A Dictionary of American Sign Language on Linguistic Principles*. Silver Spring, MD: Linstok Press.

21 Analysis of the Speech of Multilingual Children with Speech Sound Disorders

Shelley E. Scarpino and Brian A. Goldstein

Languages mentioned: *English (General American and African American), French, German, Spanish, Turkish*

Speech-language pathologists (SLPs) traditionally rely on the use of standardized assessments to determine whether a child has a speech sound disorder. Standardized assessments provide an established set of norms that may include the age at which specific sounds or sound classes are typically acquired, expected level of phonetic inventory development for a specific age and expected substitution patterns or developmental patterns by age (Dinnsen *et al.*, 1990; Smit, 1993; Smit *et al.*, 1990). These data are extensive for monolingual speakers of a variety of languages (see McLeod, 2010); however, these norms cannot be applied to bilingual speakers. For example, of the few studies investigating bilingual Spanish-English acquisition, results indicate that there are some similarities in the acquisition of phonology between monolingual and bilingual children, but there also appear to be differences (Gildersleeve-Neumann & Davis, 1998; Goldstein & Washington, 2001). Therefore, the use of normative data based on Spanish and English monolinguals could result in over- or under-diagnosis of disorders in bilingual children.

When assessing the speech of multilingual children, SLPs are faced with the task of determining whether children whose speech patterns deviate from typical developmental patterns are exhibiting a speech sound *disorder* or *difference*. Unfortunately, there is limited information available to SLPs to assist them in understanding whether or not a multilingual child's phonology is developing typically. The establishment of a set of norms based on the child's age is more problematic for multilingual children than it is for monolingual children. When developing such norms, it is presumed that the phonological systems of children acquiring the same language should, at a given age, look more alike than different. Of course, these norms take into account individual learning differences and varied language experiences, but for the most part, children of the same age are generally expected to have achieved similar levels of linguistic competency. However, the same conclusions cannot necessarily be drawn about multilingual children because some, for example, may speak and hear multiple languages at home, whereas others may speak and hear only one language at home and do not begin speaking another language until they enter school. Therefore, at the time of assessment, it is plausible that a multilingual child who lives in Germany is more advanced in the acquisition of one phonological system (e.g. Turkish) than the other (e.g. German).

Currently, the most widely accepted theory with regard to how a bilingual child's phonological system is acquired and stored is the Interactional Dual Systems Model (Paradis, 2001). According to the Interactional Dual Systems Model, bilingual language learners separate their two language systems from birth, but there is interaction and interdependence between the two systems. This model is based on research conducted by Paradis (2001), which showed that stress patterns of French influenced the stress patterns of English in her French-English bilingual participants. Additional support for this theory can be found in Barlow (2002), who found that bilingual Spanish-English-speaking children (ages 2–4) all exhibited sounds present in one of their phonetic inventories that did not occur in the other, reflecting two separate phonological systems. In addition, phonotactic rules were respected in each of the target languages (i.e. voiceless stops occurred in the word-final position of words in English, but never in Spanish words), providing further evidence of separate systems. On the other hand, Barlow noted that each of her participants occasionally produced a Spanish phone in an English word, which indicated that although there was evidence for two separate systems, these systems likely operated in an interdependent manner.

Theoretical constructs have important clinical implications with regard to the diagnosis of speech sound disorders in bilingual children. Production errors observed in a bilingual child may not reflect an underlying phonological disorder, but may be attributed to interaction between his or her two languages. For example, because the English phoneme /ɹ/ does not exist in Spanish, a Spanish-English-speaking child who has not yet acquired that sound may substitute the Spanish trill /r/ for it in English words. This type of substitution would not be considered an error, but rather a reflection of the interdependence of the child's two phonological systems.

SLPs must determine if perceived error patterns in the speech of a bilingual child reflect the interaction of the child's two phonological systems, which would be considered a speech and language *difference*; or, if the patterns indicate a developmental speech sound *disorder*. Distinguishing between phonological differences and phonological disorders is an essential skill for SLPs in order to prevent over- or under-diagnosis and to ensure that bilingual children receive the appropriate services to assist them in the acquisition of their two languages.

Until recently, little research has been conducted on the phonological development of bilingual children (see Goldstein & McLeod, Chapter 10). Of the research studies investigating the phonological skills of Spanish-English bilinguals, indications are that the acquisition of a phonological system at both the phoneme and syllable levels in each language occurs at about the same rate as it does for monolingual children (Goldstein & Gildersleeve-Neumann, 2007). There are some notable sound and syllable patterns that can be classified as linguistic universals, since they occur during speech development in a variety of languages (McLeod, 2010). Universally, children tend to produce stops, nasals and glides along with front vowels first and these sounds tend to occur primarily in CV, V and CVCV syllable shapes (Locke, 1983). Vihman (2002) found that while the rate of acquisition is similar between bilingual and monolingual children, there may be differences in each of the phonological systems of the bilingual children as compared to their monolingual peers, and typically developing bilingual children sometimes do produce errors that differ from those of monolingual children of the same age. For example, while most monolingual children are quite competent at producing the vowels of their language early in development, Kehoe (2002) found that German-Spanish bilingual children exhibit greater variability in vowel production. Kehoe found that bilingual children had difficulty producing vowel length contrasts, particularly in the language with the greatest number of vowel phonemes, whereas vowel acquisition in the language with the lesser amount of vowel contrasts was comparable to that of monolingual children of the same age. Kehoe's participants, Spanish-German bilingual children, experienced greater difficulty acquiring the more marked German vowel contrasts than the Spanish system. Since the English and German vowel systems are similar, it would be expected that Spanish-English bilinguals might have similar difficulty acquiring the vowel contrasts in English.

Goldstein and Washington (2001) found that monolingual and bilingual children typically acquire liquids, affricates and fricatives by 3–4 years of age and that by preschool age, bilingual Spanish-English children have phonetic and phonemic inventories similar to their monolingual peers. However, they also found that while the production errors may be similar to those of their monolingual peers, they tend to occur more frequently. For example, Goldstein and Washington (2001) found that bilingual children exhibit increased frequency of cluster reduction and liquid simplification in Spanish and, at the same time, increased incidences of final consonant deletion and dentalization of /s/ and /z/ than their monolingual English peers. Overall, it was found that the greatest error rates occurred on unshared consonants between the child's two languages. According to Goldstein and Gildersleeve-Neumann (2007), this could be the result of fewer opportunities for practice in each of the two languages.

Because research suggests that production error rates and patterns may be a reflection of the two particular languages a bilingual child is acquiring, it is important that SLPs become aware of the similarities and differences between the two languages in terms of phonemes and phonotactic constraints. Knowing what the phonemes of each language are, and how a constraint or phonotactic rule in one language may influence the production of the second language is crucial for correct diagnosis and intervention.

Assessment of speech sound disorders typically involves the use of standardized assessments. However, there are currently few, if any, standardized instruments available for use by practicing SLPs with bilingual children. Therefore, SLPs must employ other means for determining whether or not a child has a speech sound disorder: phonetic inventory, vowel and consonant accuracy, phonological patterns, syllable shapes, prosody, etc.

Once the speech sample has been obtained, the data need to be analyzed to determine if a disorder exists. This analysis should satisfy the five criteria of phonological analysis outlined by Grunwell (1982) and should hold true for bilingual and monolingual speakers. (a) Describe the patterns used by the speaker. (b) Identify ways these patterns differ from typical speakers. In the case of bilingual speakers, the patterns may differ from typical monolingual speakers either because of a disorder or because of their language difference. (c) Determine the impact of any disordered patterns on communication. (d) Provide information for developing treatment goals and guidelines. (e) Provide a basis for assessing changes during treatment. A variety of analyses can be used to gain an understanding of the child's speech sound system. These analyses should be conducted utilizing the data collected for each language. A bilingual child with a speech sound disorder will exhibit characteristics of disorder in both languages, although the types of errors may differ across languages (Yavaş & Goldstein, 1998). The differences in patterns across languages usually reflect the different phonological patterns of each language (Goldstein, 2004), e.g. a higher frequency of final consonant deletion (Goldstein & Washington, 2001) in English than in Spanish.

Types of Analyses

Once the sample is collected, a variety of independent analyses (i.e. those in which a comparison is *not* made to the adult target) and relational analyses (i.e. those in which a comparison is made to the adult target) should be completed. These analyses should occur in each of the multilingual children's languages.

Independent analysis
Phonetic inventory analysis
The phonetic inventory details the repertoire of consonant sounds the child uses and their distribution according to word position (i.e. word initial

and word final). It also lists the consonant clusters used by the child in allowable word positions. By 3–4 years of age, later developing sounds, such as fricatives, affricates and liquids, appear in the phonetic inventories of monolingual (Shriberg & Kwiatkowski, 1994) as well as bilingual children (Goldstein & Washington, 2001; Holm & Dodd, 1999). Bilingual Spanish-English-speaking children have been shown to have phonetic inventories similar to their monolingual peers in each language (Gildersleeve-Neumann *et al.*, 2008; Goldstein & Washington, 2001). A vowel inventory, although not usually completed for monolingual children, might be more useful when analyzing the speech of bilingual children, especially if the inventories are disparate (Goldstein & Pollock, 2000). SLPs can use these analyses to compare the state of the inventories across the languages.

Another independent analysis that should be completed is a syllable type inventory. In this case, SLPs should list the syllable types the child is using in each language, given that those types can be markedly different from each other. For example, German and Turkish syllable structures are somewhat different from each other. In Turkish, syllable types are of the $(C_{0-1})V(C_{0-2})$ variety (Topbaş, 2007) compared to $(C_{0-3})V(C_{0-4})$ in German (Fox, 2007).

Relational analysis

Relational analyses are most common in analyzing the speech of children. Such analyses can consist of determining overall segmental accuracy, vowel accuracy, whole word accuracy and percentages-of-occurrence of phonological patterns. These analyses must be completed in reference to the children's dialect in each language.

Segmental and whole word measures

Because there are so few standardized assessments for multilingual children with speech sound disorders, SLPs must rely on other objective means for quantifying children's speech sound development. The following measures have been used regularly in the literature as a means for measuring phonological proficiency.

The Percentage of Consonants (and Vowels) Correct (PCC/PVC; Shriberg & Kwiatkowski, 1982; Shriberg *et al.*, 1986) was developed as an index of articulation accuracy and has been used to determine the severity of disorder in monolingual English speakers. More recently, the Percentage of Consonants-Revised (PCC-R) metric (Shriberg *et al.*, 1997) has been introduced as a variation of the original PCC measure. When calculating the PCC-R, only substitutions and deletions are considered errors, requiring only broad phonetic transcription. The PCC-R might be more appropriate for multilingual children because they are still in the process of acquiring multiple phonological systems, and they might be expected to produce speech sound distortions as do monolingual English speakers (Shriberg *et al.*, 1997). Also, Shriberg *et al.* suggest that because the PCC-R places emphasis on substitution and deletion errors, it shows greater sensitivity to systems that are atypical. The PCC-R has been used in several previous studies of monolingual and bilingual children (e.g. Goldstein *et al.*, 2005) and therefore allows for comparisons and contrasts between studies that have used the same measures of accuracy. The PCC measures were intended for use on connected speech samples (Shriberg & Kwiatkowski, 1982); however, Goldstein *et al.* (2005) cite its use on single word samples in past studies (e.g. Bernhardt & Stemberger, 2002) and the PCC-R derived from connected speech and single word productions has been shown to be significantly correlated (Hodson, 2004). Therefore, its use for the analysis of single word productions seems valid.

The measurement of typical phonological development has, within the past decade, shifted from analysis focused solely at the segment level to include more broad accounts that take into consideration the complexity of syllables and whole words within which the segments appear. Along these lines, Ingram (2002) suggested that phonological analyses incorporate two characteristics of whole words – whole word complexity and proximity. Ingram (2002) proposed the measure of Phonological Mean Length of Utterance (pMLU) as a means to provide a relatively quick and simple way to evaluate the syllabic and segmental complexity of a child's utterances. The pMLU is used to compare the complexity of a child's utterances to the adult target. This measure takes into consideration the number of segments in the child's word production and the number of correct consonants in that production.

To compute the pMLU, each vowel and consonant in a child's production, regardless of whether it is correct when compared to the adult target, receives one point. Then, each correct consonant receives an additional point. The doubling of the point values of correct consonants takes into account the fact that consonants, especially when they occur in clusters, add more to the complexity of the word than vowels. As words become more complex, they become longer, resulting in a larger pMLU. For example, the child who produces the word *black* correctly as [blæk] would receive a score of 7, whereas the child who produces the word as [bæk] would receive a score of 5.

The pMLU measure, unlike the PCC measure, differentiates consonant deletions and substitutions. A child who exhibits frequent consonant deletions will be expected to have a lower pMLU than a child who exhibits more consonant substitutions. For example, a child who produces /blæk/ as [bwæk] would receive a score of 6, one point for each vowel and consonant, regardless of correctness, and then two additional points for the two correct consonants [b] and [k]. The child who produces a pattern of substitutions rather than deletions would receive a higher score for attempting to maintain the complexity of the syllable. The mean pMLU can be calculated across an entire speech sample, either a spontaneous sample or a single word articulation test, to determine whether a child is attempting to use simple or complex syllable shapes.

A second whole word measure proposed by Ingram (2002) is the Proportion of Whole-Word Proximity (PWP), a measurement of how closely the utterance matches the adult target. The PWP is calculated using the pMLU to derive a score that reflects the degree to which the child's attempted word matches the adult target. The PWP is calculated by first computing the pMLU of a target word, then dividing it into the pMLU of the child's production. Therefore, the child who correctly produces *black* in the above example would receive a score of 1.00 (7/7). However, the child who produces [bæk] would receive a score of 0.71 (5/7), whereas the child who produces [bwæk] would receive a score of 0.86 (6/7). The pMLU and PWP have been shown to be valid in bilingual (and monolingual) children. For example, in a group of typically developing Spanish-English bilingual children, Ingram (2002) found them to be similar to monolingual peers. Burrows and Goldstein (2010) found no significant difference in either the pMLU or PWP between Spanish-English bilingual children with speech sound disorders and monolingual peers with speech sound disorders.

The pMLU has been shown to be highly correlated with severity ratings of speech sound disorders (Flipsen *et al.*, 2005), and the PWP, according to Ingram (2002), can be seen as an indirect measure of intelligibility. SLPs are often asked to make judgments regarding severity of involvement and intelligibility as part of a speech and language evaluation. These judgments are usually subjective and can vary among different SLPs. The pMLU and PWP measures hold promise for use as a means to objectively categorize a child's level of severity and intelligibility, eliminating much of the variability associated with subjective ratings.

Phonological pattern analysis

The phonological pattern analysis looks for errors that cut across sound classes. When analyzing the speech of multilingual children, it is important to consider the fact that phonological patterns used in typically developing children differ across languages in both type and frequency of occurrence (Goldstein & Washington, 2001). Children with speech sound disorders exhibit these patterns with a higher frequency of occurrence than do typically developing children. Additionally, patterns indicative of disorder are unusual or idiosyncratic processes (e.g. initial consonant deletion), systemic sound preferences and persisting normal processes (Grunwell, 1985).

Shriberg and Kwiatkowski (1980) advocate the use of a limited number of 'natural processes' for the analysis of phonological patterns. The eight processes they suggest are (a) final consonant deletion, (b) velar fronting,

(c) stopping, (d) palatal fronting, (e) liquid simplification, (f) cluster reduction, (g) assimilation and (h) unstressed-syllable deletion. They advocate examining these processes as they serve to change more complex structures to less complex, they occur across a variety of languages, they occur frequently in children with delayed speech development and they are able to be reliably scored by SLPs. The use of phonological patterns has been examined relatively extensively in multilingual children (see Goldstein & McLeod, Chapter 10 for a detailed review).

Influence of Dialect

The independent and (especially) relational analyses described above need to be considered in light of the dialect spoken by the child. In a study of African American school-age children, Haynes and Moran (1989) found that it was typical for children speaking that dialect to delete final consonants, a pattern of speech production that would likely result in a referral to an SLP in a child who spoke Standard American English. Cole and Taylor (1990) found that in children who spoke African American English, approximately half of their participants were misdiagnosed because dialect was not taken into account and dialectical variations from the norm were considered to be in error. Therefore, it is imperative that SLPs be aware of the dialects of each language the child is exposed to in school and also in the home, in order to determine if the child is developing similarly to the peers in his or her community (Goldstein & Iglesias, 1996). For example, a child who is living in a particular location in Wales will acquire the voiced and voiceless variants of the trill, whereas those in other parts of the country will acquire only the voiced one (Ball *et al.*, 2001). Goldstein and Iglesias (2001) found that when their participants' Puerto Rican dialectical differences were taken into account, the number of consonant errors and the number of phonological processes was less than would have been reported using standard Spanish phonological norms. They report that nearly 75% of their sample would have been misdiagnosed as having a phonological disorder if differences due to the Puerto Rican dialect were not taken into account. Therefore, it is of utmost importance that during the diagnostic process, a bilingual child's speech not only be evaluated in each of his or her two languages, but that dialectical differences of each language be taken into consideration prior to making a diagnosis of disorder (Goldstein & Iglesias, 2001; Toohill *et al.*, 2010).

Conclusion

Analyzing the phonological skills of multilingual children is relatively complex given the absence of standardized assessments. Thus, making a differential diagnosis must be done using other analyses. These analyses should include a variety of independent and relational measures. Utilizing a variety of such analyses will help to ensure a reliable and valid assessment and a more direct link to subsequent intervention goals for those multilingual children who are diagnosed with a speech sound disorder.

References

Ball, M.J., Müller, N. and Munro, S. (2001) The acquisition of the rhotic consonants by Welsh-English bilingual children. *The International Journal of Bilingualism* 5, 71–86.

Barlow, J.A. (2002) Error patterns and transfer in Spanish-English bilingual phonological development. In B. Skarabela, S. Fish and A.H-J. Do (eds) *Boston University Conference on Language Development 26 Proceedings* (pp. 60–71). Somerville, MA: Cascadilla Press.

Bernhardt, B. and Stemberger, J. (2002) Intervocalic consonants in the speech of English-speaking Canadian children with phonological disorders. *Clinical Linguistics and Phonetics* 16, 199–214.

Burrows, L. and Goldstein, B. (2010) Whole word measures in bilingual children with speech sound disorders. *Clinical Linguistics and Phonetics* 24, 357–368.

Cataño, L., Barlow, J. and Moyna, M. (2005, November) Phonetic inventory complexity in the phonological acquisition of Spanish. Presented at American Speech-Language-Hearing Association Convention, San Diego, CA.

Cole, P. and Taylor, O. (1990) Performance of working class African-American children on three tests of articulation. *Language, Speech, and Hearing Services in Schools* 21, 171–176.

Dinnsen, D., Chin, S., Elbert, M. and Powell, T. (1990) Some constraints on functionally disordered phonologies: Phonetic inventories and phonotactic constraints. *Journal of Speech and Hearing Research* 33, 28–37.

Fabiano, L. and Goldstein, B. (2005) Phonological cross-linguistic effects in bilingual Spanish–English speaking children. *Journal of Multilingual Communication Disorders* 3, 56–63.

Flipsen Jr, P., Hammer, J.B. and Yost, K.M. (2005) Measuring severity of involvement in speech delay: Segmental and whole-word measures. *American Journal of Speech-Language Pathology* 14(4), 298–312.

Fox, A. (2007) German speech acquisition. In S. McLeod (ed.) *The International Guide to Speech Acquisition* (pp. 386–397). Clifton Park, NY: Thomson Delmar Learning.

Genesee, F. (1989) Early bilingual development: One language or two? *Journal of Child Language* 16, 161–179.

Gildersleeve-Neumann, C. and Davis, B. (1998) Learning English in a bilingual preschool environment: Change over time. Paper presented at the American Speech-Language-Hearing Association Convention, San Antonio, TX.

Gildersleeve-Neumann, C.E., Kester, E.S., Davis, B.L. and Peña, E.D. (2008) English speech sound development in preschool-aged children from bilingual English-Spanish environments. *Language, Speech, and Hearing Services in Schools* 39, 314–328.

Goldstein, B. (2004) Phonological development and disorders. In B.A. Goldstein (ed.) *Bilingual Language Development and Disorders in Spanish-English Speakers* (pp. 259–285). Baltimore, MD: Paul H. Brookes.

Goldstein, B. (2007) Phonological skills in Puerto Rican and Mexican Spanish-speaking children with phonological disorders. *Clinical Linguistics and Phonetics* 21, 93–109.

Goldstein, B., Fabiano, L. and Washington, P. (2005) Phonological skills in predominantly English-speaking, predominantly Spanish-speaking, and Spanish-English bilingual children. *Language, Speech, and Hearing Services in Schools* 36, 201–218.

Goldstein, B. and Gildersleeve-Neumann, C. (2007) Typical phonological acquisition in bilinguals. *Language Learning and Education* 14, 11–16.

Goldstein, B. and Iglesias, A. (1996) Phonological patterns in normally developing Spanish-speaking 3- and 4-year-olds of Puerto Rican descent. *Language, Speech, and Hearing Services in Schools* 27, 82–90.

Goldstein, B. and Iglesias, A. (2001) The effect of dialect on phonological analysis: Evidence from Spanish-speaking children. *American Journal of Speech-Language Pathology* 10, 394–406.

Goldstein, B. and Pollock, K. (2000) Vowel errors in Spanish-speaking children with phonological disorders: A retrospective, comparative study. *Clinical Linguistics and Phonetics* 14 (3), 217–234.

Goldstein, B. and Washington, P. (2001) An initial investigation of phonological patterns in typically developing 4-year-old Spanish-English bilingual children. *Language, Speech, and Hearing Services in Schools* 32, 153–164.

Grunwell, P. (1982) *Clinical Phonology*. Rockville, MD: Aspen Systems.

Grunwell, P. (1985) *Phonological Assessment of Child Speech*. San Diego, CA: College Hill Press.

Guitart, J. (1976) *Markedness and a Cuban Dialect of Spanish*. Washington, DC: Georgetown University Press.

Haynes, W.O. and Moran, M.J. (1989) A cross-sectional developmental study of final consonant production in southern Black children from preschool through third grade. *Language, Speech, and Hearing Services in Schools* 20, 400–406.

Hodson, B. (2004) *Hodson Assessment of Phonological Patterns* (3rd edn). Austin, TX: Pro-Ed.

Hoffman, C. (1991) *An Introduction to Bilingualism*. London: Longman.

Holm, A. and Dodd, B. (1999) A longitudinal study of the phonological development of two Cantonese-English bilingual children. *Applied Psycholinguistics* 20, 349–376.

Ingram, D. (2002) The measurement of whole-word productions. *Journal of Child Language* 29, 713–733.

Kehoe, M. (2002) Developing vowel systems as a window to bilingual phonology. *International Journal of Bilingualism* 6, 315–334.

Locke, J. (1983) *Phonological Acquisition and Change*. New York: Academic Press.

McLeod, S. (2010) Laying the foundations for multilingual acquisition: An international overview of speech acquisition. In M. Cruz-Ferreira (ed.) *Multilingual Norms* (pp. 53–71). Frankfurt: Peter Lang.

Oller, D.K. and Delgado, R.E. (1990) Logical International Phonetics Program (LIPP) (Version 1.4) [Computer software]. Miami, FL: Intelligent Hearing Systems.

Paradis, J. (2001) Do bilingual two-year-olds have separate phonological systems? *International Journal of Bilingualism* 5, 19–38.

Shriberg, L., Austin, D., Lewis, B., McSweeney, J. and Wilson, D. (1997) The percentage of consonants correct (PCC) metric: Extensions and reliability data. *Journal of Speech, Language, and Hearing Research* 40, 708–722.

Shriberg, L.D. and Kwiatkowski, J. (1980) *Natural Process Analysis*. New York: Wiley.

Shriberg, L.D. and Kwiatkowski, J. (1982) Phonological disorders III: A procedure for assessing severity of involvement. *Journal of Speech and Hearing Disorders* 47, 256–270.

Shriberg, L.D. and Kwiatkowski, J. (1994) Developmental phonological disorders I: A clinical profile. *Journal of Speech and Hearing Research* 37, 1100–1126.

Shriberg, L.D., Kwiatkowski, J., Best, S., Hengst, J. and Terselic-Weber, B. (1986) Characteristics of children with phonologic disorders of unknown origin. *Journal of Speech and Hearing Disorders* 51, 140–161.

Smit, A.B. (1993) Phonologic error distributions in the Iowa-Nebraska Articulation Norms Project: Consonant singletons. *Journal of Speech and Hearing Research* 36, 533–547.

Smit, A., Hand, L., Freilinger, J., Bernthal, J. and Bird, A. (1990) The Iowa articulation norms project and its Nebraska replication. *Journal of Speech and Hearing Disorders* 55, 779–798.

Topbaş, S. (2007) Turkish speech acquisition. In S. McLeod (ed.) *The International Guide to Speech Acquisition* (pp. 566–579). Clifton Park, NY: Thomson Delmar Learning.

Toohill, B., McLeod, S. and McCormack, J. (2011, in press) Effect of dialect on identification and severity of speech impairment in Indigenous Australian children. *Clinical Linguistics and Phonetics*.

Vihman, M. (2002) Getting started without a system: From phonetics to phonology in bilingual development. *The International Journal of Bilingualism* 6, 239–254.

Yavaş, M. and Goldstein, B. (1998) Phonological assessment and treatment of bilingual speakers. *American Journal of Speech-Language Pathology* 7, 49–60.

22 Translation to Practice: Acoustic Analysis of the Speech of Multilingual Children in Korea

Minjung Kim and Carol Stoel-Gammon

Languages mentioned: Cantonese, Japanese, Korean, Mandarin, Russian, Tagalog, Vietnamese

Background

Over the past years, there has been a rapid increase in international and interracial marriages in South Korea, and multicultural families now account for approximately 2% of the total population (Statistics Korea, 2007). Approximately 90% of school-aged children from these families have mothers from China, Vietnam, Japan, the Philippines or Mongolia (Korean Ministry of Education, Science and Technology, 2008). Although the label *multicultural* is often associated with these families (see Lim, 2007; Seoul Global Center, 2009), it is difficult to determine if children in these families are actually being raised in a multicultural setting. For the purposes of this chapter, what is important is that the children are raised by mothers who are not native speakers of Korean. According to the Korean Ministry of Gender Equality and Family (2007), 96% of these mothers communicate to their children in Korean, and over 40% have concerns about rearing their children using Korean. In a recent master's thesis, Lim (2008) studied multicultural mothers and their Korean-learning children and reported that about 25% of the children were bilingual or were exposed to a bilingual environment. Currently, little is known regarding speech development among these children. Because maternal language input influences early linguistic development (Liu *et al.*, 2003), the likelihood of speech and language delay among children learning Korean is a social concern. The Seoul Global Center (2009) reported that language testing showed that approximately 75% of the children whose mothers are immigrants demonstrated language delay compared to their peers. With no standardized tests available in Korea for children from families in which the mother is a non-native speaker of Korean, there is a need for a better understanding of speech and language development among these children and for the development of an appropriate tool for assessment and intervention when needed.

Korean has an unusual system in terms of phonation types for obstruents. Whereas most languages use a voicing contrast to distinguish among obstruents produced at the same place of articulation, Korean obstruents are characterized by a three-way contrast among stops and affricates (lenis /p, t, k, tɕ/-aspirated /pʰ, tʰ, kʰ, tɕʰ/-fortis /p*, t*, k*, tɕ*/) and a two-way fricative contrast (lenis /s/-fortis /s*/). All are voiceless in word-initial position. Currently, there are no acoustic studies on the acquisition of Korean in children whose mothers are non-native speakers. This chapter describes the acquisition of Korean as it relates to the acoustic properties of Korean produced by these mothers.

Korean Obstruents: Acoustic Characteristics

Korean has nine word-initial stops (listed above) distinguished by multiple acoustic parameters, including voice onset time (VOT), fundamental frequency (f_0) and the amplitude difference between the first and second harmonics (H1-H2) of the vowel following the stop. In general, mean VOT values are shortest for fortis stops, intermediate for lenis stops and longest for aspirated stops; VOT ranges for lenis stops often overlap those for fortis or aspirated stops. Lenis stops differ from aspirated stops by significantly lower f_0 values and from fortis stops by significantly greater H1-H2. Regarding other obstruents, affricates are differentiated by frication duration, f_0 and H1-H2, and fricatives are differentiated by frication duration, aspiration and H1-H2 (Cho *et al.*, 2002; Kagaya, 1974).

Kim and Stoel-Gammon (2009) reported that Korean children, aged 2;6–4;0 years, demonstrated both universal phonetic patterns and language-specific phonetic variation in acquiring Korean stops. Acoustic analyses showed that, in the earliest stage, most stops were produced with short VOT values, regardless of the VOT of the target. In the next stage, children exhibited a bimodal VOT distribution that distinguished fortis stops from aspirated and lenis stops; they also began to vary the fundamental frequency of the vowel to differentiate between aspirated and lenis categories. Transcriptional analyses of the children's productions revealed that they acquired fortis stops/affricates first, followed by aspirated and then lenis categories (Kim & Stoel-Gammon, 2011).

Acquisition of Korean by Children with Mothers who are Non-native Speakers

Transcription studies of Korean children whose mothers are non-native speakers have indicated the presence of errors that are uncommon among language learners from families in which the mother is a native speaker of Korean (Hwang & Kim, 2008; Park, 2006). These errors include *laxing* (substitution of lenis types for fortis targets) and *deaspiration* (substitution of lenis types for aspirated targets). These error patterns are likely associated with differences between the acoustic-phonetic characteristics of Korean obstruents and the obstruents of the mothers' native languages, most of which have a two-way contrast – either voiced vs. voiceless (e.g. Japanese, Vietnamese, Tagalog, Russian) or unaspirated voiceless vs. aspirated voiceless (e.g. Mandarin, Cantonese) (Keating *et al.*, 1983). Prior studies have reported that second language learners of Korean often exhibit errors in differentiating lenis obstruents from fortis and aspirated targets. Park (2001) found that adult Chinese speakers learning Korean produced higher f_0 for the lenis category and lower f_0 for aspirated stops than Korean speakers. The diminished distinction of f_0 between lenis and aspirated types in Chinese speakers learning Korean is likely related to the acoustic characteristics of unaspirated-aspirated voiceless types, both realized with higher f_0 in Mandarin and Cantonese than voiced types (Francis *et al.*, 2006). Adult Korean language learners whose mother tongue has a voicing contrast (e.g. voiced-voiceless), on the other hand, may exhibit errors between lenis and fortis categories by realizing fortis type with a low f_0.

In sum, the developmental patterns observed among children whose mothers are not native speakers may be linked to acoustic-phonetic features of Korean spoken by their mothers. Further research in this area, especially acoustic studies, is needed.

References

Cho, T., Jun, S-A. and Ladefoged, P. (2002) Acoustic and aerodynamic correlates of Korean stops and fricatives. *Journal of Phonetics* 30, 193–228.

Francis, A.L., Ciocca, V., Wong, V.K.M. and Chan, J.K.L. (2006) Is fundamental frequency a cue to aspiration in initial stops? *Journal of Acoustical Society of America* 120, 2884–2895.

Hwang, S.-S. and Kim, W-S. (2008) A study on the phonological process patterns of children with articulation and phonological problems from multicultural families in agricultural areas. *Korean Journal of Special Education: Theory and Practice* 9, 329–348.

Kagaya, R. (1974) A fiberscopic and acoustic study of the Korean stops, affricates and fricatives. *Journal of Phonetics* 2, 161–180.

Keating, P., Linker, W. and Huffman, M. (1983) Patterns in allophone distribution for voiced and voiceless stops. *Journal of Phonetics* 11, 277–290.

Kim, M. and Stoel-Gammon, C. (2009) The acquisition of Korean word-initial stops. *Journal of the Acoustical Society of America* 125, 3950–3961.

Kim, M. and Stoel-Gammon, C. (2011) Phonological development of word-initial Korean obstruents in young Korean children. *Journal of Child Language* 35 (2), 316–340.

Korean Ministry of Education, Science and Technology (2008) A plan of educational sponsorship for multicultural children. http://www.mest.go.kr/. Accessed 1.11.10.

Korean Ministry of Gender Equality and Family (2007) *Marriage-based Immigrants and their Families in Korea: Current Status and Policy Measures.* Seoul: Gippemsa.

Lim, J.S. (2008) A study on the relationships among multicultural mothers rearing attitudes, young children's language ability, and social ability. Unpublished MA thesis, Chonnam National University.

Liu, H.-M., Kuhl, P.K. and Tsao, F-M. (2003) An association between mothers' speech clarity and infants' speech discrimination skills. *Developmental Science* 6 (3), F1–F10.

Park, J.W. (2001) Experimental phonetic contrastive analysis of Korean-Chinese female speakers' Korean pronunciation. MA thesis, Yonsei University.

Park, S.H. (2006) The study of articulation and phonological patterns for children living in bilingual environment. *Korean Journal of Special Education: Theory and Practice* 7, 143–152.

Seoul Global Center (2009) Assessment of language development in children from multicultural families. http://global.seoul.go.kr/. Accessed 1.11.10.

Statistics Korea (2007) Results of marriage statistics. http://kostat.go.kr/. Accessed 1.11.10.

23 Translation to Practice: Phonological Analysis of the Speech of Multilingual Children in Malta

Helen Grech

Languages mentioned: *Arabic, English, French, German, Italian, Maltese*

Context

Malta has a complex language learning context because there are two national languages (Maltese and English). Thus, most children are bilingual to varying degrees in that they have some knowledge of both languages, but one of the languages may be dominant. Parental reports indicate that one of the languages may be used consistently at home while other families use both languages (Grech & Dodd, 2008). Maltese is acquired as a first language by more than 90% of the population (Borg *et al.*, 1992). Language mixing is typical in the Maltese culture with English carrying a higher social status. Therefore, child-directed speech tends to embed English words in the spoken Maltese context. Additionally, children are increasingly, and particularly at an early age, speaking Maltese with amalgamated English words, e.g. /isːɐmːɔrːʊ ʃopɪŋ/ *now we go shopping* (Gatt, 2010).

The National Minimum Curriculum (Ministry of Education, 1999) endorses bilingualism (Maltese and English) as the basis of the educational system. However, the emphasis on whether the teaching medium is English or Maltese varies depending on whether the school is managed by the state, church or independently. The latter two often prefer English for most classes. Most children are taught a third language in school, normally Italian. Sciriha (1999) reports that more than 80% of children attending church or independent schools and 10% of those in state schools are taught a fourth language, often French or German.

The Maltese Language

Maltese is a derivative of Arabic, spoken by approximately 450,000 people living on the Maltese Islands, situated in the middle of the Mediterranean Sea. Maltese emigrants, residing mainly in Australia, Canada and the USA, also speak Maltese (particularly, first generation emigrants). Borg and Azzopardi-Alexander (1997) reported that most of the Maltese language has been documented, although there are still some areas such as intonation and syntax that need to be researched further. Maltese grammar is Semitic with influences of other languages amalgamated with it, such as Italian. The Maltese lexicon is influenced by other languages, particularly English, French and Italian, which makes it a mixed vocabulary. Maltese and English are distinctively different in phonology, morphology and syntax. For example, Maltese presents a complex phonotactic structure; it is highly inflective and one sentence could be composed of one lexeme with three to four bound morphemes typically signifying gender, plurality and tense. In summary, Malta is a unique language learning environment because the population is multilingual to varying degrees and because Maltese is a semitically based language with influences of other languages.

Speech-language Pathology Services in the Maltese Islands

The main speech-language pathology service falls under the Health Division as part of Primary Health Care, although it extends to hospital wards and outpatient departments. The SLPs employed by the Health Division provide some service within mainstream educational institutions and the few remaining special schools. More recently, the Education Division started recruiting its own speech-language pathologists (SLPs). Private practice is also becoming increasingly popular in Malta. The only state university in Malta also has its own speech-language pathology teaching and research clinic that complements the state service. SLPs currently practicing in Malta are multilingual and proficient in at least Maltese and English. Thus, the use of interpreters is not required. The main challenge for Maltese speech-language pathology clinicians is the need to distinguish differences due to language learning context from disorder. Until recently, no standardised tests existed for Maltese-speaking and bilingual Maltese-English-speaking children. The SLPs depended on their adaptation of standardised English tests and their intuition. The pre-service curriculum for SLPs focuses on courses on applied and theoretical linguistics (in Maltese and English) in order to furnish practitioners with the necessary alternative tools for differential diagnosis of speech sound and language disorders.

Speech and Language Acquisition in the Maltese Context

A recent study by Grech and Dodd (2008) indicated that bilingualism is not a negative factor in Malta for speech development and, in fact, leads to faster acquisition of phonology. These data provide important information for SLPs and have clinical implications, since they disprove the claim that bilingual exposure may have negative effects on speech acquisition in the Maltese context. The study reported the speech patterns of a large cohort of Maltese children whose ages ranged between 2;0 and 6;0 years. Results of the study indicated that monolingual and bilingual children have different profiles of error patterns and rates of speech development.

Further ongoing research related to speech and language acquisition in Malta has led to the standardisation of the *Maltese-English Speech Assessment* (MESA) (Grech, Dodd, & Franklin 2011) and the *Language Assessment for Maltese Children* (LAMC) (Grech *et al.*, 2011), which have the unique function of assessing bilingual Maltese children, irrespective of their degree of proficiency in either language. MESA allows differential diagnosis of speech sound disorders, because it assesses articulation, oro-motor skills, phonology and consistency with monolingual and bilingual Maltese children. The LAMC includes a comprehension and a narrative sub-test as well as a sentence imitation task and a phonological awareness screen. Language mixing is coded and scored when administering these assessments, which leads to the identification of the child's characteristic speech and language profile, thereby distinguishing between typical acquisition, difference (due to language learning context) and disorder.

References

Borg, A.J. and Azzopardi-Alexander, M. (1997) *Maltese*. London: Routledge.

Borg, A., Mifsud, M. and Sciriha, L. (1992) The position of Maltese in Malta. Paper presented at the Meeting for Experts on Language Planning, Council of Europe, Malta.

Gatt, D. (2010) Early expressive lexical development: Evidence from children brought up in Maltese-speaking families. Unpublished PhD thesis, University of Malta.

Grech H., Dodd, B. and Franklin, S. (2011) *Maltese-English Speech Assessment (MESA)*. Malta: University of Malta.

Grech, H. and Dodd, B. (2008) Phonological acquisition in Malta: A bilingual language learning context. *International Journal of Bilingualism* 12 (3), 155–171.

Grech, H., Franklin, S. and Dodd, B. (2011) *Language Assessment for Maltese Children (LAMC)*. Malta: University of Malta

Ministry of Education (1999) *National Minimum Curriculum*. St. Venera, Malta: Klabb Kotba Maltin.

Sciriha, L. (1999) *A Sociolinguistic Survey of the Maltese Islands 111*. Msida, Malta: Cyclostyled, Department of English, University of Malta.

24 Intervention for Multilingual Children with Speech Sound Disorders

Christina Gildersleeve-Neumann and Brian A. Goldstein

Languages mentioned: Cantonese, English, Gujarati, Hawai'ian, Hindi, Italian, Punjabi, Spanish

Introduction

For all children with speech sound disorders (SSD), receiving intervention is crucial for not only improving intelligibility, but also for later academic success, because SSDs are linked to subsequent reading, writing and spelling difficulties (Stackhouse, 1997). Between 50 and 70% of school-age children with SSD in the USA exhibit academic difficulty and often require other remedial services (Gierut, 1998). Bilingual students face considerable challenges in receiving adequate intervention for SSD. Although most (school-based) speech-language pathologists (SLPs) indicate having children with SSD on their caseloads, they are more likely to provide intervention only in English and not in many children's home language (Kritikos, 2003). Across the world, SLPs tend to provide services in the language they speak rather than that of their clients (Jordaan, 2008). In a survey of SLPs who regularly delivered speech-language pathology services to bilingual clients, Jordaan (2008) found that 87% of SLPs provided only monolingual intervention to their bilingual clients. Moreover, 89% of SLPs suggested to parents that they speak only one language to their children. Finally, only 18% of respondents used interpreters in either assessment or intervention.

Although the regular delivery of intervention in one language to bilingual children with SSD is most common, it might not, in fact, be warranted by the evidence. For example, for those bilingual children acquiring English and another language, research indicates that instruction in the non-English (i.e. home) language helps rather than hinders the acquisition of English (e.g. Campos, 1995) and, in fact, leads to higher academic achievement in English (e.g. Thomas & Collier, 2003). Current best practices in the delivery of intervention for bilingual children with language disorders argue for providing intervention in the home language as well as in the second language being acquired (e.g. Gutiérrez-Clellen, 2001).

What is unknown is the effect of this mode of service delivery on the intervention of SSDs in bilingual children.

In providing intervention to monolingual children with SSDs, SLPs typically rely on transfer within a single language (i.e. intra-linguistic generalization) to produce positive outcomes for those children. Yet, it is not known if SLPs can also take advantage of transfer effects between a bilingual child's two languages (i.e. cross-linguistic generalization) to improve speech skills in both languages. An over-arching long-term goal for any speech-language therapy is to select short-term intervention targets and procedures to normalize speech production as quickly as possible. To achieve this level of efficiency, the SLP should select targets and procedures that yield the greatest amount of transfer possible in the shortest amount of time (Tyler, 2006). Such intra-linguistic generalization not only results in improved performance on targeted speech sounds and error patterns, but also improves untreated sounds in a variety of other conditions (e.g. spontaneous speech).

It remains largely unknown if the same transfer mechanisms operate between languages in bilingual children. Evidence of such cross-linguistic generalization in SSD intervention would help SLPs better meet children's long-term needs to develop communicative skill in two languages and minimize the effects of client–clinician language mismatches. The purpose of this chapter is to give an overview of providing intervention to multilingual children with SSDs. Specifically, we focus on cross-linguistic transfer, the ways in which intervention differs for multilingual and monolingual children, factors that influence intervention, multilingual intervention models and measures of intervention success.

Evidence for Transfer between Phonological Systems in Bilingual Children

Bilingual language development – speech development along with that in other domains of language – has typically been viewed as the monolingual development of two languages in one person. For this reason, SLPs examine test scores and measure results against those of monolingual children. Yet, this monolingual view is not applicable to bilinguals, who use their two languages in different situations, with different people and with different frequencies. This makes their linguistic skills stronger (or weaker) in different domains (Baker, 2001; Grosjean, 1989). While the information on all aspects of bilingual development is limited, substantial knowledge of SSD in bilinguals is particularly lacking (Holm & Dodd, 2001; Watson, 1991). Thus, SLPs (and other professionals) are at a loss as to how to interpret the speech skills of a bilingual child with low speech intelligibility and to make valid diagnoses and referrals. Thus, to understand intervention of SSD in bilingual children, it is necessary to examine the relative contributions of each phonological system and then indicate if cross-linguistic generalization occurs across the two systems.

Only a few small published studies have examined cross-linguistic generalization in the intervention of bilingual children with SSD, and their findings have been mixed. Holm *et al.* (1997) treated a 5-year-old bilingual Cantonese-English boy. The child heard and spoke Cantonese at home until the age of 3;3, when he went to school. The child was treated in English-only in two phases. The first phase targeted distorted /s/ and the second phase targeted cluster reduction. Findings indicated that English intervention on /s/ resulted in changes on /s/ in both languages. The intervention of cluster reduction improved cluster production in English but not in Cantonese. The effect of intervention for clusters in English did not affect Cantonese. Some argue that Cantonese does not have consonant clusters, rather on-glide diphthongs, making lack of cross-language effects for this error pattern difficult to interpret (Fung & Roseberry-McKibbin, 1999).

Holm and Dodd (2001), using a pre/post case study design, examined cross-linguistic generalization in one Cantonese-English-speaking child and one Punjabi-English-speaking child, both first exposed to English around the age of 3;0. In the first case (Cantonese-English), intervention initially consisted of articulation therapy in English, focusing on the child's distortion of /s/ (interdental). The authors hypothesized that generalization would occur to /s/ in Cantonese, given that the error was not language specific. Results indicated that after seven weeks of intervention, the child improved in English on the target sound and sounds not directly targeted, /ʃ/ and clusters; he also showed a decrease in gliding. Generalization occurred in Cantonese as well; the child produced /s/, /ts/ and /tsʰ/ in Cantonese with 70% accuracy (they did not indicate percentage accuracy of those segments prior to the initiation of intervention). Subsequently, the child received eight weekly sessions of phonological therapy. The child showed a decrease in cluster reduction and gliding in English after intervention. The authors noted that generalization across languages did not occur. With the second child (Punjabi-English), Holm and Dodd used a core vocabulary intervention approach to carry out English-only intervention. This approach emphasized sound production and phonological awareness skills. Results indicated increased consonant accuracy in both English and Punjabi immediately after and two weeks post-intervention.

Ray (2002) used a cognitive-linguistic intervention approach with a 5-year-old trilingual (Hindi, Gujarati and English) boy with a mild SSD. The child, born in the USA, was exposed to Hindi and Gujarati from birth and was 'formally introduced' to English when he entered school at age 4, but he had been exposed to it prior to that time. Minimal contrast therapy was used to target multiple error patterns (final consonant deletion, gliding of liquids and cluster reduction). Results indicated that intervention was effective in decreasing the percentage-of-occurrence of phonological error patterns in the child's speech in all three languages, increasing consonant accuracy in all three languages and improving the child's percentile rank on a standardized English articulation assessment.

In summary, the few published studies focusing on remediating SSD in bilingual children indicate that intervention (largely done in English) often promotes cross-linguistic generalization, although some studies suggest that the generalization is more frequent for shared phonetic than language-specific phonological properties. All of these studies show that approach to intervention must be different for bilingual children than it is for monolingual children.

How Does Intervention for Bilingual and Monolingual Children Differ?

Is providing intervention to multilingual children with SSD altogether different from providing it to monolingual children? The answer is yes and no. *Yes*, because the child must function at age-appropriate levels in two languages versus one for a monolingual. Yet, the answer is also *no* because the basic tenets of intervention hold for all children with SSD, regardless of the number of languages being acquired. An SSD in a bilingual or monolingual child is the same core impairment – difficulty in phonological representation and/or retrieval, motor planning and articulatory execution of speech. Thus, it is important *not* to forget all the things known about providing intervention to any child with an SSD (e.g. determine appropriate intervention goals based on assessment and independent and relational analyses, determine if speech perception, speech production and/or phono-logical representation areas are weak). SLPs can use what is known about intervention and apply it to multilinguals.

Most SLPs begin the process of providing intervention to multilingual children by asking, 'In what language do I treat?' That's the wrong question – at least initially. The more appropriate question is, 'When do I treat in Language A and when do I treat in Language B?' (Goldstein, 2006). The rationale for this question is (at least) three-fold. First, there are phonological structure differences between languages that will require specific intervention in each language (e.g. McLeod, 2007). For example, English contains a rhotic 'r' /ɹ/, but Spanish contains the flap /ɾ/ and trill /r/. Complex four consonant clusters are frequent in Russian; clusters are infrequent in Spanish. English has about 25 consonants; Hmong has about 60. Second, a multilingual child's phonological knowledge is distributed across their languages. For example, child speakers of Romance languages (Italian) are more accurate on multisyllabic words in comparison to speakers of Germanic languages (English) (Vihman, 1996), reflecting the phonological properties of these languages in adults. Third, we do not have a clear understanding of the specific profile of an SSD in a bilingual child. As Kohnert (2004: 319) notes, 'it is not reasonable to believe that, independent of clinical planning and appropriate scaffolding, children with language impairments will independently be able to transfer skills trained in English only to the Spanish needed to communicate with family members'. In multilingual children with SSDs, the SLP may be instrumental in affecting knowledge transfer of phonological structure in one language to the second language. Thus, it is important to choose the goal(s), choose the intervention approach and then choose the language(s) of intervention that are most effective at the current point in time. It is also important to reevaluate these decisions on a regular and frequent basis to determine if changes in the child's communication needs have resulted in needed changes in the intervention plan.

Choose the goal

In providing intervention to a monolingual English speaker with a moderate SSD, a common initial goal would be to decrease the occurrence of final consonant deletion. Such an initial goal would probably *not* be appropriate for a speaker of a Romance language, given the relatively few final consonants in those languages and the lesser need to make phonological contrasts using final consonants. A more appropriate goal in Spanish and Italian would be unstressed syllable deletion, reflecting the importance of multisyllabic words in many Romance languages.

Related to choosing the goal is determining the goal attack strategy (Fey, 1986). Fey outlines three such strategies: vertical, horizontal and cyclical. In a vertical strategy, one goal is taught at a time until a criterion is reached. A bilingual correlate might be focusing on a goal that is specific to one language, then considering how a target generalizes from one language to the other. For example, one might remediate /s/ in English and monitor it in Cantonese. In a horizontal strategy, more than one goal is addressed in each session. A bilingual correlate might be targeting one goal in Language A and another goal in Language B within the same session, although the targets would be divergent. For example, one might target final consonants in English and aspirated affricates in Hmong. In a cyclical strategy, a number of goals are addressed in a cyclical fashion, but only one goal is incorporated at a time within a session. A bilingual correlate might be to rotate not only targets, but also languages. For example, in weeks 1–4, target /s/ in Language A and clusters in Language B; in weeks 5–8, target clusters in Language A and /s/ in Language B.

Choose the approach

Another way to determine goals is to focus on language(s) in which the errors occur. A bilingual approach would focus on either elements common to both languages (e.g. errors on /s/) or errors highly occurring in both languages (e.g. cluster reduction). A cross-linguistic approach would focus on either elements unique to each language (e.g. CV syllables in Hawai'ian; CVC syllable(s) in English) or error types highly occurring in Language A and highly occurring in Language B (rhotic errors in English; trill errors in Spanish).

Choose the language of intervention

Regardless of approach, the language initially targeted depends on a number of other factors such as:

- language history or relative experience with each language;
- how frequently the child utilizes each of the languages;
- proficiency or how well the child understands and produces each language;
- environment (where and with whom the child uses each language);
- family considerations and goals;
- child's phonological skills and errors/error patterns in each of the two languages;
- feasibility of conducting meaningful intervention in the majority language at this point in time; that is, whether the child has any knowledge of the majority language and is using that language in their academic and home lives;
- supports for the child's languages at school, in the home and in the community.

When selecting the language of intervention, the SLP should consider the current uses of the child's languages as well as the language supports the child is receiving. Future uses of their languages are also important to consider: in which language(s) will the child receive her/his formal education? What language(s) do family members speak? How much time is spent with family and friends who speak in only one of the two languages?

In summary, there are two main points to keep in mind here. First, the goals for improvement in the child's overall speech intelligibility drive the language of intervention; the language of intervention does *not* drive the goals. Second, regardless of approach, the clinician must monitor generalization within and across languages.

Factors Influencing Intervention

In reality, cross-linguistic generalization in bilingual children who have been diagnosed with SSDs is likely constrained by several factors. Based on previous research focusing on the intervention of SSD, additional mitigating factors in the provision of services to this population are type and severity of the SSD, language proficiency and sociolinguistic variables (Jordaan, 2008).

A significant factor that may influence generalization is the type and severity of the disorder. For example, Holm and Dodd (2001) found that intervention targeting articulatory components of a child's SSD resulted in cross-linguistic generalization, but intervention targeting phonological organization did not. Research in the area of SSDs has indicated the necessity of controlling for severity in intervention studies. Tyler and Sandoval (1994) noted that differences in severity might result in different intervention outcomes. Williams (2000) found such an effect in the slope of change in children identified as profoundly impaired compared with those who were severely or moderately impaired.

Previous research suggests that bilingual children's skills in vocabulary (Pearson *et al.*, 1997), grammar (Gutiérrez-Clellen & Kreiter, 2003), and semantics (Peña *et al.*, 2003) vary based on factors such as language proficiency. This finding held in speech production as well. Goldstein *et al.* (2010) examined the relationship between speech skills and language proficiency in 50 typically developing Spanish-English bilingual children between the ages of 4;3 and 7;1 (mean = 5;8). Results indicated that proficiency was positively and significantly correlated with speech accuracy and significantly predicted speech accuracy in both Spanish and English.

Finally, sociolinguistic variables might mitigate cross-linguistic generalization. Romaine (1995, 1999) has asserted that bilingual children's language skills are the result of an interaction between the language of parents, the language of the community (including the language of instruction in schools) and the strategies that parents (and teachers) use in communicating with bilingual children. Thus, in providing intervention to bilingual children with SSD, it is necessary to account for community-level factors, such as dialect, socioeconomic level and immigration circumstance. Intervention goals should be based on and developed for the culture and values of the family and the child. Specifically, goals should be of primary importance to the family and modified to match the priorities of the family. Moreover, the SLP should 'involve families in the intervention process to the extent that they want to be included and continually provide the family with information about the program and the child's progress, even if they choose to be less actively involved' (Goldstein & Horton-Ikard, 2010: 50). In summary, intervention for a multilingual child with an SSD requires skills beyond those needed for a monolingual child from the majority language environment. Multilingual speech sound intervention requires determining the appropriate language(s) for intervention, carefully selecting intervention targets that will facilitate phonological skill in both languages, determining how to measure progress in both languages and determining how to facilitate transfer across languages. SLPs need to continually monitor language needs, determining when the language plan may shift based on children's shifting language needs.

If clinicians do not speak the languages of their clients, it will be necessary to determine the best person to provide language-appropriate intervention. In many countries, there are very few bilingual SLPs; those that are bilingual may not share the languages of their multilingual clients. It may not be possible for an SLP to provide direct intervention for services to their bilingual clients. In these cases, the SLP should oversee intervention, working with other professionals to ensure intervention is provided in the appropriate language(s) for the child. The primary SLP could enlist bilingual assistance to provide best services through working closely with an itinerant bilingual SLP, bilingual paraprofessionals, bilingual teaching assistants, family members or other individuals who can receive training and supervision and provide appropriate bilingual services. If an SLP accepts employment in a setting in which many of the children are from a shared bilingual or non-English language community, some feel it becomes an ethical obligation to learn the additional language well enough to communicate, if only at a basic level, with their clients and family (Chabon, 2010, personal communication).

Selecting intervention targets

There is limited research on bilingual intervention that we can use to aid in intervention target selection. However, similar principles apply in selecting targets within a single language. We should consider selecting targets that result in the greatest amount of transfer intra- and inter-linguistically in the shortest amount of time (Tyler, 2006). Intra-linguistic change will result in improvement on targets selected and can improve untreated targets in a variety of conditions.

One method for selecting intervention targets is to consider whether the potential target phoneme is shared between the child's languages or if it is unique to one of the child's languages. It is hypothesized that treating shared phonemes will result in a greater overall change in the child's phonological system. As one decides on speech targets, one method of selecting targets includes:

(1) Determining the frequency of the error rates for various phoneme or error patterns.
(2) For errors that are similar across languages, consider how important the correct production of that phoneme or word shape is within the

language. If it is important in both languages (such as /s/ production or initial consonant production in both Spanish and English), it is recommended that those errors are treated first.

(3) If a particular error occurs with differing frequency across languages, or is of differing importance in each of a child's languages (e.g. final consonants in Spanish and English), these targets may be selected for intervention next. Whether or not the errors that occur with differing frequency or differ in importance are treated earlier will depend on how important they are in each language.

(4) Finally, errors that exist in one language because of their nonexistence in the second language will typically be selected for intervention last. They are likely to have less of an impact on the child's overall phonological system. The decision order for selection of goals may change, however, based on how important each language is for the child, how much the child uses each language and how important the phonological property is in one language or the other.

As researchers continue to explore the most efficient and effective approach for treating SSDs in bilingual children, all clinicians must confirm that the intervention they are providing is working. To do so, collect intervention probes in both language environments (Olswang & Bain, 1994). Data will verify that intervention is affecting change in both languages. Probes in both languages will determine whether cross-language generalization is occurring.

Exceptions to Multilingual Intervention

Exceptions to providing intervention in both languages

There are situations in which the best intervention for a multilingual child may be intervention in only one of their languages. If a child is in a monolingual situation in a bilingual community, the SLP may choose to treat the child in the language they are currently speaking. Frequently, children in Spanish-speaking homes in the USA are exposed almost exclusively to Spanish at home, with the exposure to English not beginning until the children are in elementary school. Even though future needs of the child will include mastery of both English and Spanish phonological systems, the current needs of the child are in Spanish. Exposure to Spanish and the opportunities to practice in Spanish make intervention in the Spanish language of primary importance. The child is likely to learn quicker and apply what they learn more broadly if the targets are in their language. Possible reasons why intervention in the home language is likely to affect larger change in the child's phonological system are (a) the intervention is meaningful to the child, thus resulting in little resistance to it; (b) the intervention is meaningful to the family and family members are more likely to value and support the intervention being conducted; and (c) once stronger phonological and articulatory skills are achieved in the home language, it will be easier to transfer this knowledge and skill to the academic and community language.

If a child has a severe SSD and is in an elective multilingual environment – learning an additional language that is beyond that needed for regular functioning in the mainstream society – it may be beneficial to focus on intervention in the mainstream language first. Again, the focus on the mainstream language should bring about the greatest change in the child's phonological system. A focus on the elective language can be added once the child has made greater gains in the first language.

Application – Selection of Best Services

To illuminate the changing intervention language needs of a child, we provide a case study. Antonio (a pseudonym) was assessed by the first author when he was 3;9. Antonio was participating in a Spanish-only Head Start program (a US-based program that promotes school readiness for preschool-aged children from economically disadvantaged homes or with significant disabilities). Antonio's parents spoke only Spanish with him; he had one younger sister and relatives who also spoke only Spanish. Antonio had been diagnosed with a severe SSD at age 2;3; assessment had been conducted in Spanish and English. The SLP at Antonio's Head Start spoke English-only, and Antonio was receiving English-only intervention. Antonio's English-only SLP worked collaboratively with the first author and bilingual graduate students to provide appropriate intervention in Spanish, with the school-based English-only SLP serving as a regular supervisor for the graduate students, the first author serving as a consultant and the bilingual graduate students providing the direct services in Spanish-only for Antonio in the Head Start setting.

In Antonio's case, during the initial English-only intervention in his Spanish-speaking Head Start environment, little to no change in speech production had been noted. Our rationale for switching to a monolingual Spanish intervention plan was the lack of exposure in any environment to English, suggesting that the English therapy, with no application in the home environment, was potentially the reason for no progress. By contrast, we knew that intervention conducted in Spanish had the potential to receive carryover in home, preschool and social environments. It is also likely that the more solid the language environment in which intervention was provided, the more easily it would be carried over to the lesser known/ second language environment. Our initial goals for Antonio at 3;9 included expanding stop, nasal and glide phonemes in CVCV and CVCVCV word shapes. These are shared consonant phonemes and word shapes of Spanish and English and it was believed that work in either language would likely transfer from one language environment to the other and would provide a more widespread foundation for the child's overall phonological system. We spent more time focusing on articulatory sequencing than we might have for an English-only child, targeting functional Spanish words with CVCV and CVCVCV word shapes. These longer utterances matched the predominance of longer word shapes in Spanish and laid the groundwork for multi-word phrases in English.

The focus on Spanish intervention continued for two years while Antonio participated in a Spanish-only Head Start setting. The intervention results included increased accuracy of consonant phonemes in Antonio's word productions and greater production of multisyllabic utterances. After two years, Antonio entered a new school setting, an English-only kindergarten. For a year and a half, our university clinic lost contact with Antonio and we provided no services to him. During this period, we later learned Antonio received English-only services. Halfway through first grade, his new school SLP contacted our university clinic and asked if we would be willing to work with Antonio in a collaborative model. After consultation with the school SLP, we chose to work with Antonio in Spanish in our university clinic while his school SLP served his speech needs in English in the school setting. By this point in time, Antonio's sound inventory was complete except for later-developing language-specific sounds, including trill in Spanish and the English 'r'. In both language environments, language-specific sounds were targeted. That is, /ɹ/ and /r/ were targeted in English and Spanish, respectively. In both language environments, we focused on accuracy of stops, nasals and fricatives in longer word shapes to increase phonotactic accuracy in longer words and consonant clusters. /s/ distortion was targeted in our clinic with carryover activities for English productions included. Additionally, we focused on reinforcing the academic skills that Antonio was learning in English in his school environment. We did so in Spanish to reinforce the new skills and to provide his parents with a context to build these skills.

Thus, for a child like Antonio, who began language learning in a Spanish-only environment, we began intervention in a Spanish-only environment as well. We did so to strengthen his overall phonological system, providing a foundation for sound contrasts and productions that would apply to both languages. This focus on Spanish allowed Antonio to practice the targets we focused on more because of his almost-exclusive exposure to Spanish at that point in his life (ages 3–5). In addition, we chose this approach because of knowledge that intervention provided in the stronger language is easier to transfer to the weaker/less-used language than vice versa (Garrison & Kerper Mora, 1999). As Antonio's language environment changed, we altered his intervention approach, providing a collaborative Spanish-English model, to match his developing language needs.

Application 2 – effectiveness of bilingual therapy

Recently, we explored the response to bilingual intervention for two sequential Spanish-English bilingual 5-year-old boys with SSD, using the multiple probe design across behaviors approach (Gildersleeve-Neumann & Goldstein, 2010). Both boys were in Spanish-only home environments in which English was rarely used. These children received bilingual intervention for SSD two to three times per week for eight weeks. Intervention was provided in Spanish and English. Two intervention targets were selected for each child based on individual assessment results. Probe data were collected for target behaviors and for a third, nontreated target to monitor the effects of intervention on the overall speech system.

Intervention results were measure for three error patterns (two targeted and one control and for percent consonants and percent vowels correct). Intervention results indicate that the speech of both children improved in both languages. These improvements were observed in percent accuracy increases in intervention targets between pre- and post-intervention assessments. We also observed increases in overall accuracy, particularly percent consonants and percent vowels correct, and the index of phonetic complexity (IPC) (Jakielski, 1998). Although pilot data are promising, suggesting that bilingual intervention has a positive effect on both phonological systems of children, a more controlled study with a larger sample is needed.

Summary

Our ethical guidelines as SLPs require that we treat the child with an SSD in an evidence-based, efficient and effective manner. Bilingual children with SSD have the same needs as a monolingual child with SSD – intervention that improves their speech so that they sound like their peers and limit the ongoing academic and social impact of SSD. That intervention should be developed based on the presumed cause of the SSD. If a child has an organic cause for the speech difficulty, then the appropriate intervention for the particular organic cause – hearing loss, cleft palate, syndrome related – should be utilized. If the bilingual child has a functional SSD, and the reason for the SSD is thought to result from difficulties with acoustic-phonetic factors or phonological organization, then appropriate intervention approaches developed for these types of intervention should be utilized. There is no 'trick' to how to treat a bilingual child with an SSD; we utilized EBP guidelines developed with monolingual children to apply the intervention type that is most appropriate for the child's needs. What differs is in which language configuration the best intervention approach is applied – in L1? L2? Both? How much of each? In which order? Should intervention involve transferring information from one language to the other? How is this best done? These questions of language(s) of intervention are neither simple nor straightforward, nor have they been well studied to date. We also have needs to better understand how sociocultural, developmental and age of exposure factors affect the choice in language of intervention.

As we consider intervention for children with SSDs, we must remember that each child is unique. Our ethical obligations require us to make language of intervention decisions based on the individual needs of children at specific points in time. In addition, we must change the intervention approach as the language needs of our client changes. We can select goals based on current and future needs of the child; selecting goals that may generalize to the less used or not-yet used language. We need to monitor the effects of our speech intervention by continually collecting intervention probes in both languages throughout. If what we are doing is not working, we need to adjust intervention as necessary.

References

Baker, C. (2001) *Foundations of Bilingual Education and Bilingualism* (3rd edn). Clevedon: Multilingual Matters.

Campos, S.J. (1995) The Carpinteria preschool program: A long-term effects study. In E. Garcia and B. McLaughlin (eds) *Meeting the Challenge of Linguistic and Cultural Diversity in Early Childhood Education* (pp. 34–48). New York: Teacher's College.

Fung, F. and Roseberry-McKibbin, C. (1999) Service delivery considerations in working with clients from Cantonese-speaking backgrounds. *American Journal of Speech-Language Pathology* 8, 309–318.

Garrison, L. and Mora, J.K. (1999) Adapting mathematics instruction for English language learners: The language-concept connection. In L. Ortiz-Franco, N. Hernández and Y. De la Cruz (eds) *Changing the Faces of Mathematics: Perspectives on Latinos* (pp. 35–48). Reston, VA: National Council of Teachers of Mathematics.

Gierut, J. (1998) Treatment efficacy: Functional phonological disorders in children. *Journal of Speech, Language, and Hearing Research* 41, S85–S100.

Gildersleeve-Neumann, C.E. and Goldstein, B. (2010) Efficacy of bilingual treatment for speech sound disorder in children. Manuscript in preparation.

Goldstein, B. (2006) Clinical implications of research on language development and disorders in bilingual children. *Topics in Language Disorders* 26, 318–334.

Goldstein, B., Bunta, F., Lange, J., Rodriguez, J. and Burrows, L. (2010) The effects of measures of language experience and language ability on segmental accuracy in bilingual children. *American Journal of Speech-Language Pathology* 19, 238–247.

Goldstein, B. and Horton-Ikard, R. (2010) Diversity considerations in speech and language disorders. In J. Damico, N. Müller and M. Ball (eds) *Handbook of Language and Speech Disorders* (pp. 38–56). Malden, MA: Wiley-Blackwell.

Grosjean, F. (1989) Neurolinguists, beware! The bilingual is not two monolinguals in one person. *Brain and Language* 36, 3–15.

Gutiérrez-Clellen, V. (2001) Language choice in intervention with bilingual children. *American Journal of Speech-Language Pathology* 8, 291–302.

Gutiérrez-Clellen, V. and Krieter, J. (2003) Understanding child bilingual acquisition using parent and teacher reports. *Applied Psycholinguistics* 24, 267–288.

Holm, A. and Dodd, B. (2001) Comparison of cross-language generalisation following speech therapy. *Folia Phoniatrica et Logopaedica* 53, 166–172.

Holm, A., Dodd, B., Stow, C. and Pert, S. (1998) Speech disorder in bilingual children: Four case studies. *Osmania Papers in Linguistics* 22–23, 46–64.

Holm, A., Ozanne, A. and Dodd, B. (1997) Efficacy of intervention for a bilingual child making articulation and phonological errors. *International Journal of Bilingualism* 1, 55–69.

Jakielski, K.J. (1998) Motor organization in the acquisition of consonant clusters. Unpublished doctoral dissertation, University of Texas at Austin.

Jordaan, H. (2008) Clinical intervention for bilingual children: An international survey. *Folia Phoniatrica et Logopaedica* 60, 97–105.

Kohnert, K. and Derr. A. (2004). Language intervention with bilingual children. In B. Goldstein (ed.) *Bilingual Language Development and Disorders in Spanish-English Speakers* (pp. 311–342). Baltimore, MD: Paul H. Brookes.

Kritikos, E.P. (2003) Speech-language pathologists' beliefs about language assessment of bilingual/bicultural individuals. *American Journal of Speech-Language Pathology* 12, 73–91.

McLeod, S. (ed.) (2007) *The International Guide to Speech Acquisition*. Clifton Park, NY: Thomson Delmar Learning.

Olswang, L. and Bain, B. (1994) Data collection: Monitoring children's treatment progress. *American Journal of Speech-Language Pathology* 3, 55–66.

Pearson, B., Fernandez, S., Lewedeg, V. and Oller, D.K. (1997) The relation of input factors to lexical learning by bilingual infants. *Applied Psycholinguistics* 18, 41–58.

Peña, E., Bedore, L. and Rapazzo, C. (2003) Comparison of Spanish, English, and bilingual children's performance across semantic tasks. *Language, Speech, and Hearing Services in Schools* 34, 5–16.

Ray, J. (2002) Treating phonological disorders in a multilingual child: A case study. *American Journal of Speech-Language Pathology* 11, 305–315.

Romaine, S. (1995) *Bilingualism* (2nd edn). Oxford: Blackwell.

Romaine, S. (1999) Bilingual language development. In M. Barrett (ed.) *The Development of Language* (pp. 251–275). East Essex, UK: Psychology Press.

Stackhouse, J. (1997) Phonological awareness: Connecting speech and literacy problems. In B. Hodson and M.L. Edwards (eds) *Perspectives in Applied Phonology* (pp. 157–196). Gaithersburg, MD: Aspen Publications.

Thomas, W.P. and Collier, V.P. (2003) The multiple benefits of dual language. *Educational Leadership* 61, 61–64.

Tyler, A. and Sandoval, K. (1994) Preschoolers with phonological and language disorders: Treating different language domains. *Language, Speech, and Hearing Services in Schools* 25, 215–234.

Vihman, M.M. (1996) *Phonological Development*. Oxford: Blackwell.

Watson, I. (1991) Phonological processing in two languages. In E. Bialystok (ed.) *Language Processing in Bilingual Children* (pp. 25–48). Cambridge: Cambridge University Press.

Williams, A.L. (2000) Multiple oppositions: Case studies of variables in phonological intervention. *American Journal of Speech-Language Pathology* 9, 289–299.

25 Translation to Practice: Intervention for Multilingual Children with Speech Sound Disorders in Germany

Annette V. Fox-Boyer

Languages mentioned: English, French, German, German-French, German-Spanish, German-Turkish, Greek, Italian, Latin, Polish, Portuguese, Spanish, Turkish

Multilingual Children in Germany

The number of children growing up bilingual in Germany has been growing significantly since the 1950s. About 8–9% of the population have a foreign passport and about 10% of these are children (BAMF, 2010). Nevertheless, Germany can be considered a monolingual country, as there is only one official state language – high standard German – which is required to be used in nursery, school and official life. Multilingual people are encouraged to learn German in order to fully participate in German society, specifically to be able to participate in the German schooling system. Gogolin (1994: 30) describes this situation as the 'monolingual habitués of the multilingual school'. All children living in Germany are required to speak German at the time of school entry regardless of their home language status. Very few bilingual schools exist; the exceptions are international schools where the school languages are typically English, German-French, German-Spanish or German-Turkish. However, the majority of multilingual children are engaged in the monolingual German school system, where second, third or fourth languages are part of the curriculum, these mainly being English, French, Spanish and Latin. Language tuition in children's first languages, e.g. Turkish, Portuguese or Greek, is only provided in the afternoon or on the weekend in addition to the German school system.

Background of multilingual children living in Germany

Multilingual children living in German come from across the world. The largest group (30%) of bilingual children comes from a Turkish background, followed by 8% from an Italian background, 7% from an ex-Yugoslavian background and 6% from a Polish background (BAMF, 2010). They are either first, second or even third generation immigrants and most grow up as successive bilinguals who begin to learn their second language (German) at the age of three when they enter kindergarten.

Language competence of multilingual children

Before the year 2000, the language situation of multilingual children was mainly ignored politically, educationally and in speech-language pathology (SLP), even though in the 1980s, reports were published stating that the number of multilingual children attending special needs schools was twice as high as that for monolingual children (Klemm, 1987). Only educational reports such as Bildungsbericht (2006) or Jampert *et al.* (2005), which followed the PISA-study results (Programme for International Student Assessment-Study by the OECD) (Prenzel *et al.*, 2004), provided the first awareness of the fact that multilingual children in Germany were significantly disadvantaged regarding their educational chances.

Data from a regularly administered German-language speech and language screening, designed for monolingual children aged 3;6–6 years (Idstein language screening, ISS; Fox & Vogt, 2003), indicated that by the age of school entry (6 years), multilingual children performed about 1–2 standard deviations lower than their monolingual peers in their language comprehension and all grammatical features assessed (Fox & Vogt, 2007). These results suggest that multilingual children may initially have language difficulties in school. However, the phonology data for these children showed no difference between monolingual and multilingual children at any age assessed (Fox & Vogt, 2007).

Speech-language Pathology Research Regarding Multilingual Children

Only recently has there been limited research in the field of successive language acquisition and in multilingual children in Germany. Thus far, only one study has investigated the phonology of Turkish-German children (Uensal & Fox, 2002). These data showed that children aged 5 years had acquired all German and Turkish phonemes apart from /ʒ/ (Turkish) and /ç/ (German). The phones /s/, /z/ and /ts/ were produced interdentally by 45% of the children. However, the children showed an incomplete acquisition of clusters in German (see Table 25.1 for results). The few phonological processes produced by the children were those typically found in German- or Turkish-speaking-children (e.g. fronting of velars, fronting of sibilants, cluster reduction).

Table 25.1 Phonemic inventory in German-Turkish five-year-olds (from Uensal & Fox, 2002)

	German	*Turkish*
Consonants	m, n, ŋ	m, n
	b, p, d, t, g, k	b, p, d, t, k
	f, v, s, z, ʃ, **ç,** x	f, v, s, z, ʃ, ʒ
	l, ʁ, j, h	l, ɾ, h
	ts, pf	ʧ, ʤ
Syllable initial consonant clusters	b/p+l/ʁ	n.a.
	f+**l**/ʁ	
	t/d/**k**/g+ʁ	
	k/g+**l**	
	ʃ+p/v/**l**/ʁ/t/m/n	
	tsv	
	ʃtʁ, ʃpʁ	

Bold = not acquired.

Speech-language Pathology Provision for Multilingual Children

To date, speech and language acquisition and its disorders in multilingual children is generally not part of the curriculum of SLP training in Germany. In clinics, multilingual children are usually treated as monolingual children. Case histories do not always include a question about whether a child grows up as mono- or multilingual and if they do, usually only questions about German-language acquisition are asked. A recent dissertation dealt with the concept of a case history for multilingual children, looking at aspects that are important to multilingual children described in the literature (Kempf & Leineberger, 2010).

Typically, SLP assessments in Germany usually only focus on German due to (a) a lack of standardised assessments for multilingual children; (b) a lack of monolingual assessment material for most languages needed (i.e. Turkish); and (c) a lack of bilingual SLPs or bilingual assistants or translators. To date, two published German assessment tools are available to assess Turkish phonology (Lammer & Kalmár, 2004; Nas, 2010). The stimulus word material is culturally appropriate; all phonemes of Turkish are assessed, but these assessment tools do not provide guidelines or norms regarding how to analyse the children's data. The Russian-German and Turkish-German screening tool Screemik (Wagner, 2008) only assesses those phonemes that occur in both languages, German and Turkish and German and Russian. Here, norms are available but the assessment is only segment based.

SLP intervention in Germany is, with very few exceptions, provided in German only. SLPs are aware that their 'monolingual' behaviour does not agree with the current knowledge about best practice with bilingual children, but feel helpless with regard to the situation. To date, a request by SLPs for more knowledge about best practice with bilingual children has been observed. Following further education courses or published information, more and more therapists will try to integrate new knowledge from research in this field into their daily practice.

References

BAMF, Bundesamt für Migration und Flüchtling (2010) *Ausländerzahlen 2009* [Numbers of foreigners]. http://www.bamf.de/cln_092/nn_442496/SharedDocs/Anlagen/DE/DasBAMF/Downloads/Statistik/statistik-anlage-teil-2auslaendezahlen,templateId = raw,property = publicationFile.pdf/statistik-anlage-teil-2-auslaendezahlen.pdf. Accessed 15.9.10.

Chilla, S. (2008) *Erstsprache, Zweitsprache, Spezifische Sprachentwicklungsstörung?* [*First Language, Second Language, Specific Language Impairment*]. Hamburg: Dr. Kovac.

Fox, A.V. and Vogt, S. (2003) ISS-Idtsteiner Sprachscreening [ISS – Idstein language screening]. Unpublished Material of the Department of Speech Therapy Idstein.

Fox, A.V. and Vogt, S. (2007, June) Sprachkompetenzen mehrsprachiger Kinder [Language competences in bilingual children]. Presentation at the DBL Conference, Karlsruhe, Germany.

Gogolin, I. (1994) *Der monolinguale Habitus der multilingualen Schule* [*The Monolingual Habitus of the Bilingual School*]. Münster-NewYork: Waxmann.

Jampert, K., Best, P., Guadatiello, A., Holler, D. and Zehnbauer, A. (2005) *Schlüsselkompetenz Sprache. Sprachliche Bildung und Förderung im Kindergarten* [*Key Competence Language. Language Education and Support in Kindergarten*]. Weimar-Berlin: Konzepte, Projekte und Maßnahmen.

Kempf, S. and Leineberger, L. (2010) Möglichkeiten und Grenzen eines Anamnesebogens für den Spracherwerb multilingualer Kinder – Ergebnisse eines Fokusinterviews [Opportunities and restrictions of a designed case history for language acquisition in bilingual children]. Unpublished BSc Thesis, Fresenius University of Applied Sciences.

Klemm, B. (1987) Bildungs(be)nachteiligung ausländischer Schüler in der Bundesrepublik. *Westermanns Pädagogische Beiträge* 12, 34–40.

Konsortium Bildungsberichterstattung im Auftrag der Ständigen Konferenz der Kultusminister der Länder in der Bundesrepublik Deutschland und des Bundesministeriums für Bildung und Forschung (2006) *Bildung in Deutschland. Ein indikatorengestützter Bericht mit einer Analyse zu Bildung und Migration* [*Education in Germany. An Indicator Supported Report with an Analysis about Education and Migration*]. Bielefeld: W. Bertelsmann Verlag

Lammer, V. and Kalmár, M. (2004) *Wiener Lautprüfverfahren für Türkisch sprechende Kinder (WIELAU-T)* [*Wienase Phoneme Acquisition Assessment for Turkish-speaking Children*]. Wien: Lernen mit Pfiff.

Nas, V. (2010) *Türkisch-Artikulations-Test (TAT)* [*Turkish Articulation Test*]. Berlin Heidelberg: Springer-Verlag.

Prenzel, M., Baumert, J., Blum, W., Lehmann, R., Leutner, D., Neubrand, M., Pekrun, R., Rolff, H-G., Rost, J. and Schiefele, U. (eds) (2004) *PISA 2003. Der Bildungsstand der Jugendlichen in Deutschland- Ergebnisse des zweiten internationalen Vergleichs* [*Educational*

Levels of Adolescence in Germany-Results from the Second International Comparison]. Münster: Waxmann.

Uensal, F. and Fox, A.V. (2002) Lautspracherwerb bei zweisprachigen Migrantenkindern (Türkisch-Deutsch) [Phonological acquisition in bilingual migration children (Turkish-German]. *Forum Logopädie* 3, 10–15.

Wagner, L. (2008) *Screemik Version 2. Screening der Erstsprachefähigkeit bei Migrantenkindern. Russisch-Deutsch. Türkisch-Deutsch* [*Screening for the First Language of Migration Children. Russian-German. Turkish-German*]. Eugen: Wagner Verlag.

26 Translation to Practice: Intervention for Multilingual Hebrew-speaking Children with Speech Sound Disorders in Israel

Avivit Ben David

Languages mentioned: Amharic, English, French, Hebrew, Russian, Spanish

Context

Israel has been a multilingual and multicultural country since its establishment as an independent state in 1948, from several viewpoints. First, there are two official languages in Israel – Hebrew (also known as Israeli Hebrew or Modern Hebrew) and Arabic – each the medium of instruction in the Jewish and Arab school systems, respectively. Since second or foreign language instruction typically begins in elementary school, there are few Hebrew-Arabic bilingual children at preschool age. Second, since its inception, Israel has a large population of immigrants from numerous countries. The major groups in recent decades (between 1989 and 2007) – in order of size – come from the former Soviet Union, Ethiopia, North America, Latin America (mainly Argentina) and France (Ministry of Immigrants Absorption, 2007).[1] Thus, the main languages used by bilingual children along with Hebrew are Russian, Amharic, English, Spanish and French. Some connection has been found between country of origin, socio-economic status and school achievements, notably in the case of children of Ethiopian background, who are reported to have lower levels of educational attainment (Weissblay, 2010).

As a result of being multilingual and multicultural, Israel has numerous multilingual children, with nearly one-fifth (14.2%) of those attending grade schools in 2006 being immigrants or children of immigrants (Ministry of Immigrants Absorption, 2006). Children from immigrant families are usually sequential language learners, speaking the family language at home, with their main exposure to Hebrew beginning when they enter nursery school, around age 3. Speech-language pathologists (SLPs) in the country thus have need for research and clinical tools to help in providing clinical services to multilingual children.

Assessment

A key recommendation for assessment of multilingual children is that speech samples be obtained in both of the child's languages, since phonological acquisition typically differs in the two languages (Goldstein & Fabiano, 2007). Support for this suggestion is provided by two studies on phonological acquisition of typically developing simultaneous Hebrew-English bilingual children between ages 3;0 and 4;6 (After, 1986; Gan *et al.*, 1996). All the children (one child in After's study and six children in the Gan *et al.* study) exhibited some kind of asymmetry both in the number and variability of their phonological processes in the two languages. Some processes were language specific (that is, the child used the process in one language but not in the other), while others appeared in both languages but with different frequencies. For example, Gan *et al.* (1996) reported 22 instances of final consonant deletion in English as compared with only three in Hebrew. The authors explained that this asymmetry is because Hebrew favors word-final stress, whereas, English favors non-final stress, so that final consonants are more salient in Hebrew, and children tend to produce them more in Hebrew than in English. The authors conclude that different languages generate different processes or highly diverse use of the same processes, to the extent that they may even be indicative of two separate phonological process systems, one for each language (Paradis, 2001).

Berman (1977) analyzed the phonological processes of her simultaneous bilingual (Hebrew-English) daughter at the one-word stage. Although her purpose was not to compare the two target languages, and frequency counts were not undertaken, her analysis revealed that the same three types of processes (reduplications, transpositions and various reductions) occurred in both languages. These results are consistent with those of researchers who propose that at early stages of phonological acquisition, children have a single undifferentiated system for the two or more languages that they use, and also with Vihman's (2002) view that before the child develops a vocabulary of about 100 words, there is no phonological system at all (see Yavaş, 2007, for a brief review). Taken together, such studies underscore not only the need to assess both languages, but also to take into account the child's age and stage of acquisition.

Unfortunately, it is often difficult to assess both languages in a clinical setting. One reason is that either standardized tests of articulation or acquisition norms (or both) are either unavailable or inaccessible for some of the languages in question (e.g. Amharic and Russian). Even the construction of a standardized articulation test for Hebrew is still in progress. Besides, Israeli SLPs rarely speak the languages of their multi-lingual clients (i.e. there are no Amharic-speaking SLPs in the country), so that adequate assessment of both languages is often not feasible. In some instances, however, two SLPs of different language backgrounds collaborate to assess a bilingual child, or else they try to elicit information on the production abilities of the child in naming or imitation tasks by involving the parents or an interpreter.

In order to determine whether a bilingual child has a typical phonological acquisition, norms from monolingual children cannot be applied to bilingual children speaking the same language(s). Many studies have found differences between the phonological acquisition of bilingual and monolingual children acquiring the same languages, with bilingual children sometimes slower in acquisition and/or sometimes manifesting different types of phonological errors (see Goldstein, 2004, for a brief review). Although norms for typically developing bilingual children are important for the purpose of clinical diagnosis, there is currently only one study that compares typically developing bilingual children to monolingual Hebrew-speaking children. Or-Zach (2009) compared 20 bilingual (Hebrew-English) and 20 monolingual (Hebrew) children between the ages of 2;10 and 3;2 on the acquisition of three consonants that form part of the phonemic inventory of Hebrew: /x, ʁ, ts/ (Ben-David & Berman, 2007). She found a higher proportion of correct productions of /x/ and /ʁ/, but not /ts/ among the monolingual Hebrew-speaking children, but failed to provide normative data for the bilinguals.

All the languages used in Israel differ from Hebrew both in their segmental inventory (e.g. almost every language has a different rhotic consonant, Amharic has ejective consonants, French has nasalized and front rounded vowels) and in prosodic structure (e.g. each language manifests different stress patterns). These differences may decelerate the acquisition process. Faingold (1996) compared Berman's (1977) study to data from two simultaneous multilingual (Spanish-Portuguese-Hebrew) children who were also at the one-word stage, and concluded that the simultaneous acquisition of similar languages, such as Spanish and Portuguese, as against less-related languages, such as English and Hebrew, yielded different results. Children acquiring more similar languages tended to maintain word and syllabic structures, while children exposed to less-related languages appeared to prefer reductions to a larger extent.

The majority of the studies conducted on bilingual phonological acquisition in Hebrew have focused on Hebrew-English bilingual children, so there is a significant need for further research to derive normative data for bilinguals speaking other language combinations in Israel today. Mean-while, SLPs in Israel should bear in mind that if a slower rate of acquisition of bilinguals in their two languages occurs, it is not necessarily atypical, therefore the starting age for treatment might well be postponed in the case of children speaking more than one language.

Intervention

Until fairly recently, the common recommendation made by SLPs to parents of bilingual children with speech sound (and language) disorders was to speak only Hebrew to the child. In recent times, this approach has become less prescriptive, but it is still rare to find a bilingual child who is treated in a language other than Hebrew or in both languages – even though this has been recommended for bilinguals speaking different languages (Goldstein, 2004). Indeed, even when the SLP is familiar with both languages, the bulk of the treatment is conducted in Hebrew.

Because there are no studies on intervention with bilingual children in Israel, it is hard to know what approaches are, in practice, used with bilinguals. From the author's personal experience and on the basis of input from colleagues, Israeli SLPs evidently tend to treat error patterns and phonological processes that occur in both languages before those that are confined to Hebrew. However, SLPs could adopt recommendations derived from studies on other languages (Goldstein & Fabiano, 2007), such as deciding which language should be initially applied for intervention in terms of such factors as frequency of use, proficiency in the language, family considerations and amount of errors in each language. It is also important to monitor phonological change across the two languages. Finally, while it may be valuable to incorporate principles of assessment and intervention from studies on other languages, it is equally, if not more important to take into account the impact of language-particular patterns on the acquisition process in making clinical decisions.

Acknowledgements

I would like to thank Professor Yishai Tobin from the Department of Foreign Literatures and Linguistics and the Department of Behavioral Sciences of Ben-Gurion University of the Negev, Professor Ruth Berman from the Linguistics Department of Tel-Aviv University and Dr Limor Adi-Bensaid from the Department of Communication Disorders in Tel-Aviv University for their critical reading and helpful comments on an earlier version of this chapter.

Notes

(1) In addition, there are also over 2000 children of foreign workers, most from the Far East, South America, Eastern Europe and Africa, and another about 1000 children of refugees, mainly from Sudan and Eritrea (Ashkenazi *et al.*, 2009; Weissblay, 2009)

References

After, G. (1986) Phonological processes in a bilingual child aged 3;5. Unpublished seminar paper, Tel Aviv University Department of Communications Disorders. [In Hebrew.]

Ashkenazi, S., Ben Shlomo, O., Levy, M., Meir, Y., Maman, N., Peleg, Y., Tzubary, Y., Kalpus, M and Schwartz, T. (2009) The characteristics of foreign workers and refugees and the intervention of MESILA (Aid and Information Center for the Foreign Community). http://www.tel-aviv.gov.il/Hebrew/Human/Foreign/Index.asp. Accessed 25.8.10.

Ben David, A. and Berman, R. (2007) Israeli Hebrew speech acquisition. In S. McLeod (ed.) *The International Guide to Speech Acquisition* (pp. 437–456). Clifton Park, NY: Delmar Thomson Learning.

Berman, R.A. (1977) Natural phonological processes at the one-word stage. *Lingua* 43, 1–21.

Faingold, E.D. (1996) Variation in the application of natural processes: Language-dependent constraints in the phonological acquisition of bilingual children. *Journal of Psycholinguistic Research* 25, 515–526.

Gan, R., Ezrati, R. and Tobin, Y. (1996) Phonological processes in Hebrew-English bilingual children (3;0–4;6). In M. Freedman and M. Lapidot (eds) *Proceedings of the International Symposium on Communication Disorders in Bilingual Populations* (pp. 247–254). Haifa, Israel: The Israel Association for Speech, Hearing and Language [DASH].

Goldstein, B.A. (2004) Phonological development and disorders. In B.A. Goldstein (ed.) *Bilingual Language Development and Disorders in Spanish-English Speakers* (pp. 257–286). Baltimore, MD: Paul H. Brookes.

Goldstein, B.A. and Fabiano, L. (2007) Assessment and intervention for bilingual children with phonological disorders. *The ASHA Leader* 12 (2), 6–7, 26–27, 31.

Ministry of Immigrants Absorption (2006) The statistics annual report on immigrants' children 2006. http://www.moia.gov.il/Moia_he/Statistics/ChildrenData/. Accessed 25.8.10.

Ministry of Immigrants Absorption (2007) Immigration data summary 1989–2007. http://www.moia.gov.il/Moia_he/Statistics/ImmigrationToIsraelPrevYears/ImmigrationData2007.htm. Accessed 25.8.10.

Or-Zach, Y. (2009) The production of the consonants /x,r,ts/ by monolingual Hebrew speaking children and bilingual English-Hebrew speaking children. Unpublished MA project, Tel Aviv University. [In Hebrew.]

Paradis, J. (2001) Do bilingual two-year-olds have separate phonological systems? *International Journal of Bilingualism* 5 (1), 19–38.

Vihman, M.M. (2002) Getting started without a system: From phonetics to phonology in bilingual development. *International Journal of Bilingualism* 6, 239–254.

Weissblaj, E. (2009) Authorities treatment of foreign workers' and refugees' children. http://www.knesset.gov.il/mmm/data/docs/m02269.doc. Accessed 25.8.10.

Weissblaj, E. (2010) *Integration of Ethiopian immigrants in the school system* [in Hebrew]. http://www.knesset.gov.il/mmm/heb/index.asp.

Yavaş, M. (2007) Multilingual speech acquisition. In S. McLeod (ed.) *The International Guide to Speech Acquisition* (pp. 69–100). Clifton Park, NY: Thomson Delmar Learning.

27 Translation to Practice: Intervention for Multilingual Children with Speech Sound Disorders in Montréal, Québec, Canada

Isabelle Simard

Languages mentioned: *Arabic, Cantonese, Creole, Czech, English, French, German, Greek, Hebrew, Italian, Korean, Mandarin, Portuguese, Romanian, Serbo-Croatian, Spanish, Vietnamese.*

Sociolinguistic Context of Montréal

Sociolinguistics of Canada, Québec and Montréal

Canada is officially a bilingual country; therefore, all Canadians can receive services in English and French, in all 10 provinces and 3 territories. In fact, 57% of Canadians speak English as their first language (L1), 22% use French and 20% count another as their mother tongue. English is spoken primarily in all provinces except Québec, where French is predominant. Indeed, 78% of Québécois are originally francophones, 8% anglophones and 12% allophones (people whose L1 is not one of the official languages). Most of the latter live in the cosmopolitan city of Montréal, where out of 3.6 million people, 64% speak French as their L1, 12% use English and 21% are native speakers of another language (Statistics Canada, 2010).

Moreover, bilinguals, who represent 51% of Montréal's population, are differentiated from multilinguals (speakers of three or more languages), constituting 16% of Montréalers. Although all children must learn English or French as a second language at school (consequently becoming bilinguals), those who are non-native speakers of the two official languages must become multilinguals because they generally live, hence attend childcare, in areas where English is dominant and are educated in French (due to provincial law). This chapter will thus focus on the multilinguals and will offer foremost a description of the French culture, over English and the other languages, in order to be congruent with the reality of the linguistic majority of the province and city.

Typical ages of introduction of languages

Montréal children typically use French as an L1 and learn English informally in daycare or preschool (4–5 years), then formally in first grade of elementary school (age 6). Most are exposed to other languages through friends, environment, entertainment or at school (if they choose to learn a third language). The native English speakers have the right to be educated in their mother tongue, if one of their parents has attended school in English (Office québécois de la langue française, 1993); these children are taught French in primary school and can pursue learning other languages in later years (although usually exposed to many at a young age). Montréal is a city in which multilingualism is omnipresent; therefore, children can acquire languages not only sequentially (in instruction-related stages), but also simultaneously (through circumstances). Due to a high level of language contact, interference and linguistic customs (involving much code-switching and code-mixing), it is not uncommon for children to become receptive bilinguals (French and English) who prefer expressing themselves in only one language (as preschoolers), later blossoming into functioning bi/multilinguals.

Features of the languages

Québec French is similar to French from France with respect to the consonants of the phonological system, yet it does present some differences in vowels: there is a clear distinction between /e/ and /ɛ/; moreover, when diphthongized and lengthened, /ɛ/ becomes a separate phone, [ɜ], e.g. *fête* (birthday) /fɛt/ → [fɜt], thereby extending the vocalic system to 17 vowels (Leclerc, 1989). Furthermore, the French speakers of Québec typically delete the word-final schwa and the last consonant of a word-final cluster. They also affricate the coronal stops /t, d/ and lax the high vowels /i, y, u/ into [ɪ, ʏ ʊ]. The features of Québec French, as well as those of Canadian English, are described in depth in Rose and Wauquier-Gravelines (2007) and Bernhardt and Deby (2007), respectively.

Speech-language Pathology Services in Montréal, Québec, Canada

In Montréal, as in the province of Québec, preschool children have free access, in French and English, to specific speech-language pathology services in Health and Social Services Centers (CSSS) and specialized services in Rehabilitation Centers (CR). In cases of physical or cognitive impairments, as well as pervasive developmental disorders, a waiting list is established (upon receipt of request) according to priority levels: urgent (within 72 hours), high (30 days for CSSS, 90 days for CR) and moderate (within 1 year) (Ministère de la Santé et des Services sociaux du Québec, 2008).

When children reach school age (5–6 years), they may receive freely dispensed services from their School Board; they are generally assessed and may benefit from a limited number of group or individual therapies. Students classified as 'handicapped' or with 'learning disabilities' are integrated into special classes, schools or receive pedagogical support in regular classrooms (Commission scolaire de Montréal, 2003).

Alternatively, private practice is an avenue that many people choose (over the public system). Waiting lists are quite variable; however, services are currently offered in 13 languages across Québec (Ordre des orthophonistes et audiologistes du Québec, 2010). Most speech-language pathologists (SLPs) in the province work in a French context (70%), compared to fewer (48%) in the city of Montréal. Although Canada is a bilingual country, only 10% of (4210 registered) Canadian SLPs provide services in the two official languages (Canadian Association of Speech-Language Pathologists and Audiologists (CASLPA), 2010); practising bilinguals are more numerous in Québec (17%), as well as in Montréal (28%). With regard to multilingualism in clinical settings, 8% of polyglot SLPs from CASLPA are scattered throughout Canada, 5% are members of Québec's Ordre des orthophonistes et audiologistes du Québec (OOAQ) and 10% of Montréal SLPs opt to practice in three or more languages.

Multilingual Speech-language Pathology Private Practice in Montréal

ORTHO FUN I: Les petits Cocos

ORTHO FUN I: Les petits Cocos is a speech-language pathology practice for multilingual children in Montréal. The first part of the name is a homophone for *orthophonie* (speech-language pathology) and the second is a term of endearment (in French) used when referring to children; the whole alludes to 'fun correcting sounds with Isabelle's little darlings'. It is set in a child-centered, family-oriented private clinic in a residential neighborhood. It was conceptualized not only to be appealing to children, but also to be interesting for their family members and friends. It contains a spacious waiting room, including a comfortable lounge, an eating area, book shelves (complete with materials in 10 different languages), live voiceless animals and a life-size castle. The latter was designed to stimulate spontaneous speech: it is embellished with costumes, puzzles, figurines, puppets, aligned with a medieval theme, in which all can join in and engage in child-directed play. The space also holds a reception, an office and a sizeable therapy room, containing numerous toys and games in many different languages, collected all over the globe (reflecting the theme). This environment was created and is managed by a polyglot speech-language pathologist, specifically trained to assess and dispense therapies in a multilingual manner, as well as counsel parents about plurilingual contexts. The clinician, also a linguist, maintains particular interests, not only in speech sound disorders (SSD), but in fluency. The languages represented among the clientele are varied beyond French and English: Spanish, Greek, Portuguese, Italian, Arabic, Mandarin, Vietnamese, Hebrew, Romanian, Creole, Korean, Serbo-Croatian Cantonese, Czech and German. Since the speech-language pathologist is not fluent in all (expressively in 5 and receptively in 12), the involvement of the significant persons is encouraged to model the languages not mastered by the clinician. Indeed, parents are actively engaged in therapeutic sessions in order to ensure proper linguistic models.

The children's languages are spoken according to several approaches:

- *One person, one language*: each parent addresses the child in his/her mother tongue and the therapist uses the third language of the child's environment; if a parent is absent, the speech-language pathologist compensates, speaking the one representing the absentee.
- *Turn taking*: ideal for fluent multilinguals, where each round of a game is played by everyone using the same language, which changes at each turn.
- *Context directed*: participants speak the language intended in a specific game, mostly determined by written language.
- *Code-switching*: this style best represents the sociolinguistic culture of Montréal, in which the child is encouraged to use spontaneous speech in the quickest accessible language, meriting a response by the adults in the chosen language.

In all communication manners, code-mixing is treated by (the clinician and/or parents) modeling the child's utterances in one or all languages.

The rich conversational environment (where spontaneous speech is favored, code-switching is allowed and cultures are respected) facilitates progress in speech, language and communication development (Simard, 2010), particularly when coupled with a unique approach (the 'Isabelle technique').

Intervention

The children, whose ages range from 3 to 18 years, receive individual intervention at the clinic, regularly (1 hour weekly) at the initial stages; as they progress, their evolution is monitored bimonthly to yearly. The predominant types of speech-language delays/disorders represented include: language disorders (32.8%), SSDs (14.5%), fluency disorders (8.1%) and combined disorders (44.6%).

Particularly, with respect to SSD, the children manifest difficulty with the following sounds (all occurring in French except when mentioned) and present the corresponding phonological processes:

/s, z/: interdental lisp and alveolar backing

/ʃ, ʒ/: lateral lisp and palatal fronting
/k, g/: velar fronting
/ʀ/ → [ʁ], [ɹ] (English), [ʀ] and [r] (Spanish): gliding and deletion
/l/: gliding and deletion
/b, d, g, v, z, ʒ/: de-voicing
/f, v, s, z, ʃ, ʒ/: stopping
/θ, ð/ (English, Greek): stopping.

A multimodal-sensory approach (the 'Isabelle technique') was developed by the speech-language pathologist and entails a demonstration of sound production, utilizing all five senses, implying looking at the clinician's mouth, listening to her producing the isolated sounds, manipulating the toys associated with them, smelling the chosen food item used to 'tickle' the children's articulators and thus engaging their taste. This method is applied to stimulate sound production where each phoneme is represented by an animal or object (in which the name generally starts with the targeted sound). The children are taught to produce the sounds while making the movements corresponding to the animals/objects, e.g.:

/s/: slithering snake (*serpent*)
/g/: jumpy frog (*grenouille*) or grasshopper
/ʀ/: roaring lion (with three different types of engines for French, English and Spanish phones)

Vocal models are used solely to demonstrate the dental fricatives. The voiced sounds are shown (by placing a hand on the throat to feel the vibration) in opposition to the voiceless. The sequence of presentation unfolds from anterior to posterior, in pairs (except the liquid and rhotic): /p-b, f-v, t-d, s-z, ʃ-ʒ, k-g, ʀ, l/. When the children are able to produce or approximate the targeted isolated sounds, their corresponding articulators are lightly touched with a long, thin, hard sweet (chocolate, lollypop or liquorice). They are then asked to manually replicate the place of articulation on a mouth puppet.

The most common phonological processes comprise: backing, fronting, gliding, de-voicing, stopping, consonant harmony, deletion and de/nasalization. Many types of deletion occur, from sound (word-initial, syllable/word-final consonant) to syllable, via cluster reduction, which are treated (as is consonant harmony) with the aid of long, fragmentable, multi-coloured animal-shaped markers: each part represents a sound within a syllable or syllable within a polysyllabic word. Often, the animals corresponding to the targeted sounds are placed on specific parts of the marker as additional visual aids. The children are encouraged to produce the sounds, syllables and ultimately words, after fragmented and whole models are provided. Finally, denasalization, as well as nasalization, is rehabilitated with the help of animal-shaped mirrors, which allow children to visualize nasal emission or lack thereof.

For all children, the first session is one of demonstration, the second of recall and, from the third onward, of application. Moreover, they respond to a pre-determined structure: pre-therapy spontaneous speech (in the castle or with a book), reviewing of the week's homework, followed by stamping as a task-specific reward (in collaboration with parents, enabling them to identify correction opportunities), ending with game playing. After each therapy (and assessment), the children's global and specific performances or effortful attempts are rewarded. Their progress is monitored closely, as the frequency of sessions decreases according to their goal attainment, until they reach levels of control, maintenance and mastery.

References

Bernhardt, B.M.H. and Deby, J. (2007) Canadian English speech acquisition. In S. McLeod (ed.) *The International Guide to Speech Acquisition* (pp. 177–187). Clifton Park, NY: Thomson Delmar Learning.

Canadian Association of Speech-Language Pathologists and Audiologists (2010) *Membership Data*. Ottawa: Author.

Commission scolaire de Montréal (2003) Politique relative à l'organisation des services aux élèves handicapés ou en difficulté d'adaptation ou d'apprentissage. http://www.csdm.qc.ca/p-2003-2. Accessed 5.10.10.

Leclerc, J. (1989) *Qu'est-ce que LA LANGUE¿* Laval: Mondia Éditeurs.

Ministère de la Santé et des Services sociaux du Québec (2008) *Plan d'accès aux services pour les personnes ayant une déficience*. Québec: La direction des communications du ministère de la Santé et des Services sociaux du Québec. http://publications.msss.gouv.qc.ca/acrobat/f/documentation/2008/08-848-01.pdf. Accessed 5.10.10.

Office québécois de la langue française (1993) Regulations respecting requests to receive instruction in English. In *Charter of the French language* (R.S.Q., c.c-11, s.80; 1993, c.40, s.30). Québec: Author.

Ordre des orthophonistes et audiologistes du Québec (2010) *Membership Data*. Montréal: Author.

Rose, Y. and Wauquier-Gravelines, S. (2007) French speech acquisition. In S. McLeod. (ed.) *The International Guide to Speech Acquisition* (pp. 364–385). Clifton Park, NY: Thomson Delmar Learning.

Simard, I. (2010, August) Multilingual intervention with preschoolers and school-aged children: Evidence from a private practice in Montréal. Poster presentation at the 28th World Congress of the International Association of Logopedics and Phoniatrics, Athens, Greece.

Statistics Canada (2010) *2006 Census of Population*. Statistics Canada catalogue No. 97-555-XCB2006007.

28 Literacy and Metalinguistic Considerations of Multilingual Children with Speech Sound Disorders

Yvette Hus

Languages mentioned: Arabic, Cantonese, Czech, Dutch, English, Finnish, French, German, Greek, Hebrew, Italian, Mandarin, Punjabi, Russian, Southern Min, Spanish, Swedish

Speech Production, Phonological Awareness and Reading

The phonology of language is inevitably a major player in reading acquisition simply because *written* languages are arbitrary representations of *spoken* languages. In hearing populations, the phonology (i.e. the sound system rules of a language) forms the foundation on which words and meanings are established (Lundberg, 2002; Stoel-Gammon, 1998). The acquisition process involves the linking of perception of sounds to the production of an ever-increasing complexity of speech patterns, and it is the use of both the accurate perception and production of speech sounds that promotes the ability to reflect on the phonological system, that is, to acquire phonological awareness (PA; Swank & Larrivee, 1998). The term *phonological awareness* is often used interchangeably with *metaphonological ability* and *phonological sensitivity* to refer to a group of skills that includes awareness, attention and intentional manipulation of the internal structure of words, such as syllables, rhymes, onsets-rimes and phonemes (Scarborough & Brady, 2004).

Reading acquisition models, no matter the orthographic structure of the language, all point to the importance of PA development in the reading process (Goswami, 2002; Hermans *et al.*, 2008; Kuo & Anderson, 2010; Vloedgraven & Verhoeven, 2007). Its critical role is in connecting reading processes to speech processes (i.e. accurate perception and production of speech sounds) that are typically already well developed when reading acquisition is initiated (Frost *et al.*, 2009). This connection has important implications for children who bring poorly developed speech processes to the reading acquisition task.

Frost *et al.* (2009) clarify the neurobiological underpinning of PA in beginning readers. Skilled PA modulates the early reading process by making 'the neuronal networks dedicated by nature and early language experience to speech, available for print processing' (Frost *et al.*, 2009: 93). In alphabetic orthographies, they note, phoneme awareness (i.e. the recognition that words and syllables are made up of individual speech sounds that can be manipulated) and knowledge of the alphabetic code form the bridging mechanisms between spoken and printed words. The study's important confirmatory finding of the role of PA in early reading acquisition was that increases in PA were related to a decrease in activation for speech and an increase in activation for print stimuli. The investigators concluded that as individuals acquire greater literacy skills, the regions common to speech and print become increasingly more dedicated to processing of print than to speech. This finding may be used to explain, first, why PA is well established as a successful predictor in early reading skill development, and reliably distinguishes between individuals with typical from atypical reading acquisition processes that constitute high risk for reading disabilities (Frost *et al.*, 2009; Hogan *et al.*, 2005); and second, why phonetic decoding rather than PA becomes the important determiner in successful word reading by about Grade 2 (Hogan *et al.*, 2005).

While the Frost *et al.* findings provide the neurobiological explanation for PA and for the importance of intact speech processes in the acquisition of PA, behavioural studies support the importance of accurate speech processes in the development of PA and specifically, phoneme awareness (Carroll *et al.*, 2003; Chiang, 2003; Sénéchal *et al.*, 2004; Thomas & Sénéchal, 1998; Webster & Plante, 1992, 1995). What are the implications of these finding for PA development in children with speech sound disorders (SSD) and, more specifically, what are the implications for bilingual children[1] with SSD?

Role of Orthography and Oral Language in PA Development

Cross-linguistic studies have shown that while PA abilities are orthography dependent when focused on the print modality of a language (Goswami *et al.*, 1998; Seymour *et al.*, 2003; Ziegler & Goswami, 2006), they are also influenced by exposure to a specific oral language (Caravolas & Landerl, 2010; Yeong & Liow, 2010). For example, differences in onset-rime awareness between monolingual English and monolingual Cantonese-speaking 4-year-olds were related to the two languages' different syllable structure. The oral language influence helped explain why children speaking Cantonese or Mandarin (both with simple open consonant–vowel syllables and no consonant clusters) are poorer in their PA skills for English, the language with the more complex syllable structure (Cheung *et al.*, 2001). This finding underscores the importance of understanding the phonological structures of the languages being acquired by bilingual children.

Interestingly, in both the Frost *et al.* (2009) and the Hogan *et al.* (2005) studies with English speakers, *elision*, the phoneme deletion task (e.g. *say ball without the /b/*), was the most sensitive measure of individual differences in metaphonological skills. A phoneme segmentation task, however, was most accurate in identifying higher PA ability in Dutch-speaking kindergarteners and lower PA ability in first graders (Vloedgraven *et al.*, 2007). The PA task sensitivity to individual differences seems to vary according to the phonological and orthographic structure of a language, an important consideration when measuring PA abilities in specific language sets or combination of languages of bilingual speakers as PA tasks with different sensitivities may be required for each of the languages in the set.

SSDs and PA

Literacy acquisition depends greatly on the intactness and efficiency of the neurobiological system (Frost *et al.*, 2009; Golestani & Pallier, 2007; Shaywitz & Shaywitz, 2009) in determining the quality of developments of its crucial elements (Wren, 2000). The sheer complexity of the reading acquisition process predicts a multifactorial explanation for reading acquisition failure rather than an underlying unitary cause. One such factor is SSD. Although SSD may be associated with organic etiologies, in a majority of cases SSD in children have no known etiology, that is, they are functional (Gierut, 1998). The focus here is on children with functional SSD.

Variables implicated in reading failure in children with SSD

Researchers agree that children with SSD represent a heterogeneous group and that *not all* fail to develop age-appropriate literacy skills (Catts & Kamhi, 2005; Dodd & McIntosh, 2008; Edwards *et al.*, 2002; Holm *et al.*, 2008; Leitão & Fletcher, 2004; Peterson *et al.*, 2009; Rvachew *et al.*, 2007; So & Dodd, 2007). Weak phonological representation[2] is often cited as an explanatory construct for the negative impact of disordered speech on PA development: SSD interferes with the establishment of strong and accurate representation of speech sounds in the mental lexicon (Storkel *et al.*, 2010; Swank & Larrivee, 1998; Yeong & Liow, 2010). Both accurate recognition or identification of speech sounds and their accurate translation into articulatory gestures are affected when weak and inaccurate representations are formed (Gierut, 1998; Swank & Larrivee, 1998). Accurate phonological representations are crucial for the development of phoneme awareness (Caravalos & Landerl, 2010; Lundberg, 2002), which in turn impacts word decoding and spelling abilities (Wang & Geva, 2003a; Yeong & Liow, 2010). Storkel *et al.* (2010) implicated SSD in the formation of weaker and less accurate phonological as well as lexical representations, and their consequent negative impact on vocabulary acquisition. Indeed, Chiang and Rvachew's (2007) study of English L1-French L2 kindergarten bilinguals without SSD showed that while vocabulary size was closely related to PA skills, expressive vocabulary was more strongly related than receptive vocabulary.

Edwards *et al.* (2002) found that children with SSD performed significantly poorer than age peers on speech perception tasks. Poor whole word discrimination, regardless of age, was significantly correlated with receptive vocabulary size and articulatory accuracy; that is, those with larger vocabularies performed more accurately on the speech perception tasks. Poor final phoneme discrimination abilities indicated that children with SSD are less able to attend to fine phonetic details in the acoustic signal when the latter is degraded compared to typically developing age peers. The results of this study show the importance of phonotactic structure (i.e. the rules for combining phonemes into words that govern each language; Velleman, 2002) and PA.

No language exists without phonotactic rules (Trask & Stockwell, 2007). The task of bilingual children with SSD is to accurately perceive and produce the speech sounds of each of their languages, as well as understand the phonotactics of each language. A bilingual French-English speaker, for example, needs to be aware of the phonotactic rule in which both sounds in a /pn/ cluster are produced in French but not in English, even though 'p' and 'n' are preserved in writing (in English in words such as *pneumonia*) because of an orthographic rule. Children's knowledge of accurate syllable or word structures or phoneme sequences is crucial because they determine meanings (Velleman, 2002). A child with phonotactic error patterns may be able to produce a variety of consonants and vowels, but exhibit difficulty in using these in the correct combinations and sequences.

Caravalos and Landerl (2010) demonstrated that the ability to focus on specific phonemes seems to be language specific and relates to the phonotactics of the language being acquired. In their study, Czech-speaking children were more aware of phonemes in onsets. German speakers, however, were more aware of phonemes in codas. Clearly, the phonological structure of the language affects the saliency of the speech sound and its consequent capacity to trigger accurate awareness. The findings from these studies have significant implications for PA development of bilingual speakers with the added load of SSD because phoneme awareness seems to be affected by receptive vocabulary size, the quality of the speech signal and by the specific phonotactic characteristics of the ambient language(s).

SSD in children results in poor PA and phonological memory development (Webster *et al.*, 1997), and poses increased risk for developing reading disorders (RD); however, children with SSD who have better PA show an increased chance of developing oral and written language at all levels of development, from early to more advanced linguistic levels (Magnusson, 1991). Peterson *et al.* (2009) attributed poor literacy outcomes to comorbidity of SSD and language impairment (LI) rather than severity. They also implicated nonverbal IQ as a player in reading outcomes. Catts and Kamhi (2005) noted that children with more severe SSD who have extensive LI and who perform poorly on PA tasks are most at risk for reading disabilities. However, Rvachew *et al.* (2007) found that consistent production of non-developmental errors rather than severity was the key predictor in PA and literacy acquisition. Holm *et al.*'s study (2008) supports the finding that error pattern type is an important variable in literacy outcomes. They classified children with SSD according to type of speech error pattern, that is, developmental or deviant, and error consistency. Those with delayed phonological development consistently produced errors typical of younger children and had no difficulty on PA measures and reading, but showed spelling issues. Some children showed inconsistent error production, that is, multiple errors of single words and connected speech but with no underlying oro-motor difficulty. Children with these types of errors had some difficulty on PA tasks, and poor performance on spelling. The inconsistent error production implied difficulty with phonotactic rules (phoneme assembly). Children with consistent production of non-developmental speech errors performed poorly on PA tasks, and on both reading comprehension and spelling tasks. They concluded that children with *consistent atypical* speech errors have poor PA and are most at risk for literacy difficulties, most probably because of inaccurate or incomplete phonological representation.

Rule-derivation issues (difficulty discriminating acceptable sound combinations from unacceptable ones, e.g. /sb/ cluster in English onsets) were also implicated in SSD with poor literacy outcomes (Dodd & McIntosh, 2008; So & Dodd, 2007). This has negative consequences for bilingual children because those without SSD are able to use the phonological skills and knowledge gained in one language in the context of the other language (i.e. they are sensitive to word structure, as shown in Kuo and Anderson's (2010) study of Mandarin and Southern Min bilingual children). The presence of SSD would therefore render them less able to note similarities and differences or to transfer skills between their languages.

Multiple Deficit View of Reading Disabilities and SSD

Peterson *et al.* (2009) and others (Hulme *et al.*, 2005) proposed that a multiple deficit view of reading disabilities (RD) best explains the relationship between SSD and consequent literacy outcomes: a phonological processing deficit is a risk for RD. However, it interacts with other risk and protective factors in the eventual reading and spelling skill outcome. Support for this *multiple deficit view of reading* is provided in the Shatil and Share (2003) longitudinal study of kindergarten Hebrew speakers, where word recognition was best explained by phonological processing, phonological memory and early literacy knowledge, but not by phonemic awareness because PA is less important in Hebrew with its simple CV syllable structure. The results of this study call attention to the importance of considering the language's orthographic transparency[3] and syllabic complexity when examining PA and RD, because children acquiring languages with transparent orthographies, such as Greek, Italian, Spanish and German, acquire accurate and fluent decoding skills earlier and with less difficulty than those acquiring languages with opaque ones, such as Dutch, French and English (Seymour *et al.*, 2003).

It is also known that PA task sensitivity for detection of RD varies across languages. A study of Italian-speaking children with RD showed that while all children had difficulty with phonological processing (as measured by naming speed), only those with a history of previous language delay presented difficulties on phonemic awareness measures (Brizzolara *et al.*, 2006). Studies of RD in Spanish speakers determined that word reading rate rather than accuracy revealed the RD (e.g. Serrano & Defior, 2008). In Chinese-English bilingual children in Grades 1–8, both Chinese rhyme detection and English phoneme elision tasks uniquely predicted English word reading (Gottardo *et al.*, 2001). Evidently, the combinations of languages being acquired are vital to understanding the development of literacy skills.

Considerations in Assessment and Treatment for Bilingual SSD Children

The findings from the various studies with SSD children have clinical implications for evaluation and intervention, and suggest the following considerations.

Comparing bilinguals to other bilinguals

It is important to construct profiles of performance in all reading elements (Wren, 2000), including the oral expressive skills[4] of *bilingual* typical readers of a specific language set, and of their peers with RD (without SSD), to facilitate early detection of RD in bilingual children with SSD from the same language combination. That is, it is best to compare bilinguals with bilinguals (Fabiano-Smith & Barlow, 2010). Comparing bilinguals to monolinguals in each of their languages may not be valid. For example, Holm and Dodd's (1999a, 1999b, 1999d) studies of phonological acquisition in Cantonese-English bilinguals showed error patterns that were atypical for each language in comparison to monolinguals, but typical in comparison to studies of bilinguals. Cross-linguistic transfer due to the interactivity of languages (Paradis & Genesee, 1996) results in interaction between the phonologies of the languages, a common phenomenon in the literacy skills of bilinguals as well. Studies with Spanish-English bilingual children's English word and pseudoword recognition test performance was predicted by the levels of both Spanish PA and Spanish word recognition (Durgunoglu *et al.*, 1993), while studies with English L1 children in French immersion programmes confirmed PA skill transfer from English to French and explained growth in French decoding skills (Comeau *et al.*, 1999; Chiang & Rvachew, 2007). Chiang (2003), for example, found evidence for reverse transfer or L2–L1 transfer of PA skills in Chinese-English bilinguals. Here, articulation training of complex sequences in children's L2 (i.e. English) facilitated PA in their L1 (i.e. Chinese). It is agreed that the degree of phonotactic similarity between languages influences the course of reading and spelling acquisition in each language (Bialystok, 2007; Bialystok *et al.*, 2005; Wang & Geva, 2003a; Yeong & Liow, 2010).

Phonological representations, the elements that underlie PA and lexical development, are clearly tied to specific languages. The task of bilingual children is to form a set of accurate phonological representations for each of their languages. The fact that particular language combinations often result in unique speech, language, metalinguistic and reading developmental trajectories (Chiang & Rvachew, 2007; Durgunoglu *et al.*, 1993; Eviatar & Ibrahim, 2000; Liow & Poon, 1998; McBride-Chang & Ho, 2005; McGregor *et al.*, 2006; Sénéchal *et al.*, 2004) provides a strong argument for comparing the literacy skills of bilinguals to bilinguals, rather than to monolinguals of each language (Grosjean, 1985).

PA and SSD assessment

Magnusson (1991) points out that it is important to differentiate between children who cannot perform on PA tasks from those who can but have disordered linguistic knowledge. It is therefore advisable to ask for nonverbal responses in measuring PA so that the child's difficulties in speech production are not mistaken for a PA deficit. Because PA task sensitivity to individual differences varies according to the phonological and orthographic structure of a language, it is vital to choose tasks that can optimally assess PA skills in each of the child's languages in order to avoid false negative results.

Assessment of the child's speech with an appropriate instrument designed for bilinguals (Holm *et al.*, 1999c) must include a determination of the error pattern subtype because it can predict PA, reading and spelling outcomes. Furthermore, because the same subtype often underlies both of the child's languages, it can facilitate matching an effective course of treatment. For example, Crosbie *et al.* (2005) found that core vocabulary therapy resulted in greater change in speech production of English monolingual children with inconsistent speech disorder, while phonological contrast therapy resulted in greater change in children with a consistent speech disorder. Both interventions would, inevitably, positively impact PA development and consequent literacy acquisition in these children.

The core vocabulary approach was used in the treatment of bilingual SSD children. It was effective in significantly improving the speech production of a Punjabi-English bilingual child with inconsistent SSD in both languages. Interestingly, while he received treatment in English only, it generalised to Punjabi (Holm & Dodd, 1999b). This is a significant clinical finding as the child may not need to be burdened with unnecessary intervention sessions in both languages when one SSD subtype is involved. Similarly, Canadian English L1 French immersion students, who were high risk for reading disability when given PA skills treatment in French, their L2, showed improvement in English (in Genesee, 2007); furthermore, their high-risk factors were easily identifiable using either French or English PA tasks (MacCoubrey *et al.*, 2004).

Language and literacy assessment and intervention

Because the degree of bilingualism is important in literacy development, it is essential that both languages are thoroughly assessed (Goldstein & Fabiano, 2006). A clinical consideration in assessments of oral language and reading is the paucity of appropriate standardised tests for bilingual and culturally diverse children. Using the cognitive framework proposed by Wren (2000) to deliver a curriculum-based assessment (Aldrich & Wright, 2001) can be a viable and useful alternative so that the student's performance is not compared to that of a so-called normative local or national group. Recommendations for assessing and treating literacy issues in bilingual populations, based on Wren's (2000) work, are particularly useful for these children (Hus, 2009). For example, in oral language, syntactic structures can be evaluated using pictures, and with cloze sentences. Judgements of grammaticality can similarly be evaluated. To tease out language comprehension issues from reading comprehension, children may first be required to answer questions after a story is read to them. Reading comprehension can then be evaluated with a criterion-based test, such as a reading inventory, where the child is asked to read a passage of text that is levelled appropriately for the child's age or grade, followed by some explicit questions about the content of the text. Finally, although oral reading accuracy of sentences or passages gives insights into decoding skills and word recognition strategies, single word reading is more effective for evaluating decoding skills.

Conclusion

It is well established that bilingualism *per se* is *not* a risk factor in reading acquisition failure. Evidence from typical language development studies (Schwartz *et al.*, 2005) indicated that reading fluency was advanced in bilingual/bi-literate children (i.e. those who spoke and read in two languages) compared to bilingual monoliterates (i.e. those who spoke two languages but read in one only) and monolingual monoliterates (i.e. those who spoke and read in one language only) on all measures at the end of Grade 1, and they also had a clear advantage over monoliterate bilingual and monolingual peers on all phonological awareness tasks. The presence of SSD, however, is clearly a risk factor for PA development, in particular, and for reading acquisition, in general. However, the determination of each bilingual child's risk and protective factors (e.g. intact phonological memory, acceptable levels of nonverbal IQ development and absence of LI), and evidence-based treatment designed to address the error type and consistency of the SSD will likely facilitate their reading acquisition in both languages.

Notes

(1) The term bilingual is meant to include regular exposure to more than one language, regardless of sequence of acquisition as defined by Salameh *et al.* (2004).
(2) Phonological representation refers to the receptive ability to recognise words of a language, an ability that depends on the acquisition of a mental lexicon of the vocabulary of the ambient language.
(3) A transparent orthography refers to the one-to-one mapping of phonemes onto graphemes, while an opaque orthography implies representation of phonemes with multiple graphemes.
(4) The much-espoused Simple View of Reading (Joshi & Aron, 2000, 2004) includes decoding and listening comprehension as the pillars of reading comprehension, but neglects to consider the role of the expressive system of language, especially speech development, in metalinguistic skill acquisition and literacy. Its importance is demonstrated in PA and literacy development of bilingual children with SSD.

References

Aldrich, S. and Wright, J. (2001) *Curriculum based assessment directions and materials*. Syracuse City Schools, Teacher Centre. www.programevaluation.org/docs/cbamanall.pdf. Accessed 14.8.09.

Bialystok, E. (2007) Acquisition of literacy in bilingual children: A framework for research. *Language Learning* 57 (s1), 45–77.

Bialystok, E., Luk, G. and Kwan, E. (2005) Bilingualism, biliteracy, and learning to read: Interactions among languages and writing systems. *Scientific Studies of Reading* 9 (1), 43–61.

Brizzolara, D., Chilosi, A., Cipriani, P., Di filippo, G., Gasperini, F., Mazzotti, S., Pecini, C. and Zoccolotti, P. (2006) Do phonological and rapid automatized naming deficits differentially affect dyslexic children with and without a history of language delay? A study on Italian dyslexic children. *Cognitive and Behavioural Neurology* 19 (3), 141–149.

Caravolas, M. and Landerl, K. (2010) The influence of syllable structure and reading ability on the development of phoneme awareness: A longitudinal cross-linguistic study. *Scientific Studies of Reading* 14 (5), 464–484.

Carroll, J.M., Snowling, M.J., Hulme, C. and Stevenson, J. (2003) The development of phonological awareness in preschool children. *Developmental Psychology* 39 (5), 913–923.

Catts, H.W. and Kamhi, A.G. (2005) *Language and Reading Disabilities*. Boston, MA: Allyn & Bacon.

Cheung, H., Chen, H.C., Lai, C.Y., Wong, O.C. and Hills, M. (2001) The development of phonological awareness: Effects of spoken language experience and orthography. *Cognition* 81, 227–241.

Chiang, P.Y. (2003) Bilingual children's phonological awareness: The effect of articulation training. In A. Dahl, P. Svenonius and M. Richardsen Westergaard (eds) *Proceedings of the 19th Scandinavian Conference of Linguistics* (pp. 532–544). Amsterdam: Elsevier Science.

Chiang, P.Y. and Rvachew, S. (2007) English-French bilingual children's phonological awareness and vocabulary skills. *Canadian Journal of Applied Linguistics* 10 (3), 293–308.

Comeau, L., Cormier, P., Grandmaison, E. and Lacroix, D. (1999) A longitudinal study of phonological processing skills in children learning to read in a second language. *Journal of Educational Psychology* 91 (1), 29–43.

Crosbie, S., Holm, A. and Dodd, B. (2005) Intervention for children with severe speech disorder: A comparison of two approaches. *International Journal of Language and Communication Disorders* 40 (4), 467–491.

Dodd, B. and McIntosh, B. (2008) The input processing, cognitive linguistic and oromotor skills of children with speech difficulty. *International Journal of Speech-Language Pathology* 10 (3), 169–178.

Durgunoglu, A.Y., Nagy, W.E. and Hancin-Bhatt, B.J. (1993) Cross-language transfer of phonological awareness. *Journal of Educational Psychology* 85 (3), 453–465.

Edwards, J., Fox, R.A. and Rogers, C.L. (2002) Final consonant discrimination in children: Effects of phonological disorder, vocabulary size, and articulatory accuracy. *Journal of Speech, Language, and Hearing Research* 45 (2), 231–242.

Eviatar, Z. and Ibrahim, R. (2000) Bilingual is as bilingual does: Metalinguistic abilities of Arabic-speaking children, *Applied Psycholinguistics* 21 (4), 451–471.

Fabiano-Smith, L. and Barlow, J. (2010) Interaction in bilingual phonological acquisition: Evidence from phonetic inventories. *International Journal of Bilingual Education and Bilingualism* 1 (13), 81–97.

Frost, S.J., Landi, N., Mencl, W.E., Sandak, R., Fulbright, R.K., Tejada, E.T., Jacobsen, L., Grigorenko, E.L., Constable, R.T. and Pugh, K.R. (2009) Phonological awareness predicts activation patterns for print and speech. *Annals of Dyslexia* 59, 78–97.

Genesee, F. (2007) French immersion and at-risk students: A review of research evidence. *The Canadian Modern Language Review* 63 (5), 655–688.

Gierut, J.A. (1998) Treatment efficacy: Functional phonological disorders in children. *Journal of Speech, Language, and Hearing Research* 41, 85–100.

Goldstein, B.A. and Fabiano, L. (2006) Assessment and intervention for bilingual children with phonological disorders. *The ASHA Leader* 12 (2), 6–7, 26–27, 31.

Golestani, N. and Pallier, C. (2007) Anatomical correlates of foreign speech sound production. *Cerebral Cortex* 17, 929–934.

Goswami, U. (2002) Phonology, reading development, and dyslexia: A cross-linguistic perspective. *Annals of Dyslexia* 52, 141–163.

Goswami, U., Gombert, J.E. and Barrera, L.C. (1998) Children's orthographic representations and linguistic transparency: Nonsense word reading in English, French, and Spanish. *Applied Psycholinguistics* 19 (1), 19–52.

Gottardo, A., Yan, B., Siegel, L.S. and Wade-Woolley, L. (2001) Factors related to English reading performance in children with Chinese as a first language: More evidence of cross-language transfer of phonological processing. *Journal of Educational Psychology* 93, 530–542.

Grosjean, F. (1985) The bilingual as a competent but specific speaker-hearer. *Journal of Multilingual and Multicultural Development* 6 (6), 467–477.

Hermans, D., Knoors, H., Ormel, E. and Verhoeven, L. (2008) Modeling reading vocabulary learning in deaf children in bilingual education programs. *Journal of Deaf Studies and Deaf Education* 13 (2), 155–174.

Hogan, T.P., Catts, H.W. and Little, T.D. (2005) The relationship between phonological awareness and reading: Implications for the assessment of phonological awareness. *Language, Speech, and Hearing Services in School* 36, 285–293.

Holm, A. and Dodd, B. (1999a) Differential diagnosis of phonological disorder in two bilingual children acquiring Italian and English. *Clinical Linguistics and Phonetics* 13 (2), 113–129.

Holm, A. and Dodd, B. (1999b) An intervention case study of a bilingual child with phonological disorder. *Child Language Teaching and Therapy* 15 (2), 139–158.

Holm, A. and Dodd, B. (1999d) A longitudinal study of the phonological development of two Cantonese–English bilingual children. *Applied Psycholinguistics* 20, 349–376.

Holm, A., Dodd, B., Stow, C. and Pert, S. (1999c) Identification and differential diagnosis of phonological disorder in bilingual children. *Language Testing* 16 (3), 271–292.

Holm, A., Farrier, F. and Dodd, B. (2008) Phonological awareness, reading accuracy and spelling ability of children with inconsistent phonological disorder. *International Journal of Language and Communication Disorders* 43 (3), 300–322.

Hulme, C., Snowling, M., Caravolas, M. and Carroll, J. (2005) Phonological skills are (probably) one cause of success in learning to read: A comment on Castles and Coltheart. *Scientific Studies of Reading* 9 (4), 351–365.

Hus, Y. (2009) Literacy in multilingual learners: What is broken and how can we fix it? Proceedings for the Third International Symposium on Communication Disorders in Multilingual Populations, Agros, Cyprus. http://ialp.info/joomla/index.php?/Selected-papers-of-the-Cyprus-Symposium-November-2009.html.

Joshi, M. (2004) Diagnosis and remediation of reading disabilities: A pragmatic solution. In M. Joshi (ed.) *Dyslexia: Myths, Misconceptions, and Some Practical Applications* (pp. 63–82). Baltimore, MD: The International Dyslexia Association.

Joshi, M. and Aaron, P. (2000) The component model of reading: Simple view of reading made a little more complex. *Reading Psychology* 21, 85–97.

Kuo, L.J. and Anderson, R.C. (2010) Beyond cross-language transfer: Reconceptualising the impact of early bilingualism on phonological awareness. *Scientific Studies of Reading* 14 (4), 365–385.

Leitão, S. and Fletcher, J. (2004) Literacy outcomes for students with speech impairment: Long-term follow-up. *International Journal of Language and Communication Disorders* 39, 245–256.

Liow, R.S.J. and Poon, K.K.L. (1998) Phonological awareness in multilingual Chinese children. *Applied Psycholinguistics* 19 (3), 339–362.

Lundberg, I. (2002) The child's route into reading and what can go wrong. *Dyslexia* 8 (1), 1–13.

MacCoubrey, S.J., Wade-Woolley, L., Klinger, D. and Kirby, J.R. (2004) Early identification of at-risk L2 readers. *The Canadian Modern Language Review* 61, 11–28.

Magnusson, E. (1991) Metalinguistic awareness in phonologically disordered children. In M.S. Yavaş (ed.) *Phonological Disorders in Children: Theory, Research, and Practice* (pp. 87–120). New York: Routledge.

McBride-Chang, C. and Ho, C.S.H. (2005) Predictors of beginning reading in Chinese and English: A 2-year longitudinal study of Chinese kindergartners. *Scientific Studies of Reading* 9 (2), 117–144.

McGregor, K.K., Marian, V. and Sheng, L. (2006) Lexical-semantic organization in bilingual children: Evidence from a repeated word association task. *Journal of Speech, Language, and Hearing Research* 49, 572–587.

Paradis, J. and Genesee, F. (1996) Syntactic acquisition in bilingual children: Autonomous or interdependent? *Studies in Second Language Acquisition* 18, 1–25.

Peterson, R.L., Pennington, B.F., Shriberg, L.D. and Boada, R. (2009) What influences literacy outcome in children with speech sound disorder? *Journal of Speech, Language, and Hearing Research* 52, 1175–1188.

Rvachew, S., Chiang, Pi-Yu and Evans, N. (2007) Characteristics of speech errors produced by children with and without delayed phonological awareness skills. *Language, Speech, and Hearing Services in Schools* 38, 60–71.

Salameh, E.K., Hakansson, G. and Nettelbladt, U. (2004) Developmental perspectives on bilingual Swedish-Arabic children with and without language impairment: A longitudinal study. *International Journal of Language and Communication Disorders* 39(1), 65–91.

Scarborough, H.S. and Brady, S. (2004) Toward a common terminology for talking about speech and reading: A glossary of the 'phon' words and some related terms. In M. Joshi (ed.) *Dyslexia: Myths, Misconceptions, and Some Practical Applications*. Baltimore, MD: The International Dyslexia Association.

Schwartz, M., Leikin, M. and Share, D. (2005) Bi-literate bilingualism versus mono-literate bilingualism: A longitudinal study of reading acquisition in Hebrew (L2) among Russian-speaking (L1) children. *Journal of Written Language and Literacy* 8 (2), 179–206.

Sénéchal, M., Ouellette, G. and Young, L. (2004) Testing the concurrent and predictive relations among articulation accuracy, speech perception, and phoneme awareness. *Journal of Experimental Child Psychology* 89 (3), 242–269.

Serrano, F. and Defior, S. (2008) Dyslexia speed problems in a transparent orthography. *Annals of Dyslexia* 58, 81–95.

Seymour, P., Aro, M. and Erskine, J.M. (2003) Foundation literacy acquisition in European orthographies. *British Journal of Psychology* 94, 143–174.

Shatil, E. and Share, D.L. (2003) Cognitive antecedents of early reading ability: A test of the modularity hypothesis. *Journal of Experimental Child Psychology* 86, 1–31.

Shaywitz, B.A. and Shaywitz, S.E. (2009) Brain imaging in studies of reading and dyslexia. *Encyclopaedia of Language and Literacy Development* (pp. 1–6). London, ON: Canadian Language and Literacy Research Network. http://www.literacyencyclope-dia.ca/SSDfs/. Accessed 14.9.10.

So, L.K.H. and Dodd, B. (2007) The phonological awareness abilities of Cantonese-speaking children with phonological disorder. *Asia Pacific Journal of Speech, Language and Hearing* 10, 189–204.

Stoel-Gammon, C. (1998) Sound and words in early language acquisition: The relation-ship between lexical and phonological development. In R. Paul (ed.) *Exploring the Speech-Language Connection* (pp. 25–52). Baltimore, MD: Paul H. Brookes.

Storkel, H.L., Maekawa, J. and Hoover, J.R. (2010) Differentiating the effects of phonotactic probability and neighborhood density on vocabulary comprehension and production: A comparison of preschool children with versus without phonolo-gical delays. *Journal of Speech, Language, and Hearing Research* 53, 933–949.

Swank, L.K. and Larrivee, L.S. (1998) Phonology, metaphonology, and the development of literacy. In R. Paul (ed.) *Exploring the Speech-Language Connection* (pp. 253–295). Baltimore, MD: Paul H. Brookes.

Thomas, E.M. and Senechal, M. (1998) Articulation and phoneme awareness of 3-year old children. *Applied Psycholinguistics* 19, 363–391.

Trask, R.L. and Stockwell, P. (2007) *Language and Linguistics: The Key Concepts* (2nd edn). New York: Routledge.

Velleman, S.L. (2002) Phonotactic therapy. *Seminars in Speech and Language 23* (1), 43–55.

Vloedgraven, J.M.T. and Verhoeven, L. (2007) Screening of phonological awareness in the early elementary grades: An IRT approach. *Annals of Dyslexia* 57 (1), 33–50.

Wang, M. and Geva, E. (2003a) Spelling acquisition of novel English phonemes in Chinese children. *Reading and Writing: An Interdisciplinary Journal* 16, 325–348.

Webster, P.E. and Plante, A.S. (1992) Effects of phonological impairment on word, syllable, and phoneme segmentation and reading. *Language, Speech, and Hearing Services in Schools* 23, 176–182.

Webster, P.E. and Plante, A.S. (1995) Productive phonology and phonological awareness in preschool children. *Applied Psycholinguistics* 16, 43–57.

Webster, P.E., Plante, A.S. and Couvillion, M. (1997) Phonologic impairment and prereading: Update on a longitudinal study. *Journal of Learning Disabilities* 30 (4), 365–376.

Wren, S. (2000) *The Cognitive Foundations of Learning to Read: A Framework*. Southwest Educational Development Laboratory. http://www.sedl.org/reading. Accessed 16.10.09.

Yeong, S. and Liow, S.J. (2010) Phonemic representation and early spelling errors in bilingual children. *Scientific Studies of Reading* 14 (5), 387–406.

Ziegler, C. and Goswami, U. (2006) Becoming literate in different languages: Similar problems, different solutions. *Developmental Science* 9 (5), 429–453.

29 Translation to Practice: Metalinguistic Considerations for Cuban Spanish-English Bilingual Children

Ruth Huntley Bahr and Felix Matias

Languages mentioned: American English, Cuban Spanish

The Link between Speech Production and Reading

Spanish-English bilingual children in the USA are faced with mastering receptive and expressive competence in two languages while frequently learning to read only in English. To accomplish these tasks, the bilingual child must develop strong phonological representations (Storkel *et al.*, 2010) in each language, along with language-specific phonotactic knowledge in order to develop the vocabulary (Demuth, 2011) necessary to read. The child must be able to parse the incoming linguistic signal into meaningful words and sounds before he/she can begin to decode and comprehend written language. As such, competence at the phonological level forms the base for speech intelligibility and reading proficiency. Testing the child's knowledge of contrastive and non-contrastive features across languages can assist in developing treatment programs that result in a change in underlying linguistic knowledge and not just the surface behavior (Johnston, 1988). Such interventions should result in greater generalization of trained structures (Gierut, 2005). This chapter will present a detailed analysis on a bilingual child of Cuban heritage as he is acquiring literacy skills in English.

Cuban Spanish

Bilingual children in the USA can speak a number of different dialects of Spanish. One such variety is Cuban Spanish. It is similar to other Caribbean dialects of Spanish in its treatment of syllable and word-final /s/, in that they either drop the /s/ or substitute an [h] (Goldstein, 2004; Hualde, 2005). Other features may include palatalization of 'n' (final /n/ goes to [ɲ]), deletion of final intervocalic /d/ (so that *acabado* (finished) /aka'vaðo/ becomes [aka'vao]), doubling consonants when an 'r' (i.e. flap) is before them (so that *parque* (park) /parke/ becomes ['pakke]), and 'r' (flap) becoming [l] in certain situations (so that *vivir* (to live) /bi'bir/ becomes [bi'bil]) (how-to-learn-any-language.com, 2010). In the sample used in this chapter, the child frequently substituted a velar fricative for /r/, i.e. *porque* (because) /porke/ became [poxke]. Anecdotally, this substitution has been noted in other speakers of Cuban Spanish in Florida.

Case Presentation

Juan, a 5-year, 1-month-old male was seen because of parental concerns about speech fluency. No other developmental concerns were noted. Juan speaks Spanish at home and attends school in west central Florida, USA, where instruction is in English. He was verbal and communicated using both Spanish and English during the evaluation, although he demonstrated a preference for English and frequently code-switched between languages. Table 29.1 displays Juan's speech and language abilities in both Spanish and English.

The *Preschool Language Scale* (4th edn) (PLS-4; Zimmerman *et al.*, 2002) scores in English suggest that Juan has the language skills of a 3-and-a-half-year-old child. This finding is substantiated by a standard score of <55 on the *Expressive One Word Picture Vocabulary Test: Spanish-Bilingual Edition* (EOWPVT-S; Brownell, 2000) and an age equivalency of 2 and a half years. Given these scores, the clinician should consider how the vocabulary deficit contributes to noted speech sound disorders (Stoel-Gammon, 2011). Speech sound testing in both languages revealed numerous misarticulations in single word testing. Scores on the *Goldman-Fristoe Test of Articulation-2* (Goldman & Fristoe, 2000) were low (standard score = 87; percentile = 21; age equivalency = 3.6). A phonological deviancy score of 32.4 and a moderate severity rating were obtained on the *Assessment of Phonological Processes-Spanish* (APP-S; Hodson, 1986). Closer examination of the deficiencies indicated difficulty with consonant sequences, lateral /l/ and tap/trill 'r' in Spanish. Analysis of Juan's 346-word spontaneous sample

Table 29.1 Standard scores and percentile rankings for Juan's performance on the Preschool Language Scales-4 (PLS-4)

| | Spanish | | English | |
	Standard Score	Percentile	Standard Score	Percentile
Auditory comprehension	75	5	70	2
Expressive communication	79	8	60	1
Total language	73	4	61	1

gathered in Spanish evidenced code-switching to English 16% of the time and suggested the presence of a vocabulary deficit (number of different words (NDW) = 0.39). Interestingly, Juan's initial phonetic inventory, including basic vowels, was age appropriate in Spanish (see Table 29.2). He was only missing /w/, which was noted in English word productions, and the affricate /tʃ/, which did not occur in this sample. He used [t, d, k, f, s, n, l, h] in his final phonetic inventory. His percentage of consonants correct (PCC, Shriberg *et al.*, 1997) in Spanish was 0.84. However, when dialectal variations (i.e. /s/ and /r/) were not counted as errors, the PCC rose to 0.91. These levels of intelligibility were somewhat surprising given the articulation test scores and the difficulty that the clinician experienced in understanding Juan in conversation in both Spanish and English.

When considering all of the evaluation results, Juan's communication inefficiency is related to several factors. First, he evidenced word-finding difficulties. There was also the presence of numerous disfluencies, primarily part word and whole word repetitions, which could be suggestive of the type of processing difficulties young children have as they learn language (Kohnert, 2004). Finally, syllable reduction, while often dialectal, [taba] for *estaba* (was) /estaba/ and diphthong reduction, [tene] for *tiene* (I have) /tiene/, were often noted to interfere with intelligibility in running speech. Closer examination of the syllable shapes used by Juan indicated that he preferred monosyllables and disyllables (88%) to longer words (12%). He was capable of accurately producing longer words in English, like *Spiderman* and *rollercoaster*, but tended to reduce some Spanish words in running speech (Table 29.3). This finding was unexpected because the APP-S noted syllable reduction as occurring 5% of the time.

Given the noted difficulties with phoneme accuracy, phonotactics and vocabulary breadth, Juan was believed to be at high risk for reading difficulties. Testing with the *Comprehensive Test of Phonological Processing*

Table 29.2 Juan's phonetic inventory for the initial position of words in Spanish

	Bilabial	*Dental*	*Alveolar*	*Palatal*	*Velar*	*Glottal*
Plosives	p, b		t, d		k, g	
Fricatives		f, (ð)*	s	(ʃ)	x	(h)
Nasals	m		n			
Liquids			l ɹ			
Glides			j			

*Phonemes in parentheses occurred in English words produced while code-switching.

Table 29.3 A brief sample of Juan's conversational speech

Child Production	*Adult Target*	*Translation*
[no el ba asi depueh a ki asi əgɛn əgɛn]	/no el ba asi despues a ki asi əgɛn əgɛn/	No, he goes like this, then that, like this again again.
[Pero eja taba mui skɛɚ komo komo taba fæst el el ɹoləˑkostəˑ eja taba skɛɚ]	/Pero eja estaba mui skɛɚd komo komo estaba fæst el el ɹoləˑkostəˑ eja estaba skɛɚd/	But she was very scared like, like it was fast the the rollercoaster, she was scared.
[Pero a natali le gusta montax el grande komo se jama ese ples ke tene leones]	/Pero a natali le gusta montar el grande komo se jama ese ples ke tiene leones/	But Natalie like to ride the big, like, what is the name of that place that has lions?

(CTOPP; Wagner *et al.*, 1999) revealed the following composite scores: phonological awareness (91; 27th percentile), phonological memory (97; 42nd percentile) and alternate rapid naming (49; <1st percentile). While none of these scores are particularly strong, the rapid naming score, which is indicative of word retrieval difficulties, is by far the lowest. This finding is supported by the low language and vocabulary scores listed above. Word retrieval difficulties are compounded by the presence of weak phonological representations and unstable knowledge of phonotactic structure, as illustrated in the phonological analysis. Specific difficulties were noted in isolating phonemes in the initial and final positions, performing elision tasks (like 'say *time* without saying the /m/', taken from the CTOPP), blending words ([nu] for *moon* /mun/), blending nonwords ([ʃɪp] *ship* for the nonword /ʃɪb/ and nonword repetition ([biledos] for /blɛlidoʤ/). A tendency to produce real words instead of monosyllable nonwords and as part of longer nonwords was noted. While it is difficult to determine the exact reasons for these errors, it would appear that vocabulary deficits and inadequate knowledge of the phonemic and phonotactic differences between English and Spanish contribute to his difficulties (Edwards & Beckman, 2008; Edwards *et al.*, 2011).

Conclusions

A comprehensive assessment of Juan's metalinguistic knowledge revealed weak phonological representations that adversely affected vocabulary development, production of conversational speech and phonological awareness. These findings suggest that language impairment and speech sound impairment underlie Juan's difficulty with phonological processing tasks (Peterson *et al.*, 2009). Treatment goals should focus on vocabulary building within new phonotactic patterns. Phonological representations could be strengthened by helping the child discover the contrastive and non-contrastive features of his two languages. Perceptual tasks could target the fine phonetic details of words in each language, like initial and final consonants, as well as activities that target parsing of running speech, like syllable and word identification tasks. All activities should stress the integration of the perceptual, articulatory and phonological aspects of words that underlie the vocabulary necessary to perform higher order phonological tasks, like phonological awareness and word recognition (Edwards *et al.*, 2011).

References

Brownell, R. (2000) *Expressive One-Word Picture Vocabulary Test*: Spanish-Bilingual Edition. San Antonio, TX: Pearson.

Cuban Spanish – why not? (n.d.) http://how-to-learn-any-language.com/forum/forum_posts.asp?TID=20894&PN=16. Accessed 14.1.11.

Demuth, K. (2011) Interactions between lexical and phonological development: Cross-linguistic and contextual considerations – A commentary on Stoel-Gammon's 'Relationships between lexical and phonological development in young children'. *Journal of Child Language* 38, 69–74.

Edwards, J. and Beckman, M.E. (2008) Methodological questions in studying consonant acquisition. *Clinical Linguistics and Phonetics* 22, 937–956.

Edwards, J., Munson, B. and Beckman, M.E. (2011) Lexicon–phonology relationships and dynamics of early language development – A commentary on Stoel-Gammon's 'Relationships between lexical and phonological development in young children'. *Journal of Child Language* 38, 35–40.

Gierut, J.A. (2005) Phonological intervention: The how or the what? In A.G. Kamhi and K.E. Pollock (eds) *Phonological Disorders in Children: Clinical Decision Making in Assessment and Intervention* (pp. 201–210). Baltimore, MD: Paul H. Brookes.

Goldman, R. and Fristoe, M. (2000) *Goldman-Fristoe Test of Articulation-2*. Bloomington, MN: Pearson Assessments.

Goldstein, B.A. (2004) Phonological development and disorders. In B.A. Goldstein (ed.) *Bilingual Language Development and Disorders in Spanish-English Speakers* (pp. 259–285). Baltimore, MD: Paul H. Brookes.

Hodson, B.W. (1986) *Assessment of Phonological Processes-Spanish*. San Diego, CA: Los Amigos Research Associates.

Hualde, J.I. (2005) *The Sounds of Spanish*. Cambridge: Cambridge University Press.

Johnston, J.R. (1988) Generalization: The nature of change. *Language, Speech, and Hearing Services in Schools* 19, 314–329.

Kohnert, K. (2004) Processing skills in early sequential bilinguals. In B.A. Goldstein (ed.) *Bilingual Language Development and Disorders in Spanish-English Speakers* (pp. 53–76). Baltimore, MD: Paul H. Brookes.

Peterson, R.L., Pennington, B.F., Shriberg, L.D. and Boada, R. (2009) What influences literacy outcome in children with speech sound disorder? *Journal of Speech, Language and Hearing Research* 52, 1175–1188.

Shriberg, L.D., Austin, D., Lewis, B.A., McSweeny, J.L. and Wilson, D.L. (1997) The percentage of consonants correct (PCC) metric: Extensions and reliability data. *Journal of Speech, Language, and Hearing Research* 40, 708–722.

Stoel-Gammon, C. (2011) Relationships between lexical and phonological development in young children. *Journal of Child Language* 38, 1–34.

Wagner, R., Torgesen, J. and Rashotte, C. (1999) *Comprehensive Test of Phonological Processing*. San Antonio, TX: Pearson.

Zimmerman, I.L., Steiner, V.G. and Pond, R.E. (2002) *Preschool Language Scale* (4th edn). San Antonio, TX: Pearson.

30 Multilingual Children with Speech Sound Disorders: An Epilogue

Brian A. Goldstein and Sharynne McLeod

The purpose of *Multilingual Aspects of Speech Sound Disorders in Children* was to translate research into clinical practice for speech-language pathologists (SLPs) working with multilingual children with speech sound disorders. The book explored both multilingual and multicultural aspects of children with speech sound disorders. To that end, 44 authors from 16 countries reported on 112 languages in 30 chapters. The book included two types of chapters. First, research chapters summarized previous research in a particular topic area, including a section on how that research translated into clinical practice. Second, translation chapters focused on translating research into practice by providing vignettes for specific geographical or linguistic contexts. A number of themes can be discerned from both the research and translation chapters in the book.

The book provides a baseline for where the profession is now relative to multilingual children and their families. The historical assumption is that little is known about speech acquisition of multilingual children. This volume belies that notion. Although there are significant gaps in our understanding of speech acquisition in multilingual children, the authors in this book show that a rather robust knowledge base already exists.

There is a range of reasons as to why people are multilingual. They may be multilingual by circumstance (e.g. both parents speak two languages), relocation and international mobility, or by necessity (e.g. they are refugees). These differences result in diverse ways that children become multilingual. Those differences are likely to result in disparate patterns of language use and language proficiency and thus impact how speech-language pathology services are delivered to multilingual children.

In most countries, there are relatively large numbers of languages spoken. However, data are sparse on multilingual populations and SLPs are still having difficulty providing services to multilingual children. That is, the status of languages is not identical across countries. For example, Cantonese is more widely spoken in daily communication in Hong Kong, although both Cantonese and Putonghua are commonly taught in schools. SLPs might not even encounter a speaker of low incidence languages (e.g. Australian indigenous languages and Zapotec in Mexico) because speakers of those languages might not routinely access speech-language pathology services. Such languages were highlighted in this book to indicate how SLPs should show respect for languages such as Jamaican, Icelandic and sign languages, which are not commonly written about.

Issues faced by SLPs around the world are relatively similar: lack of normative data on typically developing children and those with speech sound disorders, lack of multilingual assessment tools and a lack of intervention materials. Therefore, SLPs must use alternate means to assess and treat speech skills in multilingual children; e.g. parent report, dynamic assessment and interpreters and translators. It is also evident that there are significant gaps in our knowledge base. For example, the effect of language (i.e. phonological) loss on children's speech acquisition is unknown as there are no studies addressing this issue in children. Thus, although significant progress has been made to address multilingual speech acquisition, there are numerous areas in significant need of research.

Taking a long-range view, speech acquisition in multilingual children is similar, although not identical, to that of monolingual children. Assuming enough experience in and with each language, multilingual children will become competent speakers of more than one ambient language. Speech acquisition is most often measured by children's success in producing speech sounds (i.e. segments). Speech acquisition, however, is more than how children produce speech sounds. Although (almost) all chapters have some focus on speech sounds, authors in the volume summarized other aspects, such as babbling, phonotactics, perception, prosody and literacy. Moreover, multilingual children might not show exactly the same skills in all their languages because those skills are not evenly distributed across their languages. Languages interact with one another and change. Such language contact results in code-switching, code-mixing and borrowing. Code-switching, code-mixing and borrowing are expected for multilinguals; in phonological terms, they are the unmarked condition. Finally, individual and societal variables shape speech acquisition, just as they do for other domains of language. Accounting for specific context, community, family and linguistic (e.g. dialect, use, proficiency) variables helps to account for individual variation and thus results in less-biased assessment and intervention.

When providing speech-language pathology services to multilingual children, it is important not to forget what is already known about best practices in the area. Thus, although providing speech-language pathology services to multilingual children is not identical to that afforded monolingual children, it is not altogether different either. SLPs receive training in phonetics, phonology, speech acquisition, assessment and intervention. This basic knowledge and principles can be leveraged when providing services to all children – monolingual and multilingual.

Providing speech-language pathology services to multilingual children is challenging and often complex. The authors in this volume have provided at least some groundwork and a roadmap toward lowering barriers in the provision of such services. Although that journey is far from complete, we are farther down the road given the points on the map provided by the information in this volume.

Appendix A

THE INTERNATIONAL PHONETIC ALPHABET (revised to 2005)

CONSONANTS (PULMONIC)

	Bilabial	Labiodental	Dental	Alveolar	Postalveolar	Retroflex	Palatal	Velar	Uvular	Pharyngeal	Glottal
Plosive	p b			t d		ʈ ɖ	c ɟ	k ɡ	q ɢ		ʔ
Nasal	m	ɱ		n		ɳ	ɲ	ŋ	N		
Trill	B			r					R		
Tap or Flap		ⱱ		ɾ		ɽ					
Fricative	ɸ β	f v	θ ð	s z	ʃ ʒ	ʂ ʐ	ç ʝ	x ɣ	χ ʁ	ħ ʕ	h ɦ
Lateral fricative				ɬ ɮ							
Approximant		ʋ		ɹ		ɻ	j	ɰ			
Lateral approximant				l		ɭ	ʎ	L			

Where symbols appear in pairs, the one to the right represents a voiced consonant. Shaded areas denote articulations judged impossible.

CONSONANTS (NON-PULMONIC)

Clicks		Voiced implosives		Ejectives	
ʘ	Bilabial	ɓ	Bilabial	ʼ	Examples:
ǀ	Dental	ɗ	Dental/alveolar	pʼ	Bilabial
ǃ	(Post)alveolar	ʄ	Palatal	tʼ	Dental/alveolar
ǂ	Palatoalveolar	ɠ	Velar	kʼ	Velar
ǁ	Alveolar lateral	ʛ	Uvular	sʼ	Alveolar fricative

OTHER SYMBOLS

ʍ   Voiceless labial-velar fricative

w   Voiced labial-velar approximant

ɥ   Voiced labial-palatal approximant

ʜ   Voiceless epiglottal fricative

ʢ   Voiced epiglottal fricative

ʡ   Epiglottal plosive

ɕ ʑ   Alveolo-palatal fricatives

ɺ   Voiced alveolar lateral flap

ɧ   Simultaneous ʃ and x

Affricates and double articulations can be represented by two symbols joined by a tie bar if necessary.

k͡p   t͡s

VOWELS

	Front		Central		Back
Close	i • y		ɨ • ʉ		ɯ • u
		ɪ Y		ʊ	
Close-mid	e • ø		ɘ • ɵ		ɤ • o
				ə	
Open-mid	ɛ • œ		ɜ • ɞ		ʌ • ɔ
		æ		ɐ	
Open		a • ɶ			ɑ • ɒ

Where symbols appear in pairs, the one to the right represents a rounded vowel.

SUPRASEGMENTALS

ˈ   Primary stress

ˌ   Secondary stress

ˌfoʊnəˈtɪʃən

ː   Long   eː

ˑ   Half-long   eˑ

˘   Extra-short   ĕ

| Minor (foot) group

‖   Major (intonation) group

.   Syllable break   ɹi.ækt

‿   Linking (absence of a break)

DIACRITICS   Diacritics may be placed above a symbol with a descender, e.g. ŋ̊

̥	Voiceless	n̥ d̥	̤	Breathy voiced	b̤ a̤	̪	Dental	t̪ d̪
̬	Voiced	s̬ t̬	̰	Creaky voiced	b̰ a̰	̺	Apical	t̺ d̺
ʰ	Aspirated	tʰ dʰ	̼	Linguolabial	t̼ d̼	̻	Laminal	t̻ d̻
̹	More rounded	ɔ̹	ʷ	Labialized	tʷ dʷ	̃	Nasalized	ẽ
̜	Less rounded	ɔ̜	ʲ	Palatalized	tʲ dʲ	ⁿ	Nasal release	dⁿ
̟	Advanced	u̟	ˠ	Velarized	tˠ dˠ	ˡ	Lateral release	dˡ
̠	Retracted	e̠	ˤ	Pharyngealized	tˤ dˤ	̚	No audible release	d̚
̈	Centralized	ë	̴	Velarized or pharyngealized	ɫ			
̽	Mid-centralized	e̽	̝	Raised	e̝	(ɹ̝ = voiced alveolar fricative)		
̩	Syllabic	n̩	̞	Lowered	e̞	(β̞ = voiced bilabial approximant)		
̯	Non-syllabic	e̯	̘	Advanced Tongue Root	e̘			
˞	Rhoticity	ɚ a˞	̙	Retracted Tongue Root	e̙			

TONES AND WORD ACCENTS

LEVEL				CONTOUR			
e̋	or ˥	Extra high	ě	or ↗	Rising		
é	˦	High	ê	↘	Falling		
ē	˧	Mid	e᷄	↗	High rising		
è	˨	Low	e᷅	↗	Low rising		
ȅ	˩	Extra low	e᷈	↗	Rising-falling		
↓		Downstep	↗		Global rise		
↑		Upstep	↘		Global fall		

The International Phonetic Alphabet may be freely copied on condition that acknowledgement is made to the International Phonetic Association, Department of Theoretical and Applied Linguistics, School of English, Aristotle University of Thessaloniki, Thessaloniki 54124, GREECE

Appendix B

extIPA SYMBOLS FOR DISORDERED SPEECH
(Revised to 2008)

CONSONANTS (other than on the IPA Chart)

	bilabial	labiodental	dentolabial	labioalv.	linguolabial	interdental	bidental	alveolar	velar	velophar.
Plosive		p̪ b̪	p̪͆ b̪͆	p̪ b̪	t̼ d̼	t̪͆ d̪͆				
Nasal			m̪͆	m̪	n̼	n̪͆				
Trill					r̼	r̪͆				
Fricative median		f̪ v̪	f̪͆ v̪͆	f̪ v̪	θ̼ ð̼	θ̪͆ ð̪͆	h̪͆ ɦ̪͆			fŋ
Fricative lateral+median								ʪ ʫ		
Fricative nareal	m̃							ñ̥	ŋ̃	
Percussive	w̪						ʭ			
Approximant lateral					l̼	l̪͆				

Where symbols appear in pairs, the one to the right represents a voiced consonant. Shaded areas denote articulations judged impossible.

DIACRITICS

↔	labial spreading	s̪	"	strong articulation	f̬	ˮ	denasal	m̃
͏	dentolabial	v̪	ˏ	weak articulation	v̬	˵	nasal escape	v̂
͏	interdental/bidental	n̪͆	\	reiterated articulation	p\p\p	ˮ	velopharyngeal friction	s̃
=	alveolar	t̪	,	whistled articulation	s̩	↓	ingressive airflow	p↓
~	linguolabial	d̼	→	sliding articulation	θs̩	↑	egressive airflow	!↑

CONNECTED SPEECH

(.)	short pause
(..)	medium pause
(...)	long pause
f	loud speech [{f laʊd f}]
ff	louder speech [{ff laʊdə ff}]
p	quiet speech [{p kwaɪət p}]
pp	quieter speech [{pp kwaɪətə pp}]
allegro	fast speech [{allegro fast allegro}]
lento	slow speech [{lento sloʊ lento}]
crescendo, ralentando, etc. may also be used

VOICING

ˬ	pre-voicing	ˬz
˯	post-voicing	zˬ
₍ˬ₎	partial devoicing	z̬
₍ˬ	initial partial devoicing	̬z
ˬ₎	final partial devoicing	z̬
₍ᵕ₎	partial voicing	s̬
₍ᵕ	initial partial voicing	̬s
ᵕ₎	final partial voicing	s̬
=	unaspirated	p=
h	pre-aspiration	hp

OTHERS

(◯),(C̶),(V̱)	indeterminate sound, consonant, vowel	Ʞ	velodorsal articulation
(P̱l.v̱ls̱),(Ṉ)	indeterminate voiceless plosive, nasal, etc	¡	sublaminal lower alveolar percussive click
( )	silent articulation (ʃ), (m)	‼	alveolar and sublaminal clicks (cluck-click)
(( ))	extraneous noise, e.g. ((2 sylls))	*	sound with no available symbol

© ICPLA 2008

Reproduced with permission from International Clinical Phonetics and Linguistics Association

Appendix C

VoQS: Voice Quality Symbols

Airstream Types

Œ	œsophageal speech	И	electrolarynx speech
Ю	tracheo-œsophageal speech	↓	pulmonic ingressive speech

Phonation types

V	modal voice	F	falsetto
W	whisper	C	creak
V̰	whispery voice (murmur)	V̰	creaky voice
Vʰ	breathy voice	C̣	whispery creak
V!	harsh voice	V!!	ventricular phonation
V̰!!	diplophonia	V̰!!	whispery ventricular phonation
V̟	anterior or pressed phonation	W̲	posterior whisper

Supralaryngeal Settings

L̝	raised larynx	L̞	lowered larynx
Vœ	labialized voice (open round)	Vʷ	labialized voice (close round)
V↔	spread-lip voice	Vᶹ	labio-dentalized voice
V̺	linguo-apicalized voice	V̻	linguo-laminalized voice
V˺	retroflex voice	V̪	dentalized voice
V̱	alveolarized voice	V̱ʲ	palatoalveolarized voice
Vʲ	palatalized voice	Vˠ	velarized voice
Vˠ	uvularized voice	Vˤ	pharyngealized voice
V̡ˤ	laryngo-pharyngealized voice	Vʜ	faucalized voice
Ṽ	nasalized voice	Ṽ	denasalized voice
J̞	open jaw voice	J̝	close jaw voice
J˂	right offset jaw voice	J˃	left offset jaw voice
J̟	protruded jaw voice	Θ	protruded tongue voice

USE OF LABELED BRACES & NUMERALS TO MARK STRETCHES OF SPEECH
AND DEGREES AND COMBINATIONS OF VOICE QUALITY:

[ˈðɪs ɪz ˈnɔɹməl ˈvɔɪs {3V! ˈðɪs ɪz ˈveɹi ˈhɑɹʃ ˈvɔɪs 3V} ˈðɪs ɪz ˈnɔɹməl ˈvɔɪs wʌns
ˈmɔɹ {L̞ 1V! ˈðɪs ɪz ˈlɛs ˈhɑɹʃ ˈvɔɪs wɪθ ˈlouəd ˈlæɹɪŋks 1V!L̞}]

© 1994 Martin J. Ball, John Esling, Craig Dickson

Index